Recent Advances in Primary Care

Recent Advances in Primary Care

Edited by **Dr Mayur Lakhani** & **Dr Rodger Charlton**

With Forewords by **Prof Richard Baker** & **Sir Donald Irvine**

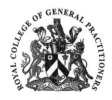

The Royal College of General Practitioners was founded in 1952 with this object:

"To encourage, foster and maintain the highest possible standards in general practice and for that purpose to take or join with others in taking steps consistent with the charitable nature of that object which may assist towards the same."

Among its responsibilities under its Royal Charter the College is entitled to:

"Diffuse information on all matters affecting general practice and issue such publications as may assist the object of the College."

British Library Cataloguing-in-Publication Data
A catalogue record for this book is available from the British Library

© Royal College of General Practitioners, 2005

Published by the Royal College of General Practitioners 2005
14 Princes Gate | Hyde Park | London SW7 1PU

Cover and text designed and typeset by the Typographic Design Unit, Newcastle-upon-Tyne
Printed by J W Arrowsmith Ltd, Bristol
Indexed by Carol Ball

ISBN 085084 292 1

Forewords

THE PACE OF PROGRESS – and other changes – in primary care is breathtaking. In almost every clinical field new treatments are being explored and new research is improving our understanding of disease processes. And there is more to come. The first few advances from the study of the human genome are just beginning to influence clinical practice, and in the next few years the way we regard many conditions is liable to change. At the same time, health care policy is being swept along by a flood of new ideas and initiatives. In almost every country in the developed world, policymakers are promoting new ways to structure and manage services as solutions to the problems of rising costs and increasing numbers of people with chronic conditions.

For the doctor or nurse working in primary care, it is very difficult to keep up. Yet despite the extraordinary rate of change, some things remain the same. Patients who are ill, or are worried they may be ill, need to be able to consult a health care professional they can trust. Most such consultations still take place with doctors and nurses in general practices, but even though some consultations now take place in walk-in centres, or are conducted by telephone or email, the fundamental nature of clinical practice is the same. The patient trusts that the doctor or nurse will possess the necessary knowledge and skills, and will apply those attributes in the best interests of the patient. The chapters that follow have much to say about the knowledge and skills required by doctors and nurses working in primary care, and will be an invaluable resource in remaining up-to-date. But the chapters present more than mere facts. The attentive reader will find that they stimulate reflections on the qualities needed of the primary care doctor, nurse or other type of professional that may provide care in the future.

The opening chapters remind us that the professional of the future must have an explicit and expanded moral code of professionalism, based on ethical principles and accepting of accountability and openness. Subsequent chapters raise questions about the degree of scientific expertise that will be needed by at least a proportion of primary care professionals of the future. As we learn more about the nature of disease, it is increasingly clear that the underlying mechanisms and approaches to treatment are complex. Increased knowledge is not making for increased simplicity. It follows that if a greater proportion of care is to be delivered in primary care, the level of scientific expertise in primary care needs to increase. Primary care will require a growing number of extensively trained clinician scientists who both deliver care to patients with particularly complex problems and take the lead in evaluating new treatments. Together with policymakers, the leaders of doctors and nurses in primary care need to begin to explore ways to bring together geneticists and other laboratory scientists with primary care clinician scientists. Most patients are managed in primary care, and as this book shows, most advances in care are delivered or have consequences in primary care, and an increasing number of clinical advances will arise from primary care. Therefore, doctors and nurses who read this book will regard the future of their disciplines with new optimism, and will look forward to the many exciting advances yet to come.

Prof Richard Baker OBE FRCGP
Professor of Quality in Healthcare, University of Leicester

WHEN SICKNESS STRIKES we all need doctors. People everywhere know that the quality of medical care can affect the outcome and possible consequences of illness, and at times make the difference between life and death. Illnesses can make patients frightened and vulnerable, and bring their defences down. These are the reasons why all patients want good doctors who are knowledgeable, fully skilled, and fully up-to-date: doctors who really know what they are doing. At the same time they want doctors who will respect their dignity, their privacy and their right to decide about their treatment, doctors with whom they can empathise, doctors whose personal integrity is beyond question. Patients need and are entitled to doctors who have all these attributes. Such doctors they would regard as thoroughly patient-centred and therefore thoroughly professional. Such doctors they can trust. And such trust is vital to them. After all, in terms of diagnosis and treatment they have no one else to turn to, nowhere else to go.

This places an awesome responsibility on individual doctors and on the medical profession. In fact most doctors are deeply conscientious in discharging this responsibility through their own idealism, sense of service and self-discipline, literally self-regulation.

The vast majority of patients, if pressed to prioritise the attributes of their doctor, will nominate technical knowledge and clinical skill together as their first choice. It makes sense – when people are feeling ill the first thing they want to know is what is wrong with them. Then they want to know that they will get the right treatment. In fact diagnosis is at the heart of medicine. The science and the art of diagnosis is primarily what distinguishes doctors from other health professionals. 'Clinical acumen' is a quality much admired and prized amongst doctors themselves.

Diagnosis can be especially difficult in general practice because, in the earliest stages of illness, symptoms are undifferentiated and ill-defined, as every family doctor knows. This, and the broad spectrum of clinical problems which is characteristic of primary care, presents general practitioners with a real and never-ending professional challenge. It is to their great credit that so many rise to the challenge so successfully.

In this new book the College lends a helping hand. Experienced – and expert – general practitioners and others have come together to produce an excellent 'state-of-the-art' account of recent advances in general practice. The book reflects the importance the College continues to give to clinical general practice. And in a world obsessed with targets and management-speak it gives a timely reminder of what really matters to patients. It should be of real value and practical help to every general practitioner.

Sir Donald Irvine
SEPTEMBER 2004

Preface

WE NEVER CEASE to be amazed by how rapidly medicine is changing. In a generalist discipline such as primary health care, it can sometimes be difficult to keep up-to-date and be aware of key developments in the many different clinical areas that comprise family medicine. Of course, family medicine is more than just a summation of clinical areas – it is a distinct discipline with its own academic base. Therefore, this book includes not only key developments in the major clinical areas of family medicine but also in health service policy, ethics and team working.

Our aim in publishing this book is to offer a compendium of the best available evidence interpreted by key clinical leaders. We are aware that there are many sources of information out there – this book is not intended to replace these. The purpose of this book is to provide a single publication – a 'one stop shop' – that busy GPs can access to learn about key advances as identified by experts in the field. We did not want to offer just primary evidence but evidence that has been assessed, analysed and interpreted for its impact on clinical practice. The chapters are not intended to be a systematic review of the subject – many high quality reviews exist already in the literature. We wanted to produce a book that is accessible and useful.

To make the book relevant we have briefed chapter authors to capture the essence of their subject and to work to an overall template. A degree of selection, and some overlap is therefore necessary and inevitable. Some of these chapters have appeared in the *British Journal of General Practice*.

We are aware that this project might be criticised on the basis that some of the material soon becomes out-of-date as new literature emerges. Despite this, we believe that having such a compendium is valuable as it captures concepts, strategic developments and ideas. For readers who want a more in-depth account, other sources of information can be consulted. Where drug therapy is concerned, readers are always urged to consult the most current authoritative guidance such as the British National Formulary.

We hope that this book will be useful for continuous professional development and that it will stimulate debate, encourage local innovation and implementation. It should help GPs prepare for appraisal, clinical governance and revalidation. We would welcome feedback and suggestions for improvement, as it is our intention to make this a biannual publication.

Dr Mayur K Lakhani FRCGP FRCPE
Dr Rodger Charlton MD FRCGP FRNZCGP

Contents

About the authors

Nigel Starey

Nigel Starey has been a GP for over 20 years. He worked in a rural dispensing practice for ten years, where he was a GP trainer and lead fund-holding partner. After three years as medical adviser to a health authority he founded the centre for primary care at Derby University and returned to active general practice in Swadlincote. He has published and worked with The Kings Fund and the DoH on primary care development, the future of general practice, and the development of genetics.

Ann Orme Smith MA FRCGP

Dr Orme-Smith has been a GP principal, trainer and VTS course organiser. Her keen interest in the ethical challenges that present to GPs led her to a master's degree in Medical Law and Ethics. She has served on the RCGP ethics committee as well as the research ethics committee of the Royal Marsden Hospital. She is co-author of *Ethics in General Practice*.

JA Muir Gray CBE DSc MD FRCPSGlas

Muir Gray has worked in public health for 25 years. For the last ten years his principal interests have been screening and knowledge management, and as director of R&D for Anglia and Oxford he supported the UK Cochrane Centre in its early days and in addition developed a number of initiatives to promote evidence-based decision making. As director of the National Screening Committee in the UK he works with groups in Oxford involved in many different aspects of communication with patients and informed decision-making. He is also director of the National Electronic Library for Health Project. He is author of the book *Evidence-based Healthcare* and joint author of *The Oxford Handbook of Public Health Practice*. His most recent book is *The Resourceful Patient*.

Dr Lindsay Smith MD FRCGP FRCP

Lindsay Smith has been a full-time Somerset rural GP and primary care researcher for 16 years, with many publications on women's health. His other interests are quality of care and education. He has been a member of, or adviser to, a number of national organisations and groups.

Anthony Harnden MSc FRCGP FRCPCH
Anthony is a university lecturer and principal in general practice and a governing body Fellow of St. Hugh's College, Oxford. He has a clinical interest in paediatrics and a research interest in childhood infection. He is a member of the Immunisation and Infectious Disease Committee of the Royal College of Paediatrics and Child Health and examines for the diploma in child health.

Sarah Jarvis BM BCh DRCOG FRCGP
Sarah Jarvis is a full-time inner-city GP in London and GP trainer. She is the women's health spokesperson for the RCGP and writes extensively for the medical and lay press. She has been medical adviser to the television series The Maternity Guide, and is the author of *A Younger Woman's Diagnose-It-Yourself Guide to Health* and the forthcoming *Pregnancy for Dummies*.

Anna Graham PhD MRCP MRCGP
Dr Graham has been a part-time GP for the last ten years. She has combined this with research in the field of sexual health. She is currently a member of the National Committee for the Sexually Transmitted Infections Foundation course as well as an adviser to Brook.

Azhar Farooqi FRCGP
Dr Farooqi is a graduate of Manchester Medical School and a Fellow of the Royal College of General Practitioners. He is a full-time GP and executive partner in a busy city practice in Eastern Leicester. He has a special interest in primary care research and particularly in diabetes and CHD. This has led to many publications in peer-reviewed journals over the past few years.

Steven Levene MB BChir FRCGP
Dr Levene has been a full-time inner-city GP in Leicester since 1986, with several publications on diabetes. His other interests include training and pain management.

Tom Fahey MD MSc FRCGP MFPH
Tom Fahey is a professor of primary care medicine at the University of Dundee and a part-time GP at Taybank Medical Practice, Dundee. His interests include cardiovascular disease and applied clinical research in primary care.

Knut Schroeder MD MSc PhD DCH DRCOG MRCP MRCGP

Knut Schroeder is a clinical senior lecturer at the Academic Unit of Primary Health Care at the University of Bristol and a part-time GP at Whiteladies Health Centre, Bristol. He has special interests in adherence to health care interventions and pragmatic primary-care based research.

Hilary Pinnock MB ChB MRCGP

Dr Pinnock is principal in general practice in Whitstable, Kent and holds a Clinical Research Fellowship with the University of Edinburgh. She has written and lectured widely on the delivery of care for people with respiratory disease. She is a committee member of the General Practice Airways group, and on the Steering Committee of the British Thoracic Society/Scottish Intercollegiate Guideline Network British Asthma Guideline.

Subrata Ghosh MD(Edin.) FRCP FRCP(E)

Subrata Ghosh trained in gastroenterology in Bristol, Tokyo and Edinburgh and took up the position as consultant gastroenterologist at the Western General Hospital, Edinburgh in 1995. As a part-time senior lecturer with the University of Edinburgh he published over 150 articles in peer-reviewed journals. In 2002 he took up the chair in gastroenterology at Imperial College, Hammersmith Hospital. Professor Ghosh is currently the secretary of the British Society of Gastroenterology IBD Committee and a member of the British Society of Gastroenterology Research Committee. He sits on the editorial board of *Gut, Clinical Science* and *British Medical Bulletin*. Professor Ghosh also acts as a referee for a number of medical charities, and sits on the research awards committee of *NACC*.

R Chaudhury MB BChir MRCP

Dr Chaudhury completed his MB BChir at Cambridge University where he also acquired a BA in Natural Sciences with particular interest in immunology and medical genetics. He has worked in and around London for most of his house officer and SHO posts. He obtained his MRCP in 1999 before acquiring a specialist registrar rotation in North West London. Dr Chaudhury is currently a Clinical Research Fellow in Gastroenterology at Imperial College, Hammersmith Hospital focusing on inflammatory bowel disease and mechanisms of action of biological agents in IBD.

Leone Ridsdale MD PhD FRCP

Dr Ridsdale has worked in general practice for over 20 years, and is a consultant neurologist. Her aims and interests include increasing access to neurology services for people in the community through teaching, innovation and research.

Andrew J Dowson MBBS MRCGP

After graduating from Guys Hospital Medical School, London, Dr Dowson became involved in headache research. In 1991 he established a headache research unit and in 1996 was appointed director of The Kings Hospital Headache Service at Kings College, London. He is interested in developing tools to enable primary care clinicians to deliver headache care effectively. Dr Dowson is chairman of the Migraine in Primary Care Advisors (MIPCA), secretary of Headache UK, medical advisor to the Migraine Action Association, and council member of The British Association for the Study of Headache. He has lectured widely, written several books and is author or co-author of approximately 100 original articles or reviews and over 100 abstracts at international meetings.

Greg Rogers MB ChB MSc[epilepsy] DRCOG MRCGP

Dr Rogers is a GP in East Kent who also spends two days a week as a GP with a Special Interest in Epilepsy. He has had an interest in epilepsy for many years and is determined to raise the medical profile of epilepsy in general practice.

Graham Davenport MA MSc MB BChir DRCOG MRCGP

Dr Davenport has been a single-handed rural GP in Wrenbury, Cheshire for 20 years. His interests are in rheumatology and postgraduate education and he is a trainer, course organiser and GP appraiser. He is president of the Primary Care Rheumatology Society and is involved in several educational and research initiatives as well as advisor to various national bodies and organisations.

Alan Cohen FRCGP

Dr Cohen was a GP for 25 years in Mitcham, prior to joining Kensington and Chelsea PCT in April 2004, as clinical director. Dr Cohen also works as director of primary care at the Sainsbury Centre for Mental Health, a national mental health charity, and also chairs the London Development Centre for Mental Health, one of the eight regional development centres of the National Institute of Mental Health in England (NIMHE). He continues in active general practice in North Kensington.

Steve Iliffe FRCGP

Dr Iliffe has been an inner-city general practitioner in London for 25 years, and is also reader in general practice at the Royal Free & UCL Medical School, with a research programme around health in later life. He is co-director of the Centre for Ageing Population Studies within the department of Primary Care & Population Sciences at RFUCLMS, and a member of the editorial boards of *Geriatric Medicine, Aging & Mental Health* and the *Journal of Dementia Care.*

Danielle Harari FRCP

Dr Harari is a consultant physician in general and geriatric medicine, and senior lecturer in elderly medicine at Guy's, King's, St. Thomas' School of Medicine, King's College, London. Her research interests include health risk appraisal in older people, and urinary and faecal incontinence.

Cameron Swift PhD FRCP

Cameron Swift is professor and head of the department of health care of the elderly at Guy's, King's & St Thomas' School of Medicine, King's College, London, and is also professor of health care of the elderly at the University of Kent, Canterbury, UK. He is an honorary consultant physician at King's College Hospital, London. His research interests include the clinical pharmacology of ageing and clinical and health services R&D related to ageing.

David Weller MBBS MPH PhD FRACGP MRCGP

Dr Weller graduated from the University of Adelaide Medical School in 1982, and has a background in academic and clinical general practice. He undertook PhD studies in Adelaide and Nottingham, and from 1995 to 2000 was senior lecturer in the department of general practice, Flinders University of South Australia. He has been professor of general practice at the University of Edinburgh since 2000 and leads the Primary Care Clinical Studies Development Group for the National Cancer Research Institute. Current research interests include primary care oncology and medically unexplained symptoms in primary care.

Alex Nicholson

After training in general practice in the North East Alex is now a specialist registrar in palliative medicine at the Severn Hospice, Shrewsbury. He recently completed a Cochrane Systematic Review, 'Methadone for Cancer Pain' and has contributed with Christina Faull to a volume on the clinical history of opioid use in cancer.

Christina Faull BMedSci MBBS MD FRCP
After nine years as the consultant in palliative medicine in Birmingham, Dr Faull is now in Leicestershire. With her co-editors she won the BMA book of the year in 1999 with the *Handbook of Palliative Care*, aimed at primary care, and with her co-author won this award again in 2003 for *Palliative Care: An Oxford Core Text*, aimed at medical students.

Rosemary Cook MSc PG Dip RGN PN Cert
Rosemary Cook has a background in primary care nursing, and was nursing officer for primary care in the Department of Health from 1999 to 2001. She now works for the NHS Modernisation Agency.

CHAPTER 1

Primary Care Health Policy

Nigel Starey

▶ **KEY MESSAGES**
- General practice is changing.
- Practices and practitioners need to ensure they remain 'fit for purpose'.
- Being part of a NHS means adapting to the needs of the service and the community.
- Clinical policy issues and policies are driven by political, economic, sociological and technological issues.

RECENT ADVANCES ▼

- Initiatives such as *foundation trusts*, access, choice, financial flows, commissioning general practice through to the new GP contract.
- Realising the potential of advancements in genetic technology to the NHS.
- Local Improvement Financial Trust (LIFT) arrangements for providing capital investment in primary care.
- General practitioners with special interests (GPwSIs) providing services to a wider population than the practice.
- New services in the community – such as substance misuse clinics, children's centres and smoking cessation services.

Introduction

This chapter discusses primary care health policy, in particular its relevance to general practice and some of the challenges it is facing.[1] Key questions considered include:

- ▶ What are the current and evolving responsibilities of general practice and primary care?

- ▶ How should they relate with other parts of the health service?

- ▶ Why does primary care, as a sector, and general practice within that sector, behave the way it does?[2]

In addition, the chapter will consider what is meant by health policy, the consequences of current policies, and their implications for practices and practitioners. This chapter does not pretend to offer a comprehensive guide to current policy across the whole range of clinical situations affecting practitioners, but offers a few examples to illustrate the way that all such policies are evolving and impacting on current practice. Recent policy developments will be examined with reference to implications for the future role of GPs and general practice[1] such as:

- ▶ local contracting for practice-based services via the new GMS contract

- ▶ foundation trusts

- ▶ financial flows

- ▶ access and choice

- ▶ NHS Direct and minor injury units.

Context

General practice has changed a great deal since the origin of the NHS in the 1940s. Table 1.1 provides some illustration of these changes, but the question remains: does its current design make it 'fit for purpose'?

Table 1.1 **Characteristics of general practice over the first fifty years of the NHS**

50s	60s	70s	80s	90s
Epidemics	Partnerships	GP training	Deputising	Fundholding
Infection	1966 contract	H_2 blockers	Practice manager	PMS
Single-handed GP	Antibiotics	NSAIDs	Nursing homes	1990 contract
Poor facilities	Health centres	Benzodi-azepines	Prevention	Himp (Health improvement prog)
No staff	Dispensing	Secretaries/ nurses	Teams	Co-ops
3000 patients per GP	2500 patients per GP	2300 patients per GP	2000 patients per GP	1800 patients per GP
Women = 5% of GPs	Women = 10% of GPs	Women = 25% of GPs	Women = 33% of GPs	Women = 50% of GPs
The family doctor	Pill	Family planning	Divorce rate rising	TOP (termination of pregnancy)

At the same time, the primary care sector has also evolved and changed. Table 1.2 illustrates some of these organisational and service changes.

Table 1.2 **Evolution and organisation of the primary care sector over the first fifty years of the NHS**

Pre-NHS	50s	60s	70s	80s	90s	00+
County nursing association	Ministry of Health		DHSS	DoH		
Local Authority	Exec council		Area and district health authority		Community Trust Health Authority	
					PCG	PCT
Health visiting			Family planning clinic		FHSA	
Private GP						
Home births		Hospital delivery			Midwife-led care	
Family care of the elderly		Geriatric units		Nursing homes		
Mental institutions		Psychiatric hospitals		Community care		
TB hospitals		Antibiotics	Antibiotic resistance		MRSA	

During the latter half of the 20th century, the range of services provided in general practice has mushroomed, driven by shorter length of stay in hospital, new home-based treatments, better organisation of general practice and changing social circumstances. Contraception, disease prevention, counselling and systematic care for chronic conditions were not issues in the early years of the fledgling NHS. As circumstances have changed, so too has:

▶ *the role of the GP* – from the Dr Finlay caricature to the modern primary care physician

▶ *the organisation providing care* – from the single-handed solo practitioner, to the primary care team through to the corporate primary care trust (PCT)

▶ *the surgery*, from the doctor's dining room, via the health centre to the one-stop primary care centre.

Primary care

There have been many different definitions of *primary care* over the first 50 years of the NHS, reflecting the different perspectives of those defining it and the evolving pattern of the 'out of hospital care' it provides. Definitions have focussed on the *provider* of care (GP-based care), the *location* of care (home-based care), or the *type of service* provided (generalist services). However it is defined, primary care in the UK is internationally recognised for the extent to which it underpins the whole health service and ensures that high quality, cost-effective health care is provided to the whole population.

Currently accepted definitions of primary care view it as a sector of care compared with *secondary* care (district hospital-based specialist care), *tertiary* care (national or regional specialist care), *emergency*, or *social* care. Primary care has evolved as the *first point of contact* between individuals with perceived health needs and those charged with addressing those needs. Barbara Starfield, an American Professor of Health Policy, with an interest in the effectiveness of health care provision, described the sector in the UK as being well developed and characterised by:[3]

- ▶ its accessibility
- ▶ the continuity of care it offers
- ▶ the biographical nature of that care
- ▶ the undifferentiated nature of that care
- ▶ the holistic approach to synthesising physical, emotional, psychological and spiritual elements.

This all implies that the primary care sector is *reactive* – meaning that:

- ▶ it reacts to what it is presented with
- ▶ it is non-judgemental
- ▶ it is free at the point of use
- ▶ it is not rationed
- ▶ it is almost sponge-like in its capacity to absorb whatever demands individuals and the community make on it.

Box 1.1 **Key characteristics of UK general practice in the second half of the 20th century**

- **registration** of the whole population and the associated lifelong medical record, transferred with registration

- **expert generalism** – management of all medical problems except when specialist intervention is required

- **gate keeping and referral** – controlling access to, and co-ordinating the activity of, specialist practice

- **independent contractor status and professional partnership** – self-employed, owner, employer, director and clinical practitioner – not subject to the constraints of being an employee, largely autonomous and self-directed

- **continuity of care** – by a personal doctor to an individual

If these features hark back to and evolved in a world where:

▶ dependence on charity and patronising paternalism characterised the doctor–patient relationship

▶ queuing for most necessities – such as fuel and food, was a widespread and normal part of everyday life

▶ families comprised two parents and were supported by an extended local network of family and friends

▶ employment often meant lifelong servitude

▶ education was a privilege

then we have to ask whether the design of general practice remains appropriate for its current and developing responsibilities within a society with very different characteristics. In addition, we need to ask whether the underpinning characteristics of the UK's general practice approach to providing medical services in primary care remain appropriate in a modern, consumerist, post-family society.

As the environment around it changes, so must the whole primary care sector – and that part of it which constitutes general practice needs to reflect on the significance of the changes to its own power, its responsibilities, its relationships and its behaviour. The sector has to learn lessons and adapt to the changing circumstances, otherwise it risks losing the confidence of the community.

Key features of future general practice might include those outlined in Box 1.2 opposite.

Box 1.2 **Key features of future general practice**

- personal care and advice to a defined population

- co-ordination of all health care for that population, including working with other providers to agree pathways of care

- care and maintenance of a lifelong health record, available to all carers wherever they are providing care

- provider of systematic, quality-assured health care within agreed service frameworks

- accountable to the community for the service it provides via peer review, a local contracting process and non-executive director involvement

- organised as a multi-professional care team, with defined rights and responsibilities as agreed and monitored by the local community

- management, ancillary, information, specialist services staff employed by the community – PCT or local authority

It is apparent that modern health care is far less dependent on institutions, such as hospitals, for its delivery – much more care is provided in the community, either in the patient's home or in community settings such as care homes for older people. As new technologies have helped reduce the duration of patient stay in hospital, so the proportion of treatment provided in the home setting has grown.

This does not mean that all that *home-based* care is properly defined as *primary care* as described above. The first real distinction is between:

▶ primary care as a provider of specialist services: redefining primary care so as to include specialist care provided in the home or community setting – such *home-based* specialist care becomes the direct responsibility of PCTs

and

▶ accepting the Starfield[3] definition and recognising that specialist care provided in the community is best provided by the specialist sector – with access to the acute hospital, for example, regulated by primary care acting as a gatekeeper.

The choice is important because it will fundamentally affect future investment and development of specialist services; evidence is needed about which alternative is most effective and efficient.

It is apparent that the second real distinction is between:

▶ *generalist* care – first point of contact, holistic care, biographical and undifferentiated

and

▶ *specialist* care – referred to, focussed on the current situation and short-term.

Inevitably, current developments such as:

▶ *access and choice*, which offer patients more power and choice over where their care will be provided

▶ *financial flows*, which will redistribute resources between hospitals

▶ *foundation trusts*, which will free trusts from some aspects of central control – but also introduce some attributes of membership organisations

▶ *modernisation of care and LIFT* arrangements to provide care in modern, purpose-built premises

▶ *NHS Direct and minor injury units*, which provide alternative access to advice and treatment

▶ *diagnostic and treatment centres* located either in secondary or primary care and treating a limited range of conditions needing elective, predictable intervention, examples of which might include arthroplasty or cataract surgery, dermatology or gynaecology services, opiate detoxification and outreach treatment of those with severe mental illness

will all mould the development of the primary care sector in the UK. Inevitably the future responsibilities of the sector will be different from its past responsibilities and government policy will encourage the sector, and general practice, to remain 'fit for purpose' as that purpose changes. Over the next few years, as the NHS Plan[4] is implemented, the foundations of current general practice will be shaken and tested by these developments. The survival of the GP, general practice and all it stands for can only be assured if it meets the needs of the society it serves.

Box 1.3 **Current tools for stimulating change in general practice**

- local commissioning of services through the new GMS contract

- development of new approaches to service through PMS arrangements

- clinical leadership in, and through, PCTs

- devolved control of resources with clinicians responsible for managing 'access and choice' as well as their financial consequences

- commissioning of enhanced services, GPwSI services, intermediate care services, social and voluntary sector services for a local population rather than a practice population

- appraisal, clinical supervision, development planning and career development

Health

It is a curious fact that for the first 50 or so years of the NHS, a national disease service was in operation, designed to meet the needs of the post war 1940s population, and one defined largely within the prevailing medical model or paradigm of that time. It was designed to meet the needs of the acute and chronically ill section of the population through medical or surgical intervention supported by nursing care, rather than to prevent disease or address the health needs of the mainly healthy population in the 21st century. If health is the state of being bodily and mentally vigorous and free from disease, then a NHS should, in future, evolve to promote such a concept of health – as well as to seek to return people with disease to that state.

This implies more emphasis on health promotion, disease prevention, personal responsibility for maintaining health, more encouragement of fitness and rehabilitation and less emphasis on the traditional, medical model of care provision. In addition, the medical paradigm also needs to move on from a fixation on somatic issues – disease as a malfunction of the organs or cells – to a paradigm that includes taking account of the molecular and genetic aspects of disease where health encompasses an individual's genetic heritage and treatment takes into account the impact on relatives and future generations.

The development of genetic medicine[5] can be anticipated – its early aspects include cancer genetics and pharmacogenetics[6] – but gene therapy and reclassification of disease at molecular or genetic level, preventative treatment based on genetic prediction testing, can all be anticipated. They raise not only profound ethical dilemmas but also challenges to current thinking about the role of medicine, clinical practice and particularly what it means to be a *family* doctor.

Policy

Dictionaries define policy as a plan of action, adopted or pursued by an individual, government, party or business, for example. The NHS is characterised by having a strong central or national policy framework – but regional, local, practice and individual policies are also important. In addition, it is important to recognise that clinical policy cannot be entirely separated from other areas of policy as it is always dependent on how care is organised, for example, the environment within which clinical care is provided. Table 1.3 illustrates this by looking at the issue of smoking cessation.

Table 1.3 **Smoking cessation policy: drivers**

National	Local	Practice	Individual
morbidity	central drive (DoH)	central drive (PCT)	practice agreement
tax revenues	jobs	data – contract	values
jobs	staff education	patient education	behaviour
third world issues	services	templates/clinics	consultation skills
partners in Europe			

This should not be taken to imply that all clinical policy is dependent on the national policy intent, only that the application of any clinical policy such as smoking cessation will be influenced by national policies – such as the tax on cigarettes. This is influenced by local and practice policies, such as education initiatives and the development of specialist support clinics, and by individual characteristics, such as consultation style and personal interests.

Practitioners need to have some understanding of the forces that drive the development of health policy because all clinicians are continually affected by them, and in a highly politicised health system such as the NHS, the constraints they impose on clinicians' freedom to pursue their own individual policies are considerable. One analytical tool to develop such understanding is known as a political, economic, sociological and technological (PEST) analysis. This tool can be applied to the issue of smoking cessation as Box 1.4 demonstrates.

Box 1.4 **Forces promoting smoking cessation policy**

P	Political drivers promoting smoking cessation
	• egalitarian – rights of community over individual freedom (libertarian), e.g. right not to be harmed by the smoking habits of others • Europe-wide ban on advertising • voter antipathy to smoking – driven by, or promoted via, media messages • public awareness of serious health risks
E	**Economic drivers promoting smoking cessation**
	• choice and opportunity costs – morbidity of smoking • efficient use of resources – NICE guidelines • insurance loading • tax – amount levied will promote quitting
S	**Sociological forces promoting smoking cessation**
	• changing family structures and power dynamics – children liberated to pressurise their parents • employment – smoke-free offices, peer pressure • leisure activities – fitness clubs, sport, swimming etc • use of other alternative 'designer' or lifestyle mood-affecting drugs
T	**Technological forces promoting smoking cessation**
	• nicotine replacement – drug treatment • communications – advertising • monitoring – smoke analysers

If this analysis describes the context within which national primary care health policy is operating, then we need to consider what national policies are currently influencing practice – and their impact.

National policies determining the way practice is developing
Quality assurance

If the taxpayer is to continue to finance the NHS, and if individual users of its services are to retain their confidence in the NHS, then it is no longer sufficient to *assume* that services will all be of high quality. Quality assurance mechanisms in industry, education, construction and social services are now mirrored in the NHS and designed to ratchet up the quality of service provided. The mechanisms are tailored for both clinical and organisational arenas and include:

▶ *The Healthcare Commission* reviews and inspections. To ensure clinical governance drives care delivery by reviewing the systems underpinning clinical practice through a systematic approach to peer review

▶ *appraisal, revalidation and re-accreditation of professional practice.* Those on professional registers, such as those held by the Nursing & Midwifery Council (NMC) and General Medical Council (GMC), being required to demonstrate their continuing fitness to practise on a regular basis

▶ *commissioning of care and performance management of organisations.* Ensuring openness and sound corporate as well as clinical performance by separating responsibility for the commissioning of care from responsibility for its provision

▶ *National Service Frameworks (NSFs) and NICE guidance.* Agreed clinical action plans, developed by working groups, agreed by the service and the Department of Health (DoH) all aimed at providing fair, high quality treatment through adopting a *systematic* approach to delivering treatment.

Redefining professionalism

▶ Changes to the openness and accountability of professionals and professional bodies – the GMC for example, but also to the pharmaceutical society and NMC, so as to promote public confidence in all aspects of professional practice and behaviour.

▶ Skill substitution: policies to promote the best use of scarce professional expertise. For instance, health care assistants doing tasks previously performed by nurses and doctors and GPwSIs taking responsibility for tasks previously requiring consultant appointments. These policies mirror international trends and are consequent on the reluctance of practitioners to continue the working hours and workload expected of their predecessors and the flexible labour policies that have promoted part-time work and portfolio careers throughout all sectors of the economy.

▶ As the NHS moves towards being a health promoting service rather than a disease management service, it requires professional practitioners who measure up to this new professional paradigm: skilled educators, familiar with critical analysis and interpretation, able to motivate and work with other individuals as teams rather than patronising paternalists caring for their patients.

De-institutionalisation of care

► Promoting *self-care* at home is an essential element of the policy to advance every individual citizen's autonomy, whilst also minimising dependence on state support and welfare benefits.

► Technological advances will go hand-in-hand with reducing length of stay in hospital, avoiding admission and developing schemes for early discharge. The concept of the 'hospital at home', for example, will become a feasible alternative, with the added benefit of reducing the NHS financial burden (even if the financial burden is simply transferred to the individual family). Thus, while in the 1950s and 1960s, mothers might have stayed in hospital for a week or so after having a baby, now they are often discharged within 24 hours.

► Technology also allows the elderly to remain independent for longer – mobile phones, personal alarms and video surveillance help make this alternative to institutional care safer. This is despite the sociological forces of fragmented family support and longevity, meaning the burden on primary care and social networks is increased. One consequence of the tension between technological and sociological issues is more emergency admissions to hospitals.

Becoming patient centred

► In order to promote the extent to which individual citizens have con-fidence in the NHS and feel it is 'their' service, the management and organisation of care is increasingly focussed on the patient's perspective. This involves steps to:
  ▷ empower patients, so that they can play an influential part in their own care,
  ▷ encourage patients to use their expertise to help others and to give them greater control over the type and location of the care they receive.

► Patient participation groups (PPGs)[7] may have a long and honourable place in the history of general practice but they now need to evolve to shift away from involvement of the interested minority to engage all whose lives are affected by the service.

▶ The introduction of the patient advice and liaison service (PALS) along with reform of the NHS complaints procedure is designed to ensure that the individual patient's perspective is more influential.

▶ Access and choice arrangements, whereby patients have more choice over where their hospital care will be provided, also has major implications for how care is paid for, as choice will affect hospital income. Access programmes may refocus the care GPs provide to those who have had difficulty accessing the service, but current instruments struggle to link need (ability to benefit) with access, in a way which is generally regarded as fair.

▶ Expert patient programmes, which utilise the knowledge and experience of those with chronic diseases, recognise that patients with diabetes or those undergoing renal dialysis, for example, often know more about aspects of their disease than their doctors do.

▶ The involvement of non-executive directors in directing NHS organisations is not new in secondary care, but their place in primary care is. These people, drawn from the local community, play a part in ensuring that professional expertise is balanced, scrutinised and challenged by the community's perspective.

▶ The logical next step of this policy theme is to involve more of the community in the running of services. Membership organisations such as *foundation trusts*, with their population-based membership, derived governing councils, local autonomy and financial freedoms are an example in point.

However, foundation PCTs and practices open to scrutiny and challenge by non-executive directors or members can be anticipated.

Impact on clinical practice

If these are the four underlying policy themes influencing the development of general practice and primary care, then what will be their effect on everyday practice?

Systematic care

▶ The development of protocols and guidelines – the drive for evidence-based practice and the requirement to demonstrate that best practise is being provided – requires practitioners to adopt a much more systematic approach to caring for their patients. NSFs for coronary heart disease, diabetes, care of the elderly, mental health and cancer may have set the pace in this area, but the commissioning of secondary care – and now of general practice – has been underpinned by evidence of quality; demonstrable, target driven and quantitative it may be, but it does contribute to reducing morbidity.

▶ The focus on aspirin, statins, beta-blockers, ACE inhibitors, response times and waiting lists will lead to improvements in accountability whilst stemming idiosyncratic clinical practice. However, it may seem that personal, continuing care will suffer in this climate and the question remains as to whether the price is worth paying.

▶ Ensuring that everyone consulting a clinician receives best practice every time, as well as a sympathetic ear, an empathetic approach and a personal, tailored consultation has to be the ultimate aim; policy will only be translated into practice if it supports such an approach.

▶ Systematic care also involves understanding the system and helping patients get the best out of the system – being their advocate, as well as their medical adviser.

▶ Any system – be it for managing hypertension or delivering GCSE results – is composed of a series of linked processes and associated control elements: feedback loops, control valves or regulators. Clinicians providing *systematic* care would be well advised to understand a little of systems theory.[8] Clinicians need to appreciate how the care they provide fits in to the rest of the system and how working with the system, using it and adapting it can improve the care their patients receive. Understanding some system archetypes such as *supply induced demand* and *shifting the burden* can offer some insight.[1]

Redesigning the interface between primary and secondary care

▶ As policy encourages change in the location and approach to care provision, so redesign of the way care is provided becomes imperative. The traditional interface between primary and secondary care – outpatients, A&E, admission, discharge and domiciliary visits and the instruments operating there, such as telephone calls, referral letters and discharge summaries – too often inhibit best quality clinical practice. Delays, waiting lists, trolley waits and delayed discharge reports are everyday experiences for patients and clinicians. They need to be 'designed out' and several current policies are encouraging this.

▶ *GPwSIs* are emerging to divert referrals for specialist care, taking referrals from other GPs, often working within a care team that spans primary and secondary care and freeing up capacity in the hospital.

▶ *Specialist outreach* – often specialist nurses can help patients with chronic or acute disease to be managed at home, but provide direct admission to the hospital ward when required. This pattern has emerged in renal medicine and cancer care, but is now spreading through many areas. Poor communication with general practice has sometimes been a problem. The lack of GP involvement can cause difficulties at night, at weekends or when other, non-associated medical problems arise.

▶ *Day care* – day surgery, elderly care, hospice care or renal dialysis. All these can help free up hospital beds and encourage the development of minimally invasive care, encouraging patient independence rather than extended hospital stays. Of course, developments in this area place more of the burden of care on the family and friends of the patient, more of the cost on the patient and more of the clinical burden on the primary care clinical team.

▶ *Intermediate health care* – a loosely defined term, which often includes some of the above as well as some outreach services (such as anticoagulant monitoring), supportive care (as for those suffering from dementia), specialist mental health provision (such as assertive outreach teams).

▶ *Minor injury units* located within the community and providing an alternative to A&E attendance. For many, the delays in A&E and the variety of cases that attend mean that diverting patients and treatment closer to home is vital. Of course quality assurance matters and the provision of template driven, systematic care by nurses working with medical support should help to reduce the burden on A&E as well as support local general practice by diverting the "walking wounded" away from their treatment rooms.

▶ *Co-ordination and information management and technology* support for care will be essential to successful redesign – clinicians need access to individuals' medical records no matter where they are consulted, and patients need to have confidence that the redesigned system will provide high-quality care.

Technical and diagnostic advances

▶ New developments in fibre optics, scanning, pathology and therapeutics, make the changes to the way care is provided, legitimate – by ensuring it is safe, efficient and effective for patients to be cared for closer to home. Upper gastrointestinal endoscopy in primary care, antenatal care including ultrasound in peripheral clinics, intermediate care for anticoagulant monitoring and the use of atypical antipsychotics in the community would be current examples, but further development can be anticipated to affect most specialities and will facilitate further movement of care closer to the patient's home. Therapeutic developments in the care of patients with rheumatoid arthritis (TNF blockers), less toxic anticancer treatments, new dementia treatments and new treatments for drug dependency are all becoming available and promise improved outcomes for patients and less dependence on specialist, hospital-based care.

Investment and access to care

▶ Until recently *investment in the primary care infrastructure* has been dependent on independent contractors and it has been apparent for some years that this has been an inadequate vehicle for delivering the system reform agenda outlined here. Apart from the difficulty of raising the necessary capital and finding replacement contractors at the time of retirement, the constraints imposed by national templates such as the 'Red book' have meant that providing appropriate facilities has been problematic. New approaches to capital investment in primary care were sketched out in the Wanless report[9] and are being delivered through LIFTs arrangements. While the report's challenge of renewing 90% of the current primary care stock within ten years may be over-ambitious, the pace of change can be expected to be rapid.

▶ Reform of *access to care* arrangements has been a national policy direction for many years, particularly concerning hospital waiting times and waiting lists. Recently, this has become more of an issue for primary care to focus on. The national primary care collaborative approach to access, through a systematic approach to redesigning the GP appointment system is an example. Although it does have certain perverse effects on routine review arrangements, it can speed access for people needing more timely care. The introduction of *triage*, either by primary care clinicians 'in house', or via telephone triage (eg, NHS Direct) are also seen as tools for tackling access issues.

▶ In reality, most people do not always want, or need, immediate access to care – they need a level of access that is appropriate to their lifestyle and health needs – commuters' needs in this area are different from the isolated elderly; children's symptoms can often develop rapidly and may be frightening for them and their parents.

▶ Gate keeping by primary care clinicians, along with 24-hour support and advice, should make the primary care system work more efficiently. This may not necessarily be achieved in a way that satisfies all parties that they are receiving personal, continuing, holistic care tailored to their individual circumstances.

Quality assurance

▶ The implication of systems such as reaccreditation, revalidation, clinical supervision and personal development planning, for the autonomy and freedom of clinicians to practise are profound. If clinicians' freedom to practise is to retain the confidence of the public, then, post Shipman, openness to peer review, a willingness to justify actions and a systematic approach to learning from significant events, personal and team development, and system audit, are required. The new contracting arrangements supervised by PCTs, offer an opportunity for establishing the required supportive relationships, which can make this agenda more of an opportunity for clinicians to enrich their careers and less a threat of a punitive approach to clinical practice.

▶ At an organisational level, quality assurance through peer review of performance has spread rapidly through the NHS – *The Healthcare Commission visits, improving working lives, investors in people, HQS (Health Quality Service)* are examples – but we should anticipate that commissioning arrangements for general practice, pharmacies etc will include elements of this approach, tailored and proportionate though the approach will need to be. While the full panoply of peer review visits for every practice and chemists shop may be too inefficient, clinical freedom and continuing financial independence require that aspects of the peer review process are introduced, including the elements of *clinical and corporate governance* (see Table 1.4) so that any general practice should be expected to justify its performance and approach to a peer review team.

Table 1.4 **Peer review of independent contractor organisation**

Clinical governance	Corporate governance
Patient experience	Probity
Patient involvement	Open decision making
Risk management	Management arrangements
Clinical audit	Accounting practice
Clinical effectiveness	Standing orders
Staff management	Officer powers
Education and training	Exec/Non-exec balance
IM&T	Partnership – internal & external
Strategic capacity	

Impact on general practice

If these are the ways that policy will impact on clinical practice, how will general practice and the general practitioner be affected?

Future of GP partnership as organisational form

It will be apparent to many that the above issues and arguments provide a considerable challenge to the tradition of professional partnership as the organisational model underpinning the delivery of most general medical practice in this country. Reform will be required if the community is to retain confidence in GPs and their practices. Any reform will have to meet the agenda oulined in Table 1.4 – corporate and clinical governance issues cannot and should not be ignored. As part of these developments, an opening up of the current model to include the community in decision making and design is required. In arguing for a membership organisation or club[1,8] other models should not be ignored, such as co-operatives, workers as shareholders, housing associations and schools with tenant and parent governors; what is required is to evolve an organisation that is *fit for purpose*. The local practice – on every housing estate and in every community – has many virtues: accessibility, adapted to local circumstances, and familiarity, for example. Unless it adapts to changing circumstances, however, these virtues are put at risk.

Future of the practice as the building block

Are the inefficiencies of independent, isolated small practices worth bearing for the personal service they offer? As policy encourages more provision of medical services in the community, by practitioners offering services to larger populations, using more capital-intensive facilities and requiring the support of a range of practitioners from different professional backgrounds, so the pre-eminence of the practice is set to decline. Rather what would seem to be required are personal relationships between practitioners and patients within an organisation of sufficient capacity to deliver high-quality care across all the appropriate areas and disciplines – groups of practices as archipelagos rather than each as an island might be the best analogy. With PCTs engaging practices in local commissioning discussions, practices can be expected to develop alliances with their neighbours to support clinical network development in areas such as those illustrated in Box 1.5, but local circumstance may expand this menu through mechanisms such as PMS, GPwSI specialist services, enhanced services and intermediate care. While the distribution of practices in an area may have been the result of personality differences and accidents of history these cannot be allowed to determine future provision.

Box 1.5 **Service provision developing with local clinical networks**

• child protection
• disability services
• care in nursing and residential homes
• out of hours and emergency cover arrangements
• specialist clinics – GPwSIs and visiting consultants
• primary care diagnostic and treatment centre care
• facilities management – human resources, premises issues, staff pay
• education and training
• clinical supervision
• palliative care
• stroke services
• hospital at home and admission avoidance schemes

Career structure

With this extensive agenda for service and clinical care redesign, we have to consider what education and training will be required to equip clinicians for careers in this sector of the health system. As GPs, our experience will help us to adapt to many of the policy driven changes, but in future more emphasis will be on:

- ▶ team working

- ▶ managing change

- ▶ patient and public involvement

- ▶ governance.

These may best be delivered through a joint 'core' training programme across professions and disciplines, which can also help break down some of the historic professional boundaries that have led to tribal behaviour, and offer the opportunity for movement between professions as careers and interests develop.

In addition, alternatives to independent contractor status are becoming more widespread – with salaried status offering greater choice and flexibility to those looking to vary commitment at different stages in their career.

Registration

At present the whole population is registered with GPs but increasing numbers find this system too restrictive. Most practices have ceased to provide a personal doctor system – instead they regard registration as being with the practice rather than the GP and this is formally recognised in the new GMS contract. In addition, patients who work, particularly if they work away from home during the week, students who study away from home, refugees and travellers, all challenge the current registration system. Technological solutions to allowing registration with several practices, encouraging patient-held records and moving to a membership approach may deliver the kind of change, which is required to ensure that practice and its relationship with the community remains supportive and flexible.

Out of hours arrangements

With responsibility passing from individual GPs to the PCT for the provision of care outside normal office hours, we can anticipate most GPs withdrawing from the direct provision of such care. Nevertheless the cost to them of withdrawing, along with the lack of spare capacity to offer alternative providers means that PCTs will have little choice but to continue to contract with deputising services and GP co-operatives in the short term. Within a relatively short time we can anticipate that first-line care will transfer from GPs to paramedics, nurses and minor injury units, as these groups are likely to be more cost effective and efficient. GPs may remain associated and available as 'second' on-call providers.

Conclusion

Primary care policy in the NHS is evolving in response to an array of forces that are dramatically affecting the care general practice provides – not just what can be provided, but also how it is provided, the quality of the care, and the relationship between carer and recipient of care. The whole relationship between practitioner and patient is changing, as is the relationship between the practitioner and the health service, and the opportunity for primary care physicians to have fulfilling careers has never been greater.

References

1. Starey N. *The Challenge for Primary Care*. Oxford: Radcliffe Medical Press, 2003

2. Gillam S, Meads G. *Modernisation and the Future of General Practice*. London: Kings Fund, 2001

3. Starfield B. Is primary care essential? *Lancet* 1994; **344**: 1129–33

4. The NHS Plan. *A plan for investment. A plan for reform*. London: HMSO, 2000

5. Department of Health. *Our inheritance, our future*. London: HMSO, 2003

6. Nuffield Council on Bioethics. *Pharmacogenetics: ethical issues*. London: Nuffield Council on Bioethics, 2003

7. Heritage Z (ed). In: *Community participation in general practice*. Royal College of General Practitioners Occasional Paper No. 64. London: RCGP, 1994

8. Senge P. *The Fifth Discipline*. London: Century Business, 1990

9. Wanless D. *Securing our future health: taking the long-term view*. London: HM Treasury, 2002

10. Starey N. In: Meads G. *Future Options for General Practice*. Oxford: Radcliffe Medical Press, 1995

CHAPTER 2

Health Care Ethics

Ann Orme-Smith

▶ **KEY MESSAGES**
- The understanding of ethical principles is of fundamental importance to all those providing health care.

- Many problems presenting in general practice have an ethical dimension that must be acknowledged and addressed, using ethical principles.

- Confidence in resolving complex ethical dilemmas will be improved by reading widely on the issue and by group case discussion.

RECENT ADVANCES ▼

- The development of pre-implantation genetic diagnosis has given rise to considerable debate concerning the ethics of its use; this debate is likely to continue.

- The recognition of the importance of individual choice at the end of life is becoming more widespread, and the provision of signed advance directives to general practitioners more frequent.

- There is increasing support, in particular from the British Medical Association, for an 'opt-out' organ donation system in the UK that relies on presumed consent, in line with the policy adopted in many other European countries.

- Published guidelines for the conduct of research in children, and ongoing projects involving advance consent in the dying, are likely to enhance medical knowledge in these two important groups.

Everyone who has the clinical responsibility of advising, caring for, and treating patients is bound by a moral code of behaviour. Health care ethics is the study of that moral code, its rules, principles, and practical application.

Ethical dilemmas present to doctors daily. Satisfactory resolution of these dilemmas needs consideration of the moral and legal implications of each of the possible decisions before the final one is made. Basic ethical principles must be applied, with the aim of enhancing the wellbeing of the individual, (respect for autonomy, beneficence, and non-maleficence) without detriment to the community or the wider society (justice). Due thought must be given to the changes in emphasis in moral thinking that take place over long periods of time, and the influence of the mix of cultures and religions that make up our citizenry today.

It is important to understand that in many cases attempts to resolve complex ethical problems require wider consideration than that offered by the basic principles mentioned above. For example, endorsing an individual's autonomous decision for a specific treatment may be detrimental to the community, if funding is at stake. A balance needs to be struck between potential loss and gain.

This chapter concentrates on four main areas of recent development in health care:

- ▶ fertility

- ▶ end of life

- ▶ organ donation

- ▶ research.

The text is intentionally concise in order to introduce the reader to as much material as possible, and to provoke further investigation and discussion.

Fertility

Medically managed fertility brings with it many ethical problems with which society has to grapple. Choosing the 'right sort' of embryo for implantation, ('genethics'),[1] not only where there is hereditary disease manifest in the family but also one with potential to treat a sibling's disease, has been debated very recently.[2,3] Other recent issues include the ownership of frozen embryos and their disposal, management of errors and the identification of sperm donors. Surrogacy, payment for it and subsequent placement of the infant, is still a problem from time to time. In vitro fertilisation (IVF) still leads to more multiple births despite the reduction in the number of embryos implanted at any one time. This entails a higher morbidity in mother and infants and a greater financial burden for the NHS.[4]

Now that medical expertise can help, infertility has come to be regarded as a medical problem. More fundamentally, founding a family is understood to be a human right under the proposed European Constitution.[5] If we accept this, do we also accept that its cost is borne by the NHS? Success rates vary between centres and often several attempts are necessary before a pregnancy continues to term. The process can be very stressful for the couple involved. How many attempts would it be reasonable for a public service to fund? Ought there to be an upper age limit for assisted parenthood? If equity is a concern, ought there to be any restrictions at all to treatment for infertility?

Human cloning is a theoretical possibility. Technical advances towards successful cloning of human tissue continue; ethical opinion and the law are still in debate. Gogarty examines the legislative aspects of human reproductive cloning in his paper; in his conclusion he remarks that:

> advanced technologies such as cloning do not warrant the traditional legal paradigm of prescriptive legislation because they evolve too quickly for such legislation to respond. In such cases the emphasis should be on the separation between acceptable or unacceptable rather than on the form of procedure itself. This will assist in constructing clear boundaries between ethical and unethical research and hence create clarity in the law and assuage public distrust in reproductive medicine…[6]

There are two main ethical issues for general practice: equitable allocation of resources and whom to refer.

Equitable allocation of resources

Those who have personal funds often commit large sums to infertility treatment in the hope of gaining the child they wish for. Those that are unable to do this depend on the NHS.

There is a marked disparity between different parts of the United Kingdom in the provision of NHS funding for assisted reproduction. Some couples have free treatment, though perhaps for only one cycle; others are required to pay for their drugs but the rest of their care is free. In some areas there are strict entry criteria that exclude a number of those desiring treatment. The situation is one of rationing and this is necessary in a health care system relying on restricted funding. If we regard a 'ration' as a fair portion of the whole, we must still decide what that fair portion might be, and accept that the necessary restriction means disappointment for some.

Allocation of family resources depends on the priorities decided by the individual couple, in this case, towards the realisation of the 'right to found a family'. Allocation of NHS resources depends on priorities placed at a distance from the individual couple. Different parts of the country have differences in the health needs of their population, with many factors to be taken into account, such as age, levels of morbidity, education, levels of employment and cultural differences. There are many calls on NHS funding that may be viewed as warranting attention before anything is committed to treating those with fertility problems.

There is no simple answer to this. A fixed budget for infertility treatment is the obvious starting point. After that, ought it to be 'first come first served' or are some 'more deserving' than others?

The shortage of NHS resources for infertility treatment has led to some women taking advantage of the 'egg giving' process offered by some private clinics. Infertility treatment is offered at a discount to those women who agree to donate to others eggs harvested during their first cycle of treatment. The financial content of this process could be seen as 'trading in eggs' although no money changes hands. Recent media publicity has led the Human Fertilisation and Embryology Authority (HFEA) to consider the need for a review of this arrangement. Meanwhile, it continues.[7]

The ethical problem at the root of egg donation is similar to that underlying the sale of organs. The egg donor may be fully informed and understand the risks of ovarian hyperstimulation. But is she able to make a fully autonomous decision, knowing that if she refuses, she will have to bear the whole cost of her own treatment? There seems to be a powerful element of coercion that could distort her appraisal of the treatment and its consequences for her and her partner.[8]

Whom to refer

Any infertile couple *may* be referred for treatment, once the restrictions described above have been overcome. Every centre offering fertility treatment must comply with the Code of Practice laid down by the HFEA in 1995.[9] This requires each centre to be satisfied that any treatment would be in the interests of any resulting child. As well as taking a social and medical history from each of the prospective parents, the GP of each is asked if there is any reason why either might not be 'suitable' for treatment. The welfare of the child is held to be of the greatest importance, and the Code of Practice reflects this. It follows that although there are no *specific* exclusions from treatment, each centre must be satisfied that assessments before treatment confirm suitability for parenthood, whatever that might be.

However, there is another group of people to consider, who are not necessarily incapable of conceiving naturally. The development of pre-implantation genetic diagnosis (PIGD) of inherited conditions such as achondroplasia makes it possible to identify affected embryos at an early stage. IVF provides a route for this, where only unaffected embryos are selected for implantation, the others being discarded. Previously, prenatal diagnosis (PND) was the only possibility, and pregnancy termination was an option for the parents if the foetus was affected. Some argue that there is no ethical difference between these two situations: each involves the death of a potential human being. Others will point out the difference to the mother; a mid-trimester termination is likely to be extremely distressing, whereas PIGD gives her the knowledge that the foetus she carries is free from the condition she fears.

The most recent ethical controversy has arisen over an extended use for PIGD. Consider two scenarios in which an existing child has a serious and life threatening condition that may be cured, or at least ameliorated, by the use of compatible cord blood donated by a sibling yet to be born. In the first case, the child has thalassaemia: as an inherited condition, PIGD can be used within the law to screen for this. The HFEA gives permission for tissue typing to be carried out.[10] This gives the existing child the opportunity for rescue by the sibling's cord blood. However, in the second case, where the existing child's condition is not inherited, PIGD is deemed inappropriate: the HFEA refuses permission for pre-implantation tissue typing.[11] This is on the grounds that testing the embryos would have been primarily in another's interest (the affected child) rather than the embryos' interests.

The difference between these two cases demonstrates the difficulty that the law has in keeping up with advances in medical technology.[12] An advance is made and, at first, its wider implications are not appreciated. When they are, public debate takes place, and it is some time before opinions are crystallised. It is only after that that changes in the law come about. Many felt that the HFEA was wrong to refuse permission to the second family: yet the HFEA decided that it would have been unlawful to give permission.

The ethical basis for allowing both procedures is clear. The lives of the affected children would be protected. The welfare of the new siblings would be assured, as 'wanted' infants. In the first case, the child to be born will not have the inherited condition. The intervention of PIGD is able to provide further information that could help the existing child. There are those that might say that the child in the second case is created for someone else's sake, a means to someone else's end. PIGD is carried out on embryos, an intervention that is unnecessary for the intended child, but necessary for another. Yet the parents maintain that their intention is to have more children, and in this way, they are able to increase their family and at the same time, help an existing sick child.

The reports and discussion in the media of these two cases illustrate the level of interest that many people have in some very complex ethical issues. On the one hand, there is the human benefit provided by the new technology; on the other, there is the fear of its extension towards the creation of 'designer babies'. Ethical opinion has to consider the risks and benefits in order to provide a morally acceptable balance.

Key messages

- Is sub-fertility a medical or a social problem?

- If it is a medical problem, ought all treatment be paid for by the NHS?

- If it is a social problem, ought its treatment be paid for by the couple concerned, not by the tax payer?

- What ethical problems are posed by these questions?

End of life

It can be very difficult to broach the subject of dying to a patient nearing the end of life. Workman refers to this as 'the taboo against speaking or writing about impending death'.[13] It is easier to embrace the teaching ascribed to Epicure in ancient Greece: 'why do you worry so much about death? Where death is, you are not. Where you are, death is not.' Maybe we have already accepted this and now the fear is focussed not on death itself, but on the process of dying.

If we exclude sudden death, few people now can expect to die in their own home, although that may have been their wish.[14] Most will die in hospitals, or hospices. Palliative and terminal care are now specialist entities, with access to a large accumulation of expertise, experience, and technology. The burden of caring for the dying is often too great for family members, particularly when the quality of care is held to be superior in a hospice, for example. The GP's traditional role of attendance at the death bed has changed. The GP is now an important figure for patients in their preparation for the dying process.

The ethical issues for the GP in his or her current role in preparing the patient for dying include providing information and advance directives (living wills).

Providing information

More specifically, the GP should aim to provide the right amount of information, at the right time and with proper support for the patient and family.

The aim of good palliative care has been described as 'a good death'. It is impossible for a doctor to know by instinct exactly what each patient understands about dying and what his or her wishes are for the management of his or her own death. It could be argued that "to force patients to have what we would call a good death is inherently medically paternalistic. A good death is one that is appropriate and requested by that particular patient."[15]

Doctors have been shown to over-estimate survival times for their dying cancer patients.[16] However, by delaying any mention of death the doctor is effectively denying patients the opportunity to ask questions about dying and to crystallise their ideas about their own death. Even though the subject may seem too difficult for the doctor, it may be very important for the patients, who can only thus express their apprehension and fears about the process of dying with someone they trust. At the very least, patients need to be properly informed in good time so that they can arrange their affairs as they wish.[17]

This is where the humanity and sensitivity of the doctor are important in helping the patient to ask questions and in answering them clearly and truthfully. These are qualities that develop from the experience of caring for dying patients and ought not to have to be formally taught. If we examine the fear that doctors have that prevents them from mentioning death to a dying patient, in part it is the fear of hurting or damaging the patient in some way. If we believe that a contented untroubled mind helps a patient to overcome mental and physical pain, is it not wrong for the doctor to disturb this tranquillity? This attitude can only be valid if the patient's mind really is contented and untroubled. Only the patient will know: without gentle enquiry, others can only guess.

Advance directives ('living wills')[18]

Advance directives can be formal or informal. There is a specific form[19] that an increasing number of people are using: a copy is kept in their medical records, duly dated, witnessed and signed, with a clear indication of that person's wishes with regard to treatment in the future. As we know, a competent person can refuse treatment, however irrational that decision might seem to be. The fear is that when someone becomes incompetent, for whatever reason, their wishes are overridden – hence the advance directive.[20]

> Dear Dr...
> I would like you to know that if I became unable to look after myself, I do not wish to be kept alive with drugs, go into a hospital, or a home. If I were unable to get my shopping or work in the garden it would soon hasten my end.
>
> Yours sincerely...

This patient had written out an informal declaration in her letter to her GP. If she had merely told the GP, or a close friend or relative, of her wishes, and the GP had recorded this at the time, this could also have been helpful. And this is something people do quite frequently – 'please, please don't ever send me in to hospital'.

It is perhaps inevitable that on occasion a patient will bring up the subject of assisted suicide,[21,22] or of euthanasia.[23] This is an important and controversial topic, currently being debated. Although legal in some European countries, neither is lawful in the UK. On the surface, this takes the responsibility for tackling a very difficult ethical problem out of the doctor's hands, who cannot agree to do as the patient wishes under the current laws.

It could be argued that by refusing therapeutic treatment, as opposed to palliation, a patient is hastening his or her own death. If the patient takes an autonomous, informed decision, the doctor, by withholding such treatment, could be seen to be either respecting that autonomy or colluding with suicide, depending on one's moral stance. However, a doctor cannot force a competent patient to have treatment against his or her will, and this is a theoretical argument only.

Until recently, the form of advance directive signed by many people states that 'I am not to be subjected to any medical intervention or treatment aimed at prolonging or sustaining my life' in certain specific circumstances of illness. If we now examine the advance directive in its latest form, there is an alternative choice: 'I wish to be kept alive for as long as is reasonably possible and consent to all appropriate medical treatment'.[19]

Once a person becomes incompetent and unable to give informed consent the existence of an advance directive can be helpful in the management of the dying process. A person's best interests are paramount in such situations. As well as respecting the patient's wishes as far as possible, the aim must to be to maintain that person's dignity and minimise their suffering.

- A nonagenarian, mentally and physically frail, is cared for in a nursing home. She develops pneumonia and becomes comatose. She has twin daughters, one insisting that their mother has nursing care only, the other that her mother's pneumonia is treated energetically, in hospital if necessary. No-one is aware of the patient's own pre-morbid wishes, although each daughter has her own view, forcibly expressed.

- How can this be resolved?

Organ donation [24]

Everyone most closely involved in organ donation, recipients, donors, and their families, will at some time be registered patients in general practice. It is important for primary care professionals to be aware of the main ethical controversies that are currently unresolved and that are obstacles that must be overcome before the supply of organs for transplantation approaches the demand. A better understanding of these problems by professionals will facilitate discussion with patients and families, each of whom is a potential donor.

The demand for donated organs was created by the medical innovation of a successful kidney transplant, in 1954. Peter Medawar said in 1968, '[the] transplantation of human organs... will come about for the single and sufficient reason that people are so constituted that they would rather be alive than dead.' [25] The UK transplant programme has expanded to such an extent that in 2002–03, 2777 solid organs, including hearts, livers and kidneys, were transplanted. This figure has to be considered in the context of other more sobering figures: at the end of this period, more than 5700 people were on the national list for an organ transplant, and 368 people had already died before a new organ became available. [26] These figures do not take into account those who need transplants but are not yet on the list. There is an increasing gap between the number of organs available and the number of those needing transplants to sustain life, many of whom are young adults. Each year this gap gets wider.

There are three main ethical controversies:

When does death occur?

'A determination of death is a legal determination that a collection of living cells is no longer entitled to the rights granted to human beings.' [27]

We accept that dying is a process that takes place over a period of time. It is during the dying process that the possibility of organ donation must be considered. As soon as the process is complete, the cells in the organism begin to die and organs become unsuitable for donation. To prevent this happening, oxygenation must be maintained.

If brain stem death has occurred and been certified, [28] oxygenation happens naturally. The heart continues to beat and respiration can be maintained. After certification of death, organs in good condition for transplantation can be removed. The ethical acceptance of this relies on the acceptance that mind and body are indeed separate, and personhood depends on the active presence of the mind. In brain stem death, only the body remains. '[It] is our mental life which constitutes what we are, not the machine that supports it'.[29]

With the increasing shortage of organs, the use of non-heart-beating donors (NHBD) is a possibility.[30] The donor would be someone who had suffered a very recent (under 30 minutes) cardiopulmonary arrest. Resuscitation would have failed, and death certified. An immediate cut down into the femoral artery and perfusion of cold preservative would be started. Simultaneously, cardiac massage and elective ventilation would be maintained.

In this case there are substantial ethical problems to be resolved. First, there is the anomaly that on the one hand death has been certified, yet cardiac massage and ventilation are being carried out. Brain stem death has not been diagnosed. Is this a 'dead donor' or an 'as good as dead donor'?[31] Second, an unauthorised assault has been carried out on the insensate person that is not an emergency intervention in his or her best interests. The intention is to aid others in society, and it may be beneficial for them. Yet the individual's autonomy is not being respected; he or she is being used as a means to others' ends, not for his or her own benefit.[32]

If the individual is carrying a donor card, or is on the national donor register, these doubts may be assuaged. The law still requires an attempt to be made to discover the wishes of a near relative, if one can be found. But the main problem lies in the doubt as to whether the person is actually dead at the time that intervention began: 'This doesn't mean that [NHBD] are still alive at the moment of organ retrieval, but simply that medicine alone cannot demonstrate that they are surely dead.'[33]

Who has rights over the body and its parts?

> [The] person lawfully in possession of the body ... may authorise the removal of any part from the body for use ... if, having made such reasonable enquiry as may be practicable, he has no reason to believe (a) that the deceased had expressed an objection ... or (b) that the surviving spouse or any surviving relative of the deceased objects to the body being so dealt with.[34]

The ethical problem lies in these words. Kennedy argues that this prejudices the living in favour of the dead.[35] The law recognises that a breach may cause shock and distress to the surviving relative(s) yet there is no way that the Human Tissue Act (HTA) can be enforced, nor is there any sanction provided in case of breach. Reliance is placed on members of the medical profession adhering to the meaning behind the wording, thus avoiding bringing the profession into disrepute. Yet observance of section 1 (2) (b) of the HTA will create delay if the appropriate relative is not immediately available. Any delay reduces the viability of the donor organ and therefore increases the likelihood of transplant failure. Perhaps more importantly, there is recognition that the ante mortem wishes of an individual may be countermanded by a relative after death.[36]

This is a clear ethical conflict. Respect for the dignity of the body after death and the concept of posthumous harm to the autonomy of the individual are arguments that oppose the concept of responsibility towards the recipient whose life depends on a donated organ. There ought to be no conflict if the possible donor had, before death, expressed a desire to be a donor after death.

Many consider that we ought to go further, by introducing the 'opt-out' system.[37] There are those who consider the rights of the recipient to pre-empt all others, believing the body after death to be a vital resource. The argument that there had never been any value in the cadaver, apart from to the anatomist, until the possibility of organ transplantation has some strength. So does the view that the necessity of consent before donation is morally incorrect.[38]

The opt-out system is softer, by giving those with a real objection to becoming donors the option to declare their unwillingness. All others would be considered and consent presumed. Sensitivity to the families of potential donors would still need to be shown, and the rare possibility of refusal accepted. If the public was made more aware of their responsibility to those waiting for organs there would be less likelihood of refusal. '[The] emphasis on individual rights in medical ethics sometimes overshadows any concept of responsibilities.'[39]

Some advocate the introduction of mandated donation.[40] Public policy would provide a concerted authoritative campaign of public education and information directed in favour of donation. This may amount to legal coercion, but is ethically justifiable if we regard it as 'the promotion of social good'.

How can society balance respect for the dead with the needs of the living?

We cannot pretend that the continuing development of organ transplantation is not beneficial. Many lives are saved and for those currently on dialysis the quality of life is improved immeasurably. There is an ethical requirement to match the supply of organs with ever-increasing demand.

When we talk of 'respect for the dead' we may mean respect for the person: their philosophy, way of life, ideals, as well as achievements. We may mean continuing respect for their material legacy: their bodies. Each person's life has a value. Does it have a continuing value after death, and can that value be altered or damaged by how we treat the body?

It is reasonable to argue that the use of organs for transplantation shows supreme respect for the donor. It gives an opportunity for life for another person without damage or sacrifice on the part of the donor. Furthermore, the potential donor's ante mortem desire ought to take priority over objections by the next of kin; by objecting, they are not showing respect for their dead relative, merely satisfying their own self-directed will.

Key messages

- Some feel that the need for organ transplantation in many cases is avoidable, either by early identification and proper treatment of preventable disease or by lifestyle changes. They use this as an argument against a donor register.

- Others feel that the power assigned to the relative to deny permission for donation is wrong, and denies the possibility of life to a recipient.

- Can each of these views be justified and accommodated?

- The sale of organs is currently prohibited. Can an ethical argument be put forward for the law to be changed in its favour?

Research

Medical research performs a vital role in the development of new and better treatment. There are many elements that contribute to good research, apart from the researchers themselves. Examination of research protocols by the Research Ethics Committee (REC), access to statisticians, provision of experimental drugs, funding, and eventual publication, are all necessary. None of this would be possible without the use of human research subjects who take part in research programmes in very large numbers, thereby fulfilling a certain responsibility of the individual to society.

The role of the REC is primarily to ensure that a research protocol fulfils ethical requirements before allowing it to proceed. Amongst the issues it examines are those relating to: information provided for research subjects; retention of organs/tissue; use of children and incompetent adults as research subjects; research into care of the dying; issues of consent; research into inherited disorders and preservation of confidentiality; potentially damaging or intrusive protocols; when to stop.

There are two topics of importance in primary care; a third is added because of its potential for interesting debate.

Research using children

Use of unlicensed, or 'off label', drugs is not unusual in paediatrics. These are drugs that have only been tested adequately in adults and do not have a product licence for paediatric use. This is because there is a dearth of good research evidence for the metabolism, safety and efficacy in children of many potentially useful drugs. We can put forward two reasons for this. First, the cost of paediatric prescribing is a relatively small part of the total drug budget, and so commands a proportionately small commitment for research from the drug industry.

Second, children as research subjects require special consideration.[41] Many of them will not be competent to give consent on their own behalf, but they must still be involved in the consenting process if the research is to be conducted ethically. The parent of a very sick child may feel some pressure to consent to a research programme that they perceive as the only hope for their child's recovery. Can their consent be said to be given freely, without coercion? Are they considering the benefit for other children, and giving consent altruistically?[42]

Guidelines used by RECs for research in children make the following points:

- ▶ research in children is important and should be supported

- ▶ children have unique interests and are not mini adults

- ▶ research is only ethical in children if it cannot be done in adults equally well

- ▶ the child's agreement must be secured

- ▶ any procedure not directly benefiting the child should satisfy legal and ethical principles of minimal risk.

Research into care of the dying

There are parallels here with the question of research in children. Many of the drugs used in palliative care for the dying are used empirically, for example, those used for 'death rattle'. There has not been any research into the best form of treatment for this condition mainly because it is impossible to get consent from a patient who has reached this terminal stage, nor can consent be given by a proxy for an adult.[43]

Research being carried out in the palliative care wards at the Royal Marsden Hospital in London may change this.[44] This relies on advance consent process for entry into a trial for which the patient may be eligible at a later date, that is, when death rattle develops. The researchers state:

Research in palliative care is notoriously difficult. If generally accepted, this consent process may provide a means of increasing the number of patients in the terminal phase entering trials. This is essential if we are to improve the evidence base underpinning the practice of palliative care and improve the care of dying patients.

Testing a hypothesis

General practice is a rich source of research material. In particular, the epidemiology of disease in a defined population can be studied.[45]

A radical hypothesis has been published recently.[46] This proposes developing a combination pill (the Polypill) designed to reduce cardiovascular disease by 80%. Wald and Law conclude that:

> [the] *Polypill strategy could largely prevent heart attacks and stroke if taken by everyone aged 55 or older and everyone with existing cardiovascular disease. It would be acceptably safe and with widespread use would have a greater impact on the prevention of disease in the Western world than any other single intervention.*

Is this a hypothesis with great potential benefit to mankind, or is it yet another step towards making a large segment of the population dependent on daily medication? Without properly conducted research trials it would not be adopted; general practice is ideally suited for the conduct of such trials. It could be argued that the underlying ethical question must be answered first: what are the potential risks as well as benefits to the induction of medicalisation of large numbers of healthy people, whose only indication for 'treatment' is their age?

The excitement and sense of achievement that accompanies every new technical discovery in medicine must be tempered by the calm consideration of its potential risks and ethical consequences.

Key messages

- A drug company wishes to trial a new drug in patients with a serious, potentially fatal disease. It is to be compared with the current 'best treatment'. The company will provide all the drugs free of charge, as well as fund the researchers and pay laboratory costs. It is unlikely that the hospital will be able to fund supplies of the new drug, if it is shown to be the more effective treatment in these patients.

- What are the ethical implications that need to be discussed by the REC?

References

1. Heyd D. *Genethics: Moral Issues in the Creation of People.* London: University of California Press Ltd, 1994

2. Henderson M, Norfolk A. Birth of 'saviour sibling' stirs call for debate on fertility law. *The Times* 20 June 2003 p9

3. Dyer C. News: Couple wins right to select embryo. *BMJ* 2003; **326**: 782

4. Tindall G. Mixed blessings: ethical issues in assisted conception. *J R Soc Med* 2003; **96**: 34–5

5. Article 11–9 Part II, proposed European Constitution 2003, and Human Rights Act 1998 Article 12

6. Gogarty B. What exactly is an exact copy? And why it matters when trying to ban human reproductive cloning in Australia. *J Med Ethics* 2003; **29 (2)**: 88

7. Dyer O. News: Fertilisation authority to review 'egg giving'. *BMJ* 2003; **327**: 250

8. See reference 4

9. www.hfea.gov.uk for HFEA Code of Practice 1995 6th edition (accessed 1/03/2004)

10. This decision was challenged in the High Court. The HFEA went to the Court of Appeal which overturned the High Court ruling, see reference 3

11. In this case the parents travelled to Chicago where tissue typing was available to them. The resulting 'matched' child was born in the UK

12. See reference 6

13. Workman S R. Doctors need to know when and how to say die. [letter] *BMJ* 2003; **327**: 221

14. In a personal practice with a list size of 2300, from Feb 1995 – Feb 2000, the writer signed 20 death certificates, four per year. Eight people died in nursing homes and 12 in their own homes. There were 11 women and nine men, and the average age was 82 years, with a range of 66 to 93. Heart disease accounted for eight deaths, bronchopneumonia for seven and cancer for the remaining five

15. Jones J, Willis D. What is a good death? [letter] *BMJ* 2003; **327**: 224

16. Glare P, Virik K, Jones M, *et al.* A systematic review of physicians' survival predictions in terminally ill cancer patients. *BMJ* 2003; **327**: 195

17. Ellershaw J, Ward C. Care of the dying patient: the last hours or days of life. *BMJ* 2003; **326**: 31

18. See: www.mind.org.uk/Information/Legal/Legalbriefing+advancedirectives.htm

19. See: www.ves.org.uk

20. Irwin M. A new kind of living will. *J R Soc Med* 2003; **96**: 411

21. Hurst S A, Mauron A. Assisted suicide and euthanasia in Switzerland: allowing a role for non-physicians. *BMJ* 2003; **326**: 271–3

22. Assisted suicide and euthanasia in Switzerland. [letter] *BMJ* 2003; **327**: 51–3

23. Here defined as the act of killing someone painlessly at his or her request with the object of relieving suffering

24. This section is confined to cadaveric solid organ donation. The use of the living donor and payment for body parts are discussed in: Price D. *Legal and Ethical Aspects of Organ Transplantation* Cambridge: Cambridge University Press, 2000

25. Anyanwu A, Treasure T. Prognosis after heart transplantation. [editorial] *BMJ* 2003; **326**: 509. The quote was made by Sir Peter Medawar, Nobel Laureate and distinguished immunologist. His work demonstrated that the immunological barriers to transplantation could be surmounted, and formed the basis for the successful development of organ transplants in humans

26. Figures from UK Transplant. See: www.uktransplant.org.uk

27. Broyde M J. The diagnosis of brain death [letter] *N Engl J Med* 2001; **345**: 617 quoted in Zamperetti N, Bellamo R, Ronco C. Defining death in non-heart beating organ donors. *J Med Ethics* 2003; **29**: 182

28. Criteria for the diagnosis of brain stem death. *J R Coll Physicians Lond* 1995; **29**: 381–2

29. Savulescu J. Death, us and our bodies: personal reflections. *J Med Ethics* 2003; **29**: 127–30

30. UK Transplant reported on 24/09/02 that six trusts had been funded for NHBD programmes

31. Kerridge I, Saul P, Lowe M, *et al.* Commentary on Machado C. A definition of human death should not be related to organ transplants. *J Med Ethics* 2003; **29**: 202

32. Kant I, translated by Paton H J. *Groundwork of the Metaphysics of Morals*. London: Routledge, 1991. The categorical imperative, p78

33. See reference 27

34. www.uktransplant.org.uk Human Tissue Act 1961 Chapter 54 section 1(2)

35. Kennedy I. *Treat Me Right: Essays in Medical Law and Ethics*. Oxford: Oxford University Press, 1988, p252. He quotes Donald Longmore, saying in 1968 'We can either preserve the ancient laws that guarantee the inviolability of the dead, and the present rights of the next of kin, or we can rewrite those laws in favour of the living'

36. *Ibid* p237–56. In this essay published in 1988 he expresses disappointment that no government had at that time seen fit to change the law since 1961 in spite of repeated pressure to do so

37. English V, Sommerville A. Presumed consent for transplantation: a dead issue after Alder Hey? *J Med Ethics* 2003; **29**: 147–52

38. Emson H E. It is immoral to require consent for cadaver organ donation. *J Med Ethics* 2003; **29**: 125–7

39. See reference 37

40. Chouhan P, Draper H. Modified mandated choice for organ procurement. *J Med Ethics* 2003; **29**: 157–62

41. Royal College of Paediatrics and Child Health, Ethics Advisory Committee. Guidelines for the ethical conduct of medical research involving children. *Arch Dis Child* 2000; **82**: 177–82

42. Sutcliffe A G. Testing new pharmaceutical products in children. [editorial] *BMJ* 2003; **326**: 64–5

43. Jubb A M. Palliative care research: trading ethics for an evidence base. *J Med Ethics* 2003; **28**: 342–5

44. Rees E, Hardy J. Novel consent process for research in dying patients unable to give consent. *BMJ* 2003; **327**: 198–200

45. Pickles W. *Epidemiology in Country Practice*. London: RCGP, 1939 (out of print)

46. Wald N J, Law M R. A strategy to reduce cardiovascular disease by more than 80%. *BMJ* 2003; **326**: 1419–23

Resources

General Medical Council (GMC)

Duties of a doctor

This series of booklets published by the GMC gives clear guidance on several important areas, including the duties of a doctor, confidentiality and seeking patients' consent.

Journals

These provide the best source of writing, debate and controversy relating to current ethical issues in medicine.

Journal of Medical Ethics, the Journal of the Institute of Medical Ethics. Published bimonthly by the BMJ Publishing Group. In particular, for a comprehensive discussion of approaches to ethics see *J Med Ethics*. 2003; **29** (5)

British Medical Journal

Books

Brazier M. *Medicine, Patients and the Law*. Harmondsworth: Penguin, 1992

Dworkin R. *Life's Dominion*. New York: Vintage Books, 1994

Glover J. *Causing Death and Saving Lives*. Harmondsworth: Penguin, 1990

Harris J. *The Value of Life: An Introduction to Medical Ethics*. London: Routledge, 1985

Heyd D. *Genethics: Moral Issues in the creation of people*. London: University of California Press Ltd, 1994

Kennedy I. *Treat Me Right: Essays in Medical Law and Ethics*. Oxford: Oxford University Press, 1988

Orme-Smith A, Spicer J. *Ethics in General Practice*. Abingdon: Radcliffe Medical Press, 2001

Price D. *Legal and Ethical Aspects of Organ Transplantation*. Cambridge: Cambridge University Press, 2000

Steinbock B, Norcross A (ed). *Killing and Letting Die*. New York: Fordham University Press, 1994

Screening

Muir Gray

- All screening programmes do harm; some do good as well.

- Screening programmes are public health services that need to be managed at the level of a large population to monitor quality effectively – in the UK this is done by the National Screening Committee (NSC).

- The first task of the NSC is to use research evidence to identify programmes that do more good than harm – the second is to make policy recommendations about those programmes at reasonable cost.

- When it has been decided to introduce screening, care has to be taken to ensure that the programme is set up in a way that will minimise harm and maximise benefit.

- In policy making the evidence for screening is often limited because of the rarity of the conditions being screened for.

- Screening is a programme, not a test.

- Screening programmes, formerly called secondary prevention, should be set in the context of primary prevention and good diagnostic and treatment services; screening programmes are part of disease control programmes.

- Screening is managed on the principles of total quality management.

- The term 'screening', although deeply embedded in professional and public consciousness, is not particularly helpful in the 21st century.

All screening programmes do harm; some do good as well.

The management of screening is a public health service and consists of a limited number of tasks, notably:

▶ identifying programmes that do more good than harm

▶ estimating which programmes do more good than harm at reasonable cost

▶ ensuring that each programme is introduced and delivered at a sufficient level of quality to reproduce the levels of benefit and harm that were found in the research setting in ordinary service settings.

These are the key responsibilities of the UK NSC which has been developing a new approach to screening since its foundation in 1997.

Criteria for screening policy

The criteria developed by Wilson and Jungner[1] have stood the test of time very well and were adopted by the NSC even though it was about thirty years since they had been published (see Box 3.1).

Box 3.1 **Criteria for appraising screening developed in the 1960s**

- the condition sought should be an important health problem
- there should be an accepted treatment for patients with recognised disease
- facilities for diagnosis and treatment should be available
- there should be a recognisable latent or early symptomatic stage
- there should be a suitable test or examination
- the test should be acceptable to the population
- the natural history of the condition, including development from latent to declared disease, should be adequately understood
- there should be an agreed policy on whom to treat as patients
- the cost of case-finding (including diagnosis and treatment of patients diagnosed) should be economically balanced in relation to possible expenditure on medical care as a whole
- case-finding should be a continuing process and not a 'once and for all' project

There was, however, concern about the use of these criteria because of changing thoughts on evidence and the evaluation of programmes. The Wilson and Jungner criteria were very welcome following the hubris of the early 1960s during which multiphasic screening had been introduced in many countries without adequate evaluation. Useful though they were, these criteria did not meet the particular needs of the late 20th century because:

▶ insufficient emphasis was given to the harm caused by screening in an era in which concern about harm, and the possibility of litigation, was much higher

▶ the strength of the evidence required to support the claim of benefit was not sufficiently clear

▶ the opportunity costs of screening rather than the availability of resources had become an increasing issue as all societies were faced by the challenges posed by population ageing, new technology, and rising demand.

Because of this the NSC developed a new set of criteria focusing on four main questions (Box 3.2):

▶ do we understand the natural history of the disease

▶ is there a good screening test

▶ is there an effective treatment

▶ is the programme acceptable to the population?

Box 3.2 **Criteria for appraising the viability, effectiveness and appropriateness of a screening programme – 2003**

The condition
• the condition should be an important health problem
• the epidemiology and natural history of the condition, including development from latent to declared disease, should be adequately understood and there should be a detectable risk factor, disease marker, latent period or early symptomatic stage
• all the cost-effective primary prevention interventions should have been implemented as far as practicable
• if the carriers of a mutation are identified as a result of screening the natural history of people with this status should be understood, including the psychological implications

The test

- there should be a simple, safe, precise and validated screening test

- the distribution of test values in the target population should be known and a suitable cut-off level defined and agreed

- the test should be acceptable to the population

- there should be an agreed policy on the further diagnostic investigation of individuals with a positive test result and on the choices available to those individuals

- if the test is for mutations, the criteria used to select the subset of mutations to be covered by screening, if all possible mutations are not being tested, should be clearly set out

The treatment

- there should be an effective treatment or intervention for patients identified through early detection, with evidence of early treatment leading to better outcomes than late treatment

- there should be agreed evidence-based policies covering which individuals should be offered treatment and the appropriate treatment to be offered

- clinical management of the condition and patient outcomes should be optimised in all health care providers prior to participation in a screening programme

The screening programme

- there should be evidence from high-quality randomised controlled trials that the screening programme is effective in reducing mortality or morbidity. Where screening is aimed solely at providing information to allow the person being screened to make an informed choice (e.g. Down's syndrome, cystic fibrosis carrier screening), there must be evidence from high-quality trials that the test accurately measures risk. The information that is provided about the test and its outcome must be of value and readily understood by the individual being screened

- there should be evidence that the complete screening programme (test, diagnostic procedures, treatment or intervention) is clinically, socially and ethically acceptable to health professionals and the public

- the benefit from the screening programme should outweigh the physical and psychological harm (caused by the test, diagnostic procedures, and treatment)

- the opportunity cost of the screening programme (including testing, diagnosis and treatment, administration, training, and quality assurance) should be economically balanced in relation to expenditure on medical care as a whole (i.e. value for money)

- there should be a plan for managing and monitoring the screening programme and an agreed set of quality assurance standards

- adequate staffing and facilities for testing, diagnosis, treatment, and programme management should be available prior to the commencement of the screening programme

- all other options for managing the condition should have been considered (e.g. improving treatment, providing other services), to ensure that no more cost-effective intervention could be introduced or current interventions increased, within the resources available

- evidence-based information, explaining the consequences of testing, investigation, and treatment, should be made available to potential participants to assist them in making an informed choice

- public pressure for widening the eligibility criteria for reducing the screening interval, and for increasing the sensitivity of the testing process, should be anticipated. Decisions about these parameters should be scientifically justifiable to the public

- if screening is for a mutation the programme should be acceptable to people identified as carriers and to other family members

References

Department of Health. *Screening of pregnant women for hepatitis B and immunisation of babies at risk*. London: Dept of Health, 1998 (Health Service Circular: HSC 1998/127)

Wilson JMG, Jungner G. Principles and practice of screening for disease. Public Health Paper Number 34. Geneva: WHO, 1968

Cochrane AL, Holland WW. Validation of screening procedures. *Br Med Bull* 1971, **27**: 3–8

Sackett DL, Holland WW. Controversy in the detection of disease. *Lancet* 1975; **2**: 357–9

Wald NJ (Editor). *Antenatal and Neonatal screening*. Oxford: Oxford University Press, 1984

Holland WW, Stewart S. *Screening in Healthcare*. The Nuffield Provincial Hospitals Trust, 1990

Gray JAM. *Dimensions and definitions of screening*. Milton Keynes: NHS Executive Anglia and Oxford, Research and Development Directorate, 1996

Appraising evidence

Of central importance is the development of new thinking about evidence and for this the NSC was able to look to the broader questions surrounding evidence stimulated by the evidence-based decision-making movement and the Cochrane Collaboration. In a hierarchy of evidence, a systematic review of randomised controlled trials is usually placed at the top. Even this, however, does not resolve disputes because value judgements are involved in the selection or rejection of trials to be included in a systematic review. This point was most fiercely argued in the debate on breast cancer screening. A review in *The Lancet* said that the evidence for breast cancer screening had been biased by the inclusion of trials of low quality.[2] A vigorous exchange of letters took place in *The Lancet's* correspondence column and the issue was reviewed by the International Agency for Research on Cancer which published a report two years later.[3] The conclusion of this report was that:

> ... the trials have provided sufficient evidence for the efficacy of mammography screening of women between 50 and 69 years. The reduction in mortality

from breast cancer among women who chose to participate in screening pro-
grammes was estimated to be about 35%. For women aged 40–49 years, there
is only limited evidence for a reduction.

The limitations of randomised controlled trials

In many screening programmes, for example screening programmes which
may lead to termination as in screening for Down's syndrome, the randomised
controlled trial is not an appropriate type of study design, and other forms of
evidence including modelling are used. The most striking example of this has
been the SURUSS study, which reviewed the outcome of antenatal testing for
Down's syndrome screening and then used modelling to estimate the impact
of different screening policies.[4]

Many studies focus on the benefit of screening, but the need to focus on
harm was also emphasised by the NSC, aware of the fact that controlled trials
with enough power to identify the benefit of screening may not have sufficient
power to identify the harm.

Limited evidence about harm

Evidence about harm is now required by the NSC, but is not always clearly
stated in research studies carried out in the 1980s and 1990s.

The fact that screening is offered to people who are apparently healthy is
obviously one hallmark of the activity, but another important hallmark is the
fact that side effects can occur in people who stand no possibility of benefit.
In clinical practice the person with a health problem who seeks the help of
a clinician accepts, once it has been properly explained to them, the risks
that treatment might involve. However, in screening some people in group D
(see Figure 3.1), experience adverse effects but do not have the disease for
which they have been screened. For example, it is theoretically possible that a
person without colorectal cancer could have their colon perforated during
colonoscopy and die.

Figure 3.1 **The possibility of adverse effects of screening**

		Disease	
		Present	Absent
Adverse effects	Do not occur	A	B
	Occur	C	D

For this reason it is important to gather evidence about harm, both common psychological harm, which is usually transient, and rarer and more serious harms that occur.

The need to calculate opportunity costs

The question, 'Would you spend £35 million on breast cancer screening?' may elicit a different response from the question, 'If you had £35 million to spend on breast cancer control, would you spend it on screening?'.

The new criteria of the NSC seek to address the opportunity costs by considering whether or not the resources that might be made available for screening would be better invested in either primary prevention or treatment services. Furthermore, as the scarcest resource in health services becomes staff and not money, it is important to consider whether or not the investment of resources would not be better channelled into some other intervention designed to reduce the burden of the particular disease, or to reduce the burden of disease in the particular population that might be served by a screening programme.

The appreciation of opportunity costs forces screening programmes to identify new ways of delivering services. For example, the Newborn Hearing Screening Programme has developed a completely new type of health worker, without traditional professional qualifications, to carry out the screening test, and in primary care the receptionist could be trained to take blood samples or measure blood pressure.

New concepts in population disease control

One of the aims of screening is to control a disease at the level of the population, and when screening was developed health care largely consisted of individual consultations by clinicians working either in primary care or in hospitals, isolated and remote from other hospitals. Since that time a number of changes have taken place.

The development of clinical networks has introduced systematic thinking to clinical care, setting the consultation in the context of other levels of care, and the influential report from the Institute of Medicine called *Crossing the Quality Chasm*[5] describes four levels of care:

- ► Level 1 – the consultation
- ► Level 2 – the microsystem, for example the morning surgery

▶ Level 3 – the organisation, for example the hospital

▶ Level 4 – the world of regulations, policies and guidelines.

Screening, therefore, can now fit more clearly into a systematic approach to disease control, and the concept of disease control is one that developed in poorer countries with examples such as the 'Schistosomiasis Control Programme', or the 'Malaria Control Programme'. This type of planning, called vertical planning, was often disparaged by people, particularly in the UK, where it was felt that horizontal planning, namely organising primary care and secondary care, was more important. The truth, of course, lies somewhere in the middle. Many countries have now adopted a disease control model where, on the basis of a good platform of high-quality primary care, they are introducing disease control programmes. In England they are called National Service Frameworks. However, systematic thinking is also influencing screening within the context of disease control programmes in a number of different ways.

Reducing population risk by primary prevention

The National Service Framework for Coronary Heart Disease in England marked a shift away from the medicalisation of cardiac risk factors by emphasising that the top priority was to promote primary prevention among people who did not have heart disease.

This reflects the strategy advocated by the late Professor Geoffrey Rose in his influential book *Strategy of Preventive Medicine*.[6] Geoffrey Rose's approach would not be to seek out individuals with high blood pressure but to try to reduce the body mass index of the whole population, or even the mean weight by two or three kilograms. As most strokes occur in people not identified in high risk screening strategies, and the health benefits that would result if the mean weight of the population could be reduced by 10% are dramatic.[7]

This led to another important concept – the focus on person-based rather than risk-based screening.

Identifying people at high risk

The National Service Framework emphasised the need to identify people who already had heart disease, picking up the intriguing statement by Professor Nicholas Wald who said that: 'The best screening test for heart disease is the question "Do you have heart disease?"'.

Epidemiological evidence has been gathered to support this approach. The Heart Protection Study, for example, demonstrated that the group who benefited most from cholesterol reduction were people with heart disease, whatever their initial level of cholesterol.[8-9] The issue, therefore, was not to identify people with a single risk factor and judge intervention on the basis of that risk factor, but to identify people who would benefit from a wide range of measures to reduce risk.

This was complemented by the development of risk factor calculators that would allow the overall risk of an individual to be measured, and by suggestions that what was needed was a Polypill – namely a pill that would assume that everyone over a defined age was at risk of vascular disease and seek to reduce that risk by small amounts of active pharmacological treatments, each delivered at a dose high enough to have a beneficial effect but low enough to minimise side effects.[10] This also led the NSC to introduce a pilot project to reduce the risk of diabetes and vascular disease by using two questions as screening tests:

▶ do you have diabetes?

▶ do you have heart disease or any other form of vascular disease?

On the basis of the answers to these questions, the population could be divided into four groups. Those who have heart disease and diabetes already receive risk reduction. Those who have neither receive advice to try and change their lifestyle, although the contribution of professional advice is relatively limited. The use of these screening tests, and the two-by-two box that results from it, allows the identification of individuals at particularly high risk to be screened for diabetes, and in the pilot project the presence of a family history or a body mass index of over 25 is being used (see Figure 3.2).

Figure 3.2 **Clinical Detection and Screening Scenario** | All individuals aged 40 and over

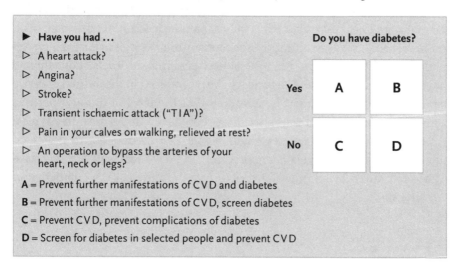

▶ Have you had ...
▷ A heart attack?
▷ Angina?
▷ Stroke?
▷ Transient ischaemic attack ("TIA")?
▷ Pain in your calves on walking, relieved at rest?
▷ An operation to bypass the arteries of your heart, neck or legs?

Do you have diabetes?

	Yes	No
Yes	A	B
No	C	D

A = Prevent further manifestations of CVD and diabetes
B = Prevent further manifestations of CVD, screen diabetes
C = Prevent CVD, prevent complications of diabetes
D = Screen for diabetes in selected people and prevent CVD

Thus this concept of screening focuses more closely on populations at risk rather than on risk factors. This concept for disease control is also relevant when screening for infectious diseases.

Chlamydia control

A proposal was made to screen for chlamydia and the initial proposal suggested that a test be offered every two years. Communicable disease control, however, is different from the control of non-communicable disease. If an individual does not have the disease on testing, there is only one way in which that person can become positive and that is by infection from a person who is positive. Thus the model of screening for non-communicable disease is not directly applicable to screening for communicable disease. The testing of asymptomatic people, piloted by the NSC in its chlamydia pilot programme which took place in two populations in England, included asymptomatic testing. This was, however, part of a broader set of measures to control the communicable disease, including the promotion of primary prevention and the effective follow-up and treatment of those who tested positive.

New concepts in management

Screening is a programme, not a test; this is one of the problems that the health service has with private sector screening where all too often an individual is offered a test, and the investigation and reassurance of those who test positive is then transferred to the NHS.

Programme management is essential to ensure quality and quality is essential to ensure that screening causes more good than harm. Screening policy is based on research findings but there is growing evidence that the level of care delivered in a research study is better than the level of care delivered in an ordinary health service setting, for the control group as well as for the intervention group. For this reason it cannot be assumed that the levels of benefit and harm achieved in a research setting will be reproduced in the ordinary service setting. Similarly, it cannot be assumed that the level of quality that was achieved by the research workers can be reproduced in practice. In a typical research study covering half a million people, a number of highly dedicated professionals achieve levels of organisation and technical skill that will have to be reproduced by a hundred times as many staff to cover a population of 50 million.

Figure 3.3 **The relationship between quality and harm and the need for explicit national standards**

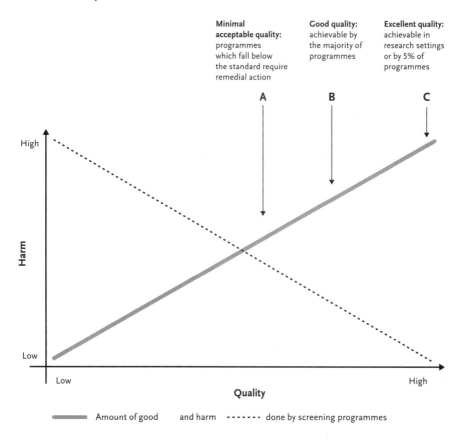

It is very difficult for any individual programme to work in this way. The balance between good and harm is very fine in screening and it is therefore essential for programmes to be able to compare their performance with the performance of other programmes. This requires national management. Nationally managed programmes have a number of common characteristics set out in Box 3.3.

Box 3.3 **Features common to all national screening programmes**

National screening programmes
• cover a defined population
• have a simple set of objectives
• develop valid and reliable criteria to measure performance and produce an annual report
• relate performance to explicit quality standards
• organise quality assurance systems to help professionals and organisations prevent errors and improve performance
• communicate clearly and efficiently with all interested individuals and organisations
• co-ordinate the management of these activities, clarifying the responsibilities of all individuals and organisations involved

The national management of a programme involving millions of people being screened and thousands of health care professionals is complicated but a core principle of the work of the NSC has been simplification. Almost all screening programmes follow the pattern below.

Figure 3.4 **Pattern of screening programmes**

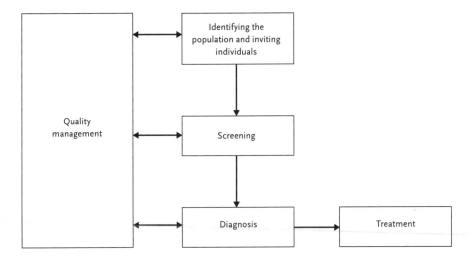

Screening programme managers are not directly responsible for the quality of treatment services. However, it is irresponsible to set up a screening programme without considering the quality of treatment and taking every possible action to make it more systematic and to improve the quality of treatment offered to those identified as having the disease.

Some screening programmes are even simpler, for example the identification of the blood pressure level leads to treatment being introduced on the basis of blood pressure measurement alone; there is no explicit diagnostic test for high blood pressure.

Figure 3.5 **Pattern of high blood pressure screening**

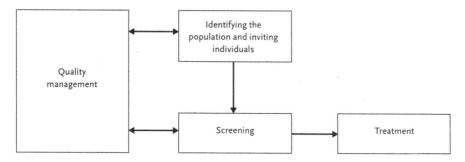

A nationally managed programme has management arrangements for programme monitoring and quality assurance. A number of other programmes take place across the country as a whole but are managed locally without national systems of quality assurance.

Quality assurance in screening

Quality assurance in screening is kept relatively simple and embraces four inter-related activities:

▶ the prevention of error by good staff training and selection and the purchase of good quality equipment

▶ the identification of errors with rapid action to minimise their adverse effects

▶ continual performance improvement on the part of professionals and screening programme teams

▶ the setting and re-setting of national standards for screening.

This systems-based approach to screening is effective in assuring quality but has been criticised for its production-line approach. It is true that the basic principles and practices are based on the techniques of quality assurance developed by the Japanese car industry but the development of this systems-based approach has been accompanied by a radical re-thinking of the philosophy of screening, with a move away from a utilitarian population-based approach to one that focuses on the needs, fears and desires of the individual.

Screening or risk management?

Screening is a public health service delivered by clinicians to individuals. From its earliest days screening has been promoted as part of the public health services and decision making has been based largely on utilitarian grounds, namely on the needs of populations and the benefits to populations. If, for example, a programme would benefit a thousand people and harm twenty, the net benefit, 980 people, would be regarded as evidence on which a programme could be considered for introduction.

An alternative scenario based on utilitarianism is that if a programme would be of benefit to only a very small number of people it would not be offered, even if those individuals felt very strongly that they would benefit. The difference between these two approaches is well described in the analysis of decision making about breast cancer in the United States and Canada.[11] Screening for rare diseases does take place and is increasing, but screening for rare diseases is based on evidence of benefit for the small number of people that would be detected. More subtle problems arise when the evidence is not so strong, as is the case for screening women under the age of 50 for breast cancer or screening for prostate cancer. The fact that there is no evidence of benefit for these populations, based on our conventional definitions of effectiveness, does not mean that an individual might not benefit. The fact that the effect on a population is too small to measure indicates the magnitude of the benefit for the population but does not exclude the possibility of benefit for the individual. This has led people to call for the introduction of screening programmes such as screening for prostate cancer because of the possibility of benefit, and the people who call for prostate cancer screening are unconvinced by the epidemiological arguments based on concepts such as lead-time bias. Even when there is clear evidence of benefit, the problem posed by the fact that some people would be harmed without a possibility of benefit has caused a re-thinking about ways in which the programmes should be presented.

References

1. Wilson J M G, Junger J J. *Principles and Practice Of Screening For Disease.* Geneva: World Health Organization, 1968

2. Gotzsche P C, Olsen O. Is screening for breast cancer with mammography justifiable? *Lancet* 2003; **355 (9198)**: 129–34

3. Vainio H, Gaudin N. Mammography screening can reduce deaths from breast cancer. International Agency for Research on Cancer (IARC) and World Health Organization. www.iarc.fr/pageroot/PRELEASES/pr139a.html (accessed 3/9/2004)

4. Wald N, Rodeck C, Hackshaw A, *et al.* First and second trimester antenatal screening for Down's syndrome: the results of the Serum, Urine and Ultrasound Screening Study (SURUSS). *Health Technol Assess* 2003; **7 (11)**: 1–88

5. Committee on Quality of Health Care in America, Institute of Medicine. *Crossing the Quality Chasm: A New Health System for the 21st Century.* Washington, D.C.: The National Academies Press, 2001

6. Rose G. *The Strategy of Preventive Medicine.* Oxford: Oxford University Press, 1993

7. Mulvihill C, Quigley R. *The management of obesity and overweight. An analysis of reviews of diet, physical activity and behavioural approaches. Evidence briefing.* Health Development Agency (HDA), 2003

8. MRC/BHF Heart Protection Study of cholesterol lowering with simvastatin in 20,536 high-risk individuals: a randomised placebo-controlled trial. *Lancet* 2002; **360 (9326)**: 7–22

9. Collins R, Armitage J, Parish S, Sleigh P, Peto R. MRC/BHF Heart Protection Study of cholesterol-lowering with simvastatin in 5963 people with diabetes: a randomised placebo-controlled trial. *Lancet* 2003; **361 (9374)**: 2005–16

10. Smith R. Polypill may be available in two years. [Editorial] *BMJ* 2003; **32** http://bmj.bmjjournals.com/cgi/content/full/327/7418/0-g (accessed 3/9/2004)

11. Tanenbaum S J. 'Medical effectiveness' in Canadian and U.S. health policy: the comparative politics of inferential ambiguity. *Health Serv Res* 1996; **31 (5)**: 517–32

CHAPTER 4

The GP and Pregnancy Care

Lindsay F P Smith

▶ KEY MESSAGES

- GPs, with suitable interest and training, can contribute to pregnancy care and pregnancy-related care.

- Care should focus on the needs of women and their partners, be evidence based and provided as part of a multidisciplinary team.

- Pregnancy-related care includes contraception, infertility management, pre-conception counselling, miscarriage care, termination of pregnancy, the promotion of breast-feeding and the detection of postnatal problems.

- Such care is a core part of the discipline of family medicine and should not be marginalised; GPs must be encouraged and enabled to undertake such care.

RECENT ADVANCES ▼

- All GPs will need to decide under the new UK 2004 GP contract whether they wish to provide any direct maternity care.

- Some GPs with special interests are likely to be commissioned at primary care trust (PCT) level to provide pregnancy-related care for patients across the PCT.

- The new NICE guidelines on routine antenatal care for low-risk pregnant women will need to be adopted and should improve care.

- Down's syndrome screening will become universal nationally by 2004 and more accurate by 2007.

- Pre-conception genetic screening is likely to be required in primary care.

- Miscarriage management will become more evidence based with women deciding on the type of care they wish.

- Non-operative infertility management will be increasingly a primary-care-based activity.

Introduction

Pregnancy and childbirth is different to almost all other forms of clinical practice. Pregnancy is not a pathological disease or process. It is a physiological event, which most women experience. The majority of pregnancies end normally and without complication.

The aim of maternity care should be to enable women to deliver a healthy baby whilst maintaining their own health and maximising their choices around and throughout this normal phase of their life. High quality maternity care can only be provided when competent professionals listen to an individual woman's wishes and assist her (and her partner) in making informed choices based on research evidence, where this is available. Women need time to reflect upon information provided and may, in addition, ask for professionals to advise them. Ultimately it is the woman's decision as to the type of care and choices that she makes. The duty of professionals is to support her (and her partner) in their decision making and in their subsequent choices (or refer them to someone who will, where the professional disagrees).

Several factors can help to achieve high quality maternity care. These include:

► good communication between professionals

► patient-held records

► clear lines of responsibility

► locally agreed guidelines

► shared governance and audit

► closer interaction and training of professionals.

Maternity care can be seen in the narrow definition of that provided when the woman is pregnant and wishing to continue her pregnancy. Much care is also provided within general practice both before and after pregnancy that should not be seen in isolation from the pregnancy per se. Such related care includes contraception, infertility management, pre-conception counselling, miscarriage care, termination of pregnancy, the promotion of breast-feeding, detection of postnatal problems beyond the traditional six-week limit and child heath services. Most women wish to have greater choice of maternity care; some also wish for greater continuity of care as part of that choice. All GPs can promote choice and some may choose to provide continuity of care whereas hospital doctors are unlikely to do so and continuity of midwifery care is variable. It is crucial that those providing pregnancy care work as a team, to agreed guidelines to which patients' representatives have contributed.[1-2]

Roles

Continuity

The roles of professional carers are closely linked to achieving continuity. Continuity is essential for women to experience high-quality care. It has been classified in various ways: informational continuity; management continuity; and relational continuity. The midwifery literature commonly refers to continuity of care (the first two) and continuity of carer (the latter). What women value most is continuity of the carer. Various midwifery staffing arrangements have been tried and assessed to try and provide better continuity for pregnant women. For example, team midwifery tries to achieve the first two continuity aspects usually at the expense of the latter. With the introduction of the progressively restrictive European Working Time Directive, increasing numbers of doctors on hospital rotas and shift-working patterns by junior obstetric staff, it is most unlikely that pregnant women will receive any continuity of personal care from hospital doctors. The recent national publication of the NICE antenatal care guidelines, linked to good multidisciplinary working at a local level, should improve informational continuity. It is now accepted by most consultant obstetricians that there is no clinical need for obstetric involvement with every pregnant woman. Also, consultants would be more cost effective if they concentrated on women with complicated pregnancies. Most also realise that not all women want to see an obstetrician.

Through all these past and likely future changes, the patient's GP can provide excellent continuity of care and of carer. GPs have always provided such valued personal care historically, not just during the pregnancy but before, during and after, and across medical, social and psychological problems and across family members. Traditionally, practice-based community midwives will also be able to provide such personal care and, indeed, together with the GP they should be able to provide excellent antenatal and postnatal continuity, including from one pregnancy to the next. Whether sufficient GPs wish to provide such antenatal and postnatal care to their patients in the future is not clear at present; it would be a great loss if they did not, not just to women but to the discipline of general (i.e. family) practice.[3-5]

Patient views

Women have the central role in maternity care: they carry their baby and give birth. Everyone else – family, carers, professionals – is in a supporting role to the woman. This can easily be forgotten. Many reports quite rightly emphasise the need for care to be woman-centred and not professional group, or institution centred.

Many, but not all, women wish their GPs to be involved in their pregnancy care. There is some evidence that the majority of women prefer to see both their GP and their midwife in early pregnancy, whereas those that only see one professional tend to be dissatisfied with such arrangements. Women want their GPs to provide:

- ► up-to-date information about choices in clinical matters

- ► continuity of care as part of a motivated, interested, successful, and harmonious maternity care team

- ► pre-pregnancy care, appropriate referral and sharing of care with adequate time to discuss anxieties

- ► home birth medical cover if desired

- ► a visit from their GP early after their return home

- ► contraceptive advice, neonatal, and feeding advice if necessary.[6-8]

The role of the GP in pregnancy care

Most GPs continue to promote choice for women by either (a) actually providing some aspect of maternity care themselves, and/or (b) ensuring choices exist for women including place of birth. Most GPs provide antenatal and postnatal care, although the degree of their involvement is not clear. In some practices it may be in name only to enable them to claim the relevant item of service fee; in others they may fully share such care with midwives and hospital doctors. Pregnancy care must be a core part of family practice in the UK. The new GP contract acknowledges this by permitting GPs to choose to provide antenatal and postnatal care; this opportunity to review their hands-on role needs to be taken.[9–11]

The role of the GP in pregnancy-related care

Ideally women should be able to choose when they wish to become pregnant i.e. to plan their pregnancies. To do so they need contraceptive advice. Most GPs provide contraception care and the majority of contraceptive services are provided by GPs. Such contraception advice should be linked to pre-conception care. Unfortunately a significant minority of couples will have problems conceiving. GPs are well placed to provide aspects of infertility care. Ten to fifteen per cent of pregnancies end in miscarriage; the GP is often consulted by a woman in early pregnancy with bleeding and/or pain. Some women become pregnant by mistake and wish to have a termination. GPs are usually consulted in such instances and have an important role in counselling, referral (both NHS and private) and subsequent follow-up especially for contraception and emotional problems.

Breast-feeding has clear health benefits for both mother and child. Despite the majority of women commencing breast-feeding only a minority do so beyond six weeks postpartum. The GP, midwife and health visitor (HV) together must provide supportive evidence-based care for breast-feeding mothers who are having problems to maximise breast-feeding rates. In particular the GP may be consulted over possible infection-causing mastitis. Postnatal depression is increasingly recognised as a major illness affecting not only the mother but also her baby and perhaps existing children. The GP and health visitor must be sensitive to such a possibility and respond appropriately to cues that the new mother may give. Child health surveillance services are provided by most GPs. This starts with the first baby check, which in future may be the province of the midwife rather than the doctor. However, the GP and HV subsequently provide such care starting with the formal six-week GP check and finishing with the four-year-old pre-school medical. An integrated programme is essential.[12]

Pregnancy-related care

Pre-pregnancy care

The idea that care before pregnancy can improve the outcome of a subsequent pregnancy is attractive both for the providers of health care and to its consumers: pregnant women and their partners. Unfortunately, there is little evidence from research that changing any aspect of a woman's pre-pregnancy medical, social, psychological, or spiritual well-being can improve outcome. With one major exception (folic acid supplementation), pre-pregnancy advice is not supported by any high-quality trial evidence and must therefore be viewed with some scepticism.

For the majority of women (those at 'low' risk of adverse pregnancy outcome), pre-pregnancy advice could be given opportunistically by the primary health care team. Practices should have an agreed policy on whom to advise and when, linked to an electronic template which can be audited. All women should stop medication if at all possible before trying to conceive. For most drugs, however, there has to be a balance between known benefits and possible but uncertain risks, such as those associated with the use of asthma inhalers and many antidepressants. All women should receive advice about the need to take folic acid and be immunised successfully against rubella and reduce their smoking and alcohol intake. All women should have a family history taken to detect inheritable disorders.

In addition, certain groups are at high risk of adverse pregnancy outcome including the 2–3% with inheritable disorders, those with previous adverse pregnancy outcome or those with chronic maternal disease. There is some evidence that pregnancy outcome for the latter group can be improved by particular pre-pregnancy care in specific specialist pre-pregnancy clinics. Adverse pregnancy outcome may be avoided for those with inherited disorders by pre-pregnancy counselling if this results in avoidance of pregnancy or subsequent screening and selective termination of affected pregnancies.

Genetic testing in advance of pregnancy is rarely undertaken but is likely to increase in the future. There are two common situations in pregnancy where advance genetic testing may be requested. These are where there is a known family history of an inheritable disease, and secondly in a situation where the parents are related, e.g. first cousins. The latter is important because it is much more likely than in a random parental match that both parents would contribute the same recessive gene to their offspring, e.g. cystic fibrosis. The recent White Paper acknowledges that primary health professionals will want to develop their knowledge of this area and the skills necessary to counsel patients and their families appropriately. It is also recognised that primary health care professionals will wish to develop an understanding of the issues surrounding testing and subsequent recording of genetic information in patient records.[13-14]

Infertility

GPs are normally involved in the care of women who are, or who believe themselves to be, infertile. Women often present to their GP because they have failed to become pregnant. The GP's subsequent action will vary upon their interest and expertise. There are basic steps which any GP should undertake which include the usual history, examination, investigations and ongoing support. Areas where GP care may well change in the future are treatment and referral. It is possible that GPs with a special interest in infertility will be commissioned by PCTs to provide care for women referred on to them by other GPs within the PCT. This is because most GPs at present do not treat infertility but refer instead. However, even at present some individual GPs can and do prescribe appropriately for infertile women, once they have established that the cause is lack of ovulation. There are two treatments which can be effective and safe in primary care.

Clomiphene is the drug of choice for women with normal FSH/LH who are not ovulating. It can be successfully used for between six and twelve cycles and its success rate is about 80% ovulation with a 25–50% pregnancy rate. It is a sensible treatment for unexplained infertility in general practice in those women who are not ovulating regularly. There is a theoretical risk of ovarian malignancy with long-term use of any treatment which stimulates ovulation; this includes clomiphene. The research evidence on whether there is a true risk is contradictory. Secondly, metformin is increasingly accepted as an effective treatment. Women who still do not ovulate can be treated with a combination of metformin and clomiphene which increases the pregnancy rate from less than 10% with clomiphene alone to between 50–65% with combined therapy.

The recent NICE guidance which instructs all PCTs to provide a minimum number of IVF treatments to infertile women may promote the development of GPs with Special Interests (GPwSIs) to provide a service up to, but not including, such specialist in-vitro fertilisation. Such care should be more cost effective than a secondary care-based service and would also free-up specialist time to provide IVF treatment which only they can provide.[15–18]

Miscarriage

First trimester miscarriage affects one in seven pregnancies and can lead to distress and clinical problems. Optimal management is uncertain. Recent evidence suggests that the *gradual and sporadic* trend to offer haemodynamically stable women more choice of their management is likely to speed up. Until the widespread introduction of early pregnancy assessment clinics (EPACs) over the last decade, expectant management had been utilised by GPs for *up to* one quarter of all miscarriages, which were managed in the community *and* without surgical intervention.

Nowadays nearly all pregnant women with early pregnancy bleeding and/or pain are referred to such EPACs. Traditionally surgical evacuation has been performed following the diagnosis of miscarriage on the basis that this would decrease the risk of subsequent gynaecological infection. However, this is not without complications such as infection, uterine perforation and cervical laceration. Although the supporting evidence base is weak, other management options (expectant or medical) have been increasingly offered to women with a miscarriage. Expectant management allows spontaneous passage of retained products of conception and medical management uses drugs to aid expulsion of retained products.

In the future women should be given sufficient information by their GP to make an informed choice about how their miscarriage should be managed. It should be for women, not their doctors, to decide.[19]

Antenatal care

Antenatal care standards

NICE published its antenatal care guidelines in October 2003. This major document should supersede the historical pattern of somewhat random antenatal care that has developed in the UK over the past half century. Produced by a multi-disciplinary group, this readable and usable document is essential reading for all those providing antenatal care. It is based on evidence where it is available and the degree of grading evidence is indicated in the document as you would expect from any document from NICE. Table 4.1 lists its recommendations that have the highest level of research evidence to support them (Grade A i.e. from randomised controlled trial(s)). The following are a few important areas from the perspective of a GP with an interest in maternity care.

Table 4.1 **NICE Guidelines – Antenatal care: Grade A evidence-based recommendations**

Guidance
Pregnant women should be offered opportunities to attend antenatal classes and have written information about antenatal care.
Midwife and GP led models of care should be offered for women with an uncomplicated pregnancy. Routine involvement of obstetricians in the care of women with an uncomplicated pregnancy at scheduled times does not appear to improve perinatal outcomes compared with involving obstetricians when complications arise.

Guidance

Antenatal care should be provided by a small group of carers with whom the woman feels comfortable. There should be continuity of care throughout the antenatal period.

Structured maternity records should be used for antenatal care.

Maternity services should have a system in place whereby women carry their own case notes.

Pregnant women should be offered an early ultrasound scan to determine gestational age (in lieu of last menstrual period (LMP) for all cases) and to detect multiple pregnancies. This will ensure consistency of gestational age assessments, improve the performance of mid-trimester serum screening for Down's syndrome and reduce the need for induction of labour after 41 weeks.

Pregnant women (and those intending to become pregnant) should be informed that dietary supplementation with folic acid, before conception and up to 12 weeks' gestation, reduced the risk of having a baby with neural tube defects (anencephaly, spina bifida). The recommended dose is 400 µg per day.

Iron supplementation should not be offered routinely to all pregnant women. It does not benefit the mother's or foetus's health and may have unpleasant maternal side effects.

There is insufficient evidence to evaluate the effectiveness of vitamin D in pregnancy. In the absence of evidence of benefit, vitamin D supplementation should not be offered routinely to pregnant women.

Pregnant women should be informed that beginning or continuing a moderate course of exercise during pregnancy is not associated with adverse outcomes.

Pregnant women should be informed about the specific risks of smoking during pregnancy (such as the risk of having a baby with low birth weight and preterm). The benefits of quitting at any stage should be emphasised.

Women who smoke or who have recently stopped should be offered smoking cessation interventions. Interventions that appear to be effective in reducing smoking include advice by physician, group sessions, and behavioural therapy (based on self-help manuals).

Women should be informed that most cases of nausea and vomiting in pregnancy will resolve spontaneously within 16–20 weeks gestation and that nausea and vomiting are not usually associated with a poor pregnancy outcome. If a woman requests or would like to consider treatment, the following interventions appear to be effective in reducing symptoms:
- Non-pharmacological: Ginger or P6 acupressure
- Pharmacological: Antihistamines

Antacids may be offered to women whose heartburn remains troublesome despite lifestyle and diet modification.

Women who present with constipation in pregnancy should be offered information regarding diet modification, such as bran or wheat fibre supplementation.

Women should be informed that varicose veins are a common symptom of pregnancy that will not cause harm and that compression stockings can improve the symptoms but will not prevent varicose veins from emerging.

A one-week course of topical imidazole is an effective treatment and should be considered for vaginal candidiasis infections in pregnant women.

Guidance

Women should be informed that exercising in water, massage therapy and group or individual back care classes might help to ease backache during pregnancy.

Routine breast examination during antenatal care is not recommended for the promotion of postnatal breastfeeding.

Psychiatric screening:
- pregnant women should not be offered routine screening, such as with the Edinburgh postnatal depression scale (EPDS), in the antenatal period to predict the development of postnatal depression
- pregnant women should not be offered antenatal education interventions to reduce perinatal or postnatal depression, as these interventions have not been shown to be effective.

Haemoglobin levels outside the normal UK range for pregnancy (that is, 11 g/dl at first contact and 10.5 g/dl at 28 weeks) should be investigated and iron supplementation considered if indicated.

Pregnant women should be offered an ultrasound scan to screen for structural anomalies, ideally between 18 and 20 weeks' gestation, by an appropriately trained sonographer and with equipment of an appropriate standard as outlined by the National Screening Committee.

Routine vaginal examination to assess the cervix is not an effective method of predicting preterm birth and should not be offered.

Pregnant women should be offered estimation of foetal size at each antenatal appointment to detect small or large for gestational age infants.

Routine formal foetal-movement counting should not be offered.

The evidence does not support the routine use of antenatal electronic foetal heart rate monitoring (cardiotocography) for foetal assessment in women with an uncomplicated pregnancy and therefore it should not be offered.

The evidence does not support the routine use of ultrasound scanning after 24 weeks' gestation and therefore it should not be offered.

The use of umbilical artery Doppler ultrasound for the prediction of foetal growth restriction should not be offered routinely.

Prior to formal induction of labour, women should be offered a vaginal examination for membrane sweeping.

Women with uncomplicated pregnancies should be offered induction of labour beyond 41 weeks.

All women who have an uncomplicated singleton breech pregnancy at 36 weeks' gestation should be offered external cephalic version (ECV). Exceptions include women in labour, and women with: a uterine scar or abnormality; foetal compromise; ruptured membranes; vaginal bleeding and medical conditions.

The organisation of maternity care will need to change. The first appointment for a pregnant woman should be longer, earlier, and provide her with much more information on the choices she has in terms of the organisation and planning of her pregnancy. This means that GPs will have to advise their reception staff to ensure that patients who contact the practice saying they are pregnant are given early appointments either with them or their mid-wives depending on local arrangements. Secondly, the frequency of appointments should be reduced to ten for nulliparous women with no problems and to seven for multiparous women. Such appointments for women at low risk should be shared equally between community midwives and GPs. This is important because the document states quite clearly that continuity enhances the quality of pregnancy care and outcome. Finally, it is stated quite clearly, that GP- and midwife-led care provides equally favourable outcomes for low-risk women compared with consultant-led care.

There is evidence-based guidance on examinations. Women should be weighed and their height measured at their first appointment to produce a body mass index (BMI) measurement, which is a good guide to later complications. Unless they are very light or very heavy there should be no further weighing of the woman for the rest of the pregnancy. Similarly routine breast and pelvic examinations are no longer recommended. Interestingly the guidance recommends that routine listening to the foetal heart at every antenatal visit is unnecessary, due to lack of evidence of associated benefit. Of course, a woman is likely to request that the midwife or doctor listen to her baby's heart because this has been traditional and may well reassure many. The other important point to note is that whenever a woman's blood pressure is taken for whatever reason her urine must be checked for proteinuria at the same time. It is not sufficient just to check the blood pressure to reassure the patient that all is well.

The guideline provides advice on the management of common symptoms but acknowledges there is, for most, little evidence upon which to base this advice. The exception is nausea and vomiting where notably the guideline recommends ginger and acupuncture as both are of proven benefit for these troubling early pregnancy symptoms. It also recommends that antiD should be offered to all rhesus-negative women at 28 and 34 weeks although issues concerning cost, organisation required at GP-level and problems with storage and access are not discussed. Regarding appropriate management NICE recommends that all women should be seen at 36 weeks and those found to be breech at that time should be routinely offered external cephalic version (ECV) at 37 weeks unless there are the usual contraindications.

In terms of appropriate investigation there are several recommendations of note. Most importantly, at the beginning of pregnancy, ultrasound should be used to date every woman's pregnancy and not her last menstrual period, even when she is certain of her dates. This will reduce inappropriate intervention. All women should be checked for asymptomatic bacteriuria in the first trimester, although NICE acknowledges that the evidence base for this is old and probably needs updating. Finally, it is recommended that routine urine testing for glycosuria should not be undertaken. Therefore practices will have to throw away their urine sticks which have both protein and glucose strips on them and just use ones with protein! Future research may change this recommendation, particularly the Hyperglycaemia and Adverse Pregnancy Outcome Study (HAPO) study. This study, funded by the US National Institutes of Health, aims to test 25,000 women for hyperglycaemia in 16 centres around the world. The objective of HAPO is to determine what level of hyperglycaemia carries a significant risk of adverse pregnancy outcome and hence establish criteria for the diagnosis of gestational diabetes.

It is important for all members of the practice including reception to be increasingly aware of the symptoms of early pre-eclampsia. Women with such symptoms may misinterpret them as being unrelated to the pregnancy and therefore pre-eclampsia may go unrecognised. Therefore the patient may present to normal surgery or even to a practice nurse so it is important that the whole team are aware of the range of symptoms that pre-eclampsia can cause. There is absolutely no point either in advising women to complete routine foetal movement charts. They are of no benefit to low-risk women whatsoever. That certain areas have been earmarked for research is laudable, although whether resources will be made available to fund such important primary care-based research is not at all clear.

In summary, these guidelines are an improvement on the existing situation, and should lead to better, more focused, more evidence-based, women-centred care. There are still problems with funding some of the suggestions. There will also be problems with achieving the cultural changes required to stop doing some things and instigate others. However, GPs should be able to use their influence not just within their practices, but also with PCTs and through Maternity Service Liaison Committees (MSLCs) to ensure that changes occur in their locality to improve the quality of care that low-risk women receive antenatally.[20]

Infections and pregnancy

Two major issues continue to generate debate in this area. These are: which infections should be screened for in pregnant women, and what to do when a pregnant woman develops a rash.

Antenatal infection screening

Screening for asymptomatic infections in pregnant women is an emotive area. For some there is clear evidence of benefit but in others there is not, however, pressure groups can be vociferous in these latter areas. As for screening for non-infective pregnancy illnesses, any screening test must be part of a comprehensive programme, which is evidence based. In particular the infection must have a latent phase, an acceptable test, known natural history, and an effective and acceptable treatment. The recommendations of the NICE antenatal care guidelines are given in Table 4.2. These agree, not surprisingly, with those of the antenatal care sub-group of the National Screening Committee. A few of the recommendations merit some explanation.

Table 4.2 **NICE – CG6 Antenatal Care – Routine care for the healthy pregnant woman: screening for infections**

Pregnant women should be offered routine screening for asymptomatic bacteriuria by midstream urine culture early in pregnancy. Identification and treatment of asymptomatic bacteriuria reduces the risk of preterm birth.

Pregnant women should not be offered routine screening for bacterial vaginosis because the evidence suggests that the identification and treatment of asymptomatic bacterial vaginosis does not lower the risk for preterm birth and other adverse reproductive outcomes.

Pregnant women should not be offered routine screening for asymptomatic chlamydia because there is insufficient evidence on its effectiveness and cost effectiveness. However, this policy is likely to change with the implementation of the national opportunistic chlamydia programme.

The available evidence does not support routine cytomegalovirus screening in pregnant women and it should not be offered.

Serological screening for hepatitis B virus should be offered to pregnant women so that effective postnatal intervention can be offered to infected women to decrease the risk of mother-to-child transmission.

Pregnant women should not be offered routine screening for hepatitis C virus because there is insufficient evidence on its effectiveness and cost effectiveness.

Pregnant women should be offered screening for HIV infection early in antenatal care because appropriate antenatal interventions can reduce mother-to-child transmission of HIV infection.

A system of clear referral paths should be established in each unit or department so that pregnant women who are diagnosed with an HIV infection are managed and treated by the appropriate specialist teams.

Rubella-susceptibility screening should be offered early in antenatal care to identify women at risk of contracting rubella infection and to enable vaccination in the postnatal period for the protection of future pregnancies.

continued overleaf

Pregnant women should not be offered routine antenatal screening for group B streptococcus (GBS) because evidence of its clinical effectiveness and cost effectiveness remains uncertain.

Screening for syphilis should be offered to all pregnant women at an early stage in antenatal care because treatment of syphilis is beneficial to the mother and foetus.

Because syphilis is a rare condition in the UK and a positive result does not necessarily mean that a woman has syphilis, clear paths of referral for the management of women testing positive for syphilis should be established.

Routine antenatal serological screening for toxoplasmosis should not be offered because the risks associated with screening may outweigh the potential benefits.

Pregnant women should be informed of primary prevention measures to avoid toxoplasmosis infection, such as: washing hands before handling food; thoroughly washing all fruit and vegetables, including ready-prepared salads, before eating; thoroughly cooking raw meats and ready-prepared chilled meals; wearing gloves and thoroughly washing hands after handling soil and gardening; avoiding contact with faeces in cat litter or in soil.

The evidence to support screening for asymptomatic bacteriuria is decades old and research trials were managed very differently in the past. It is likely that future research will affect this recommendation if high quality up-to-date trials are funded in this area. Until then, all pregnant women will need to provide a midstream specimen of urine (MSU) for culture to exclude this infection. Interestingly, the converse is true for chlamydia screening: this is not recommended but may well be in the near future as there are ongoing trials in this area. Streptococcus B screening is undertaken in many countries in Europe and in the USA. This is probably unnecessary: a large percentage of otherwise normal pregnant women carry this bacterium. Screening is invasive, many would be labelled as 'abnormal' and given antibiotics (often intravenously) without definitive proof of clinical or cost effectiveness. Finally, toxoplasmosis can have a devastating effect on the foetus if first contracted by a susceptible pregnant woman. But there are problems with establishing a certain diagnosis of first infection, unpleasant side effects of treatment which may not have definite benefit, and lack of evidence that such screening and intervention would produce benefit for the generality of pregnant women.[21]

Rash in pregnancy

Women often present to their GP or other carers with a rash in pregnancy. Such rashes can be very easy but sometimes very difficult to diagnose. The obvious rashes of impetigo, herpes simplex, atopic eczema and chickenpox can be fairly easily diagnosed. Often however, the woman simply has a non-specific rash for which there are no distinguishing features. Certain viral infections causing such rashes are of particular importance to pregnant women. These include rubella and parvovirus B19 infection.

Varicella infection in the first half of pregnancy will cause serious damage to the developing baby in less than 1% of pregnancies. Typical damage occurs to the eye, skin and brain depending on the gestation at which the primary infection is contracted by the mother. Infection in the second half of pregnancy can lead to intrauterine infection, which can lead to serious neonatal illness. Rubella contracted by the mother in pregnancy can also lead to congenital abnormality and even foetal death, especially in the first trimester with a smaller risk of limited problems, particularly deafness up to sixteen weeks. Parvovirus B19 can cause a very similar illness to rubella and a range of other viral infections in adult women as well as in children. Infection in the first half of pregnancy can lead to foetal death, or hydrops fetalis, but not permanent congenital abnormality. However, again, the infection can lead to anaemia or severe neonatal illness.

Present guidance from the Health Protection Agency (HPA) for a woman with undiagnosed rash in the first half of pregnancy has major organisational and workload implications were it ever to be fully implemented by health care professionals. It states:

▶ for those with non-vesicular rash, blood should be taken to exclude rubella and parvovirus B19 infection

▶ in addition all women who have been in contact with a person suffering from a non-vesicular illness, although they are well themselves, should be investigated for asymptomatic infection with parvovirus B19 (and rubella unless known to be immune). Contact is defined as being in the same room for fifteen minutes or face-to-face contact

▶ women with proven parvovirus B19 infection in the first half of pregnancy should have subsequent regular ultrasound scanning to detect early development of hydrops fetalis

▶ oral anti-viral treatment is advised for pregnant women who present within 24 hours of varicella in pregnancy

▶ such women should be referred to hospital for intravenous antibiotic treatment if they develop complications of varicella infection or if they become unwell for more than a week.[22]

Antenatal ultrasound scans
At present low-risk women are either offered two scans (an early dating scan

at around 12 weeks and a more detailed scan to detect foetal abnormalities at about 20 weeks) or one scan (at around 16 weeks, linked to dating for Down's syndrome screening). In the future all women will require an earlier dating scan and a second foetal anomaly scan at 20 weeks, the latter occurring in many parts of the UK already. The earlier dating scan will be used to predict the expected date of delivery (EDD) in preference to the date of the woman's last menstrual period; this approach will reduce unnecessary intervention such as induction for postmaturity. It will also be increasingly used as part of Down's syndrome screening (see below).

The 20-week scan is seen by nearly all couples as a pleasant experience from which they can obtain ultrasound pictures of their developing foetus. Women need better information about the reason for this scan being undertaken (the detection of abnormalities) but this information needs to be realistic about what can be detected. Otherwise, if a baby is subsequently born with a congenital abnormality the parents can become very angry and unhappy that it was not detected by the 'screening test' (the 20-week scan).

Table 4.3 **Estimated detection rates of 20-week scan for serious congenital abnormalities**

Congenital abnormality	Estimated detection rate
Anencephaly	99%
Spina bifida	90%
Exomphalos or gastroschisis	90%
Major limb abnormalities	90%
Major kidney abnormalities	85%
Hydrocephalus	60%
Diaphramatic hernia	60%
Down's syndrome	40%
Major congenital heart problems	25%
Cerebral palsy	0%

These figures will vary from hospital to hospital and it is therefore important that in the future hospitals publish their own figures so women can make an informed choice as to where they wish to go for their 20-week scan. Women who have already had a baby with a congenital abnormality should be referred antenatally to a foetal medicine unit by their midwife or GP; such units have higher resolution scanners and more skilled operators than are usually found in typical district general hospitals.[23]

Down's syndrome screening

Screening for this condition is still patchy in the UK. Not all hospitals provide a screening service. There exists at present a wide variety of screening programmes throughout the country. Thus the National Screening Committee antenatal care sub-group undertook a national survey and produced national guidance that all hospitals are expected to follow. This did not specify which screening test or tests to use but did specify a minimum detection rate with a maximum false–positive rate. This requirement was recently endorsed by the NICE antenatal care guidelines (Table 4.4). Hospitals have until 2005 to meet the minimum requirement of detecting at least 60% of cases antenatally with a false–positive rate of < 5%. They then have a further two years (to April 2007) to meet the higher standard of a least 75% detection with a false–positive rate of < 3%. Not all of the current screening programmes will meet the higher standard so many hospitals will have to change their facilities and staffing structures to meet these higher standards. These standards refer to a cut-off of 1 : 250 risk at term.[24–5]

Table 4.4 **Future development of the national Down's screening programme. All these tests meet the present standards but those marked with an asterisk do not meet the 2007 standard.**

Stage	Test
From 11–14 weeks	nuchal translucency (NT)*
	the combined test (NT, hCG and PAPP-A)
From 14–20 weeks	the triple test (hCG, AFP and uE3)*
	the quadruple test (hCG, AFP, uE3, inhibin A)
From 11–14 weeks and 14–20 weeks	the integrated test (NT, PAPP-A + hCG, uE3, inhibin A)
	the serum integrated test (PAPP-A + hCG, AFT, uE3, inhibin A)

Labour and postnatal care

Labour

The *National Services Framework for Children, Young People and Maternity Services*[26] was published in 2004. It sets 11 standards, of which one is for maternity services. This states that 'women should have easy access to supportive, high quality services designed around their individual needs and those of their babies.' This is consistent with past government policy, which was to promote choice and continuity as set out in the document *Changing Childbirth*.

Box 4.1 **Key issues raised in the National Service Framework for Children, Young People and Maternity Services**

care should be woman centred, enabling informed choices through easy access to information and support
integrated maternity and neonatal services
improved preconception care
direct access to midwives antenatally as first point of contact
competent identification of mental health problems by health care professionals
high quality antenatal and newborn screening
choice of appropriate place of birth, including home birth and midwife led units
Caeserian sections offered by consultant obstetricians where there is evidence of clinical benefit
skilled resuscitation personnel at every delivery with physical examination of baby soon after birth
postnatal care based on structured assessment
up-to-date breastfeeding information and support

Previously there were many GPs providing intrapartum care in the UK. This percentage has steadily fallen from about 15% of all births being under the care of the GP in 1975 to about 6% in 1988. There are no recent national figures since that time. Similarly the number of units within which GPs provide intrapartum care has fallen. In 1988 there were 65 isolated, 29 alongside and 134 integrated general practitioner maternity units. GPs have now withdrawn from nearly all of these. A recent UK survey was undertaken to establish the present provision of, and variation in, maternity units in terms of their number, type, booking options, training and governance. It found that GPs now provide intrapartum care in fewer than 1% of units.

With respect to intrapartum care the GP in theory can be involved at three levels:

1. Many GPs are not happy to take on the responsibility of, or provide, intrapartum care. However, they can agree with a woman that her choice for non-consultant care is reasonable even if they are not going to provide such care themselves (facilitate choice).

2. They can agree to be involved in care and attend the birth as a support person to her and the midwife (provide psycho-social support).

3. They can attend and provide intrapartum clinical care such as interpreting cardiotocographs (CTGs) suturing episiotomies, performing low forceps (be a 'GP obstetrician').

GPs who attend home births and those who attend hospital births in a support role only will be expected to exercise only those skills that all GPs should have. Those who choose to practice as GP obstetricians will have one or more additional obstetric skills. The exact nature of these skills will depend on their past education and training and on their continuing education. These should be made clear to women in advance, so that unrealistic expectations do not develop by default. General practitioners are principally concerned with the management of the normal and identifying those deviations from the norm that indicate the necessity to seek specialist advice if outside their competence. GP obstetricians will share with all GPs their common expertise in a) the management of normal pregnancy and in b) providing comprehensive and continuing care for the physical, psychological and social needs of their patients before, during, and after their pregnancy.

The new GP contract rightly specifically excludes intrapartum care from the core work of GPs. But it also rightly specifies such care as an enhanced service which PCTs can commission at a local level against a nationally determined service specification. Such a service could be provided by GPs for their own patients only, or for a community delivery unit. In both cases the GP would be promoting women's choices and, in the latter, perhaps enabling such a unit to remain viable. Whether PCTs act to commission such care remains to be seen; funded GP involvement in hospital births therefore is at the discretion of PCTs in the future, as GPs will have no right to claim fees for such work as they do now. Some GPs may, however, continue to attend selected home births to provide continuity, support and midwifery back up.[27–30]

Postnatal care

Postnatal care is the area of maternity care that is most criticised, and most in need of improvement. High quality postnatal care is essential to achieve targets in such areas as breast-feeding and reducing inequalities. For most GPs postnatal care has changed little over the past 5–10 years: they see the new mum and baby at the six-week check but rarely before that unless there is a problem. The routine GP home visit to a newly delivered mother and her baby soon after the birth has more or less stopped. The first baby check, which traditionally has been undertaken by a hospital junior doctor, is likely to be undertaken in future by a midwife as research has demonstrated that they do it better. There is ongoing research assessing whether the midwife can also safely undertake the six-week check, which at present is undertaken by the GP in the surgery. If this comes about nationally then the GP could be totally excluded from postnatal care.

The future GP has a choice still. They may be involved by choice or only when called upon by other health care professionals. For a minority of GPs the new GP contract will mean that the PCT commissions them to undertake the first baby check. This might occur in a community midwifery unit, or around larger consultant-led units with increasingly early hospital discharge, or in areas where there are significant numbers of home births. But for the majority of GPs in the future they may play no part in routine postnatal care of baby or mother. They must choose whether to make the effort to contact the new mother, which the author believes nearly all women would wish, or not and imply that postnatal care is no longer part of core general practice. The planned NICE guidance on postnatal care should at least improve the evidence base for all postnatal care and may clarify the role of the GP as well.[31-2]

Future considerations

Future role of the general practice

GPs will continue to provide pregnancy-related care, and this is likely to increase in areas such as pre-conception care, genetic counselling, contraception and infertility management. GPs are best placed to provide efficacious and cost-effective care for inter-current and chronic illness in women who also happen to be pregnant. GPs are best placed to provide an overview of the needs of the pregnant woman in terms of her health before, during and after the pregnancy and in terms of her medical, social and psychological care and finally in terms of her family and social circumstances. The participation of GPs in the provision of maternity care will continue to evolve, especially as the proposed new GP contract has been accepted by the profession. Many practices will wish to continue to provide antenatal and postnatal care, jointly with midwives and hospital doctors. A group of GPs with a special interest (GPwSIs) in pregnancy care are likely to develop in line with joint RCGP/DoH guidance; these GPs will provide a service to the whole primary care trust in a specific area e.g. contraception, infertility, genetic counselling. Some GPs will wish to provide a range of pregnancy care to their own patients; they should be enabled to do so where they are adequately trained, competent, undertake appropriate continuous professional development (CPD), and where their patients wish them to do so.

There is a need to clarify the relative roles of midwives, GPs, gynaecologists and obstetricians. Close integration and interaction between the groups should enable the safe development and improvement necessary to provide patient-focused, high-quality pregnancy and pregnancy-related care. Such emphasis does not mean that the health of the baby is irrelevant. What it acknowledges is that the woman is the best custodian of the 'baby's best interests'. Such negotiation must occur locally, involve women, and be flexible. The views of local women, purchasers and carers should all be considered, as well as the competencies of local midwives, GPs and obstetricians (and gynaecologists) and availability of resources such as community hospitals. For many women the GP is the only professional they know at the start of their pregnancy.

The midwife and the GP in partnership should be the main providers of core pregnancy care (the primary maternity care team). Following the appropriate education and training, between them they can provide complete care for pregnant women in the great majority of cases. To do this they will need open access to appropriate secondary care-based investigations such as scans and serum screening. They will refer women to other carers according to locally agreed guidelines that should be founded on evidence-based national guidelines in three situations:

1. when treatable complications arise outside their competencies, e.g. Caesarean section for pre-eclampsia

2. when either the midwife or the GP are not available when a woman needs care, e.g. labour care to another midwife

3. when a woman requests referral, e.g. to see a consultant.

Most importantly, GPs will need to want to provide pregnancy care in the future and their patients will need to want them to do so. It remains to be seen whether the organisation of maternity services in the UK will be flexible and patient-centred enough to enable this to happen.[33-4]

Future of research

There are many unanswered questions, the research agenda being huge. With continued poor government funding of true primary care research in the UK substantial progress remains a long way off. A selection of important questions that the author believes would improve the quality of pregnancy and pregnancy-related care that is currently available are listed below.

Box 4.2 **Questions for future research**

What is the value to women on continuity of GP care?
What added value do GPs bring to routine antenatal appointments? (e.g. dealing with ongoing health problems at one appointment).
What is the value of pre-pregnancy advice (including genetic screening) from a GPwSI compared to usual GP care?
What is the effect on the pregnancy, and on the baby, of increasing anxiety levels in those women who are unable to follow health promotion advice e.g. fail to stop smoking?
Can GPs with a special interest provide an acceptable infertility service at PCT level?
Are guidelines of any use in improving pregnancy rates?
What are the value of EPACs?
Should women who miscarry be offered a formal follow-up appointment?
Should screening for asymptomatic bacteriuria be undertaken in low-risk women in the 21st century?
Can an efficacious and acceptable method of screening and treating toxoplasmosis be found? Should the UK introduce population immunisation for varicella and/or parvovirus?
To what extent do parents give fully-informed consent to the 20-week foetal anomaly scan?
How acceptable nationally is first trimester testing?
What effect does the wait between an abnormal NT result and getting the second trimester serum result have on parents?
What is the value to women of GPs attending childbirth?
Does such provision of continuity improve outcomes such as reducing intervention?
What is the added value to women and their families of GP involvement in postnatal care?
How can breast-feeding be promoted effectively, especially in vulnerable groups?

References

1. Department of Health. *Changing Childbirth*. Part 1: Report of the Expert Maternity Group. London: HMSO, 1993

2. www.dh.gov.uk/PolicyAndGuidance/HealthAndSocialCareTopics/ChildrenServices/ ChildrenServicesInformation/fs/en (accessed 06/09/2004)

3. Haggerty J, Reid R, Freeman G, *et al*. Continuity of care: a multidisciplinary review. *BMJ* 2003; **327**: 1219–21

4. Homer CS, *et al*. Collaboration in maternity care: a randomised controlled trial comparing community based continuity of care with standard hospital care. *BJOG* 2001; **108(1)**: 16–22

5. Green JM, *et al*. Continuity of carer: what matters to women? A review of the evidence. *Midwifery* 2000; **16(3)**: 186–96

6. Smith LF. Views of pregnant women on the involvement of general practitioners in maternity care. *Br J Gen Pract* 1996; **46**: 101–04

7. Hutton E. *What women want from midwives, obstetricians, general practitioners, health visitors.* London: National Childbirth Trust, 1994

8. Jewell D, Smith LF, Young G, Zander L. *The case for community based maternity care.* 3rd Edition. The Association for Community Based Maternity Care

9. RCGP Maternity Care Group. *The Role of General Practice in Maternity Care*. Occasional Paper 72. London: Royal College of General Practitioners, 1995

10. *General Practitioners and Intrapartum Care: Draft Interim guidance England and Wales only.* GMSC. London: British Medical Association and Royal College of General Practitioners, 1997

11. Smith LF. Should general practitioners have any role in maternity care in the future? *Br J Gen Pract* 1996; **46**: 243–7

12. Jewell D, Smith LF. Community-based maternity care. In: Marsh G, & Renfrew M (editors). *Oxford General Practice Series*. Oxford: Oxford University Press, 1999

13. White Paper – Genetics. Available at: www.dh.gov.uk/assetRoot/04/01/92/39/04019239.pdf (accessed 06/09/2004)

14. Smith LFP. Pre-pregnancy counselling. In: *Maternity Services in the year 2000.* Chamberlain G, & Patel N (editors). London: Royal College of Obstetricians and Gynaecologists, 1994

15. Lord JM, Flight IHK, Norman RJ. Metformin in polycystic ovary syndrome: systematic review and meta-analysis. *BMJ* 2003; **327**: 951–5

16. Tackling polycystic ovary syndrome. *Drugs and Therapeutics Bulletin*. 2001; **39**: 1–4

17. RCOG. The initial investigation management of the infertile couple. National evidence-based clinical guidelines. London: Royal College of Obstetricians and Gynaecologists, 2002

18. Smith LFP. The role of primary care in infertility management. *Human Fertility* 2003; **6**: S9–S12

19. RCOG. The Management of early pregnancy loss. RCOG Clinical Guideline. London: Royal College of Obstetricians and Gynaecologists, 2000

20. www.NICE.org.uk/page.aspx?o=89892 (accessed 6/09/2004)

21. www.dh.gov.uk/assetRoot/04/06/61/91/04066191.pdf (accessed 6/09/2004)

22. Morgan-Caper P, Crowcroft N S. Guidelines on the management of, and exposure to, rash illness in pregnancy. London: Communicable Disease and Public Health 2002; **5(1)**: 59–71

23. Routine Ultrasound Screening in Pregnancy. Report of the RCOG Working Party, July, 2000

24. www.nelh.nhs.uk/screening/dssp/home.htm (accessed 6/09/2004)

25. Wald N J, *et al.* First and second trimester antenatal screening for Down's syndrome: the results of the Serum, Urine and Ultrasound Screening Study (SURUSS). *Health Technol Assess* 2003; **7(11)**: 1–77

26. Depart of Health, Department for education and Skills. *National Service Framework for Children, Young People and Maternity Services.* London: HMSO, 2004

    www.dh.gov.uk/PolicyAndGuidance/HealthAndSocialCareTopics/ChildrenServices/ ChildrenServicesInformation/ChildrenServicesInformationArticle/fs/en?CONTENT_ ID=4089111&chk=U8Ecln (accessed 22/11/2004)

27. Smith L F, Jewell D. Contribution of general practitioners to hospital intrapartum care in maternity units in England and Wales in 1988. *BMJ* 1991; **302**: 13–16

28. Smith L F. Provision of obstetric care by general practitioners in the south western region of England. *Br J Gen Pract* 1994; **44**: 255–7

29. Brown D J. Opinions of general practitioners in Nottinghamshire about provision of intrapartum care. *BMJ* 1994; **309**: 777–9

30. Responsibilities in Intrapartum Care – Working together. A joint statement from the RCM and the RCGP. London: RCM, 1995

31. Singh D, Newburn M. Postnatal care in the month after birth. *The Practising Midwife* 2001; **4**: 22–5

32. Dowswell T, Renfrew M J, Gregson B, *et al.* A review of the literature on women's views on their maternity care in the community in the UK. *Midwifery* 2001; **17**: 194–202

33. Department of Health and Royal College of General Practitioners. Implementing a scheme for general practitioners with special interests. London: DoH/RCGP, 2002

34. Royal College of General Practitioners and Royal College of Physicians. GPs with special interests. London: RCGP, 2001

CHAPTER 5

Paediatrics

Anthony Harnden

▶ KEY MESSAGES ▼

HUMAN METAPNEUMOVIRUS (hMPV)	• A recently discovered viral cause of respiratory infection. Epidemiology and clinical features remain to be defined but all children have serological evidence of exposure by five years of age.
MATERNAL SMOKING AND CHILD HEALTH	• Smoking in pregnancy leads to infant lung hypoplasia. Wheeze with viral infection is more likely if a household member smokes indoors or outdoors.
MENINGITIS VACCINES	• Conjugate vaccines include long-term immunological memory. Meningococcal C vaccine has been successfully introduced into the UK immunisation schedule; next in line may be a conjugated pneumococcal vaccine.
HEALTH IMPACT OF CHILDHOOD OBESITY	• There is an epidemic of childhood obesity in the developing world. Childhood obesity causes an adverse cardiovascular risk factor profile, which remains in adult life. Twenty-five per cent of four- to ten-year olds have glucose intolerance.

Human metapneumovirus

Children with respiratory infections frequently present to primary care. The diagnosis and management of these children is often straightforward – they have 'a virus' and most infections are self-limiting. Symptomatic treatment with antipyretics is the standard advice. But qualitative research suggests parents are dissatisfied with a diagnosis of 'it is just a virus' and their satisfaction with the consultation may be enhanced by a more precise diagnosis and more information about the likely course of their child's illness.

A significant recent advance in our understanding of the aetiology of viral respiratory infections in children has been the identification of a commonly acquired but newly discovered virus – human metapneumovirus (hMPV). Using classical microbiological techniques such as culture and immunofluorescence, a viral aetiology – for example, rhinovirus, adenovirus, parainfluenza, influenza, respiratory syncytial virus (RSV) – has been identified in about 60% of children with respiratory infection. Advances in genetic diagnostic techniques and in particular the use of polymerase-chain-reaction (PCR) have improved our ability to increase the percentage of children for whom we can identify a viral cause for their respiratory infection.

Figure 5.1 **Electron micrographs of human metapneumovirus**

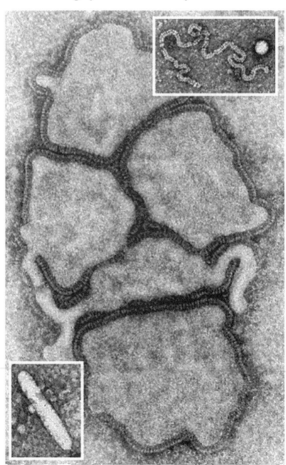

Negative-stain electron micrographs of human metapneumovirus
Reproduced by permission of the University of Chicago Press

So what is metapneumovirus and what do we know about the clinical pattern of the illness resulting from infection? Human metapneumovirus (Figure 5.1) was first reported in *Nature* in 2001 by a virology group in Holland.[1] The group discovered a paromyxovirus, closely related to avian pneumovirus (APV), in twenty-eight children with respiratory infection. Until their discovery APV, which causes rhinotracheitis in turkeys, was the sole member of the metapneumovirus genus to be identified. The larger subfamily of pneumoviruses includes amongst other viruses a major player in respiratory infection in children – RSV. What was especially fascinating about their discovery was the demonstration by serological work on stored blood specimens, taken in 1958 from people between ages 8–99 years, that hMPV has been circulating for more than 50 years and that by the age of five years nearly all children had been exposed to the virus.

Since the first report of the hMPV genus, various groups around the world have begun to document the incidence of infection and associated clinical features. Researchers from Tennessee examined 248 specimens collected between 1976 and 2001 from children with respiratory infection that had previously tested negative for known viruses.[2] Forty-nine (20%) tested positive for hMPV RNA. They concluded that 12% of respiratory infections in the children were attributable to hMPV.

For most children the virus causes a mild upper respiratory infection. In others an influenza-like illness may result with fever, mylagia and vomiting. Reports have described bronchiolitis, croup, pneumonia, conjunctivitis, otitis media, febrile seizures, diarrhoea, rash and altered liver function tests following infection. Preterm infants may be more susceptible. Serological evidence of universal exposure suggests that some infections are sub-clinical.

Exacerbations of asthma secondary to viral respiratory tract infections and viral-associated wheeze in young children, commonly present in primary care. A recent Finnish study reported human metapneumovirus in 8% of consecutive children admitted to hospital with acute respiratory wheezing.[3] In 70% of these children hMPV was the sole viral agent. Larger studies are required to determine the morbidity resulting from infection in children with asthma, but it is clear that this newly discovered virus has an important role in causing wheeze.

In addition to its close phylogeny relationship, hMPV resembles RSV in that the first infection does not seem to induce persistent immunity. Repeated infections throughout life with RSV are common. Indeed 5–25% of all upper and lower respiratory infections in the elderly are due to RSV. Despite evidence of universal exposure by the age of five, hMPV has also been documented to cause respiratory illness in young adults and in the elderly.[4]

The temporal pattern of hMPV infection is poorly defined. It certainly circulates during the winter, probably without the usual narrow monthly confines of RSV (November to January) and influenza (January to March). But we are awaiting descriptions of any seasonal peaks. Co-infection with other viruses may occur and there have been reports of significantly worsening of RSV bronchiolitis if hMPV is present as well. Before the novel coronavirus causing Severe Acute Respiratory Syndrome (SARS) was discovered, human metapneumovirus was mooted as a potential causative agent.

Human metapneumovirus is an important cause of respiratory infections in children. However, many remaining questions need to be answered before the prevalence of this virus in children with respiratory infection becomes a priority for the clinical management in UK primary care. The development of near patient tests will help improve diagnostic accuracy of common viral infections. But even if general practitioners can diagnose hMPV infection, what is the optimal treatment and what is the rate of secondary complications? How do we prevent transmission and acquisition? What is the most appropriate advice to offer parents? It is interesting that cutting-edge science has proven that another sizeable proportion of children who are diagnosed as having 'just a virus' do in fact have just another virus.

Maternal smoking and child health

There are a number of methods to assist in smoking cessation in primary care, many of which are underpinned by hard evidence. The new GP contract reflects the importance of smoking cessation advice and recognises primary care achievements that have been made in this area. However, despite the decline in the prevalence of smoking in the general population, rates in young women remain high.

Up to one third of women smoke during pregnancy. In addition to the impact this has on the woman, the impact on the child's health is significant. This section of the chapter provides an updated account of the knowledge we have of the health consequences for the child of maternal smoking, from conception onward.

Mothers who smoke have a higher incidence of obstetric complications. Both relative and absolute risks are considerable. It has been calculated that the odds ratio for ectopic pregnancy is 2.5 for women that smoke more than 20 cigarettes per day.[5] Smoking may be responsible for 15% of all preterm births. Placenta praevia, placental abruption and premature rupture of membranes are all more common in women who smoke. Smoking is a risk factor for maternal colonisation with group B streptococcus, an important cause of chorioamnionitis and neonatal sepsis. One study reported a colonisation rate of 33% amongst smokers and 16% amongst non-smokers.[6]

Two key areas in which maternal smoking has a direct impact on the child are birth weight and lung development. Smoking affects the functioning of the placenta, resulting in a reduction of oxygen diffusion and, subsequently, chronic hypoxic stress for the unborn child. It has been estimated that each cigarette per day throughout pregnancy results in a 10–15g reduction in birth weight.[7] Epidemiologists have demonstrated associations between low birth weight and hypertension, adult heart disease, diabetes and insulin resistance. It may be that there is a greater reduction in birth weight for babies born to smoking mothers who have a genetic susceptibility – polymorphisms on two maternal metabolic genes.

The growth and structural maturation of foetal lungs are dependent on foetal breathing movements. These breathing movements are reduced by maternal smoking. The resulting impairment in these movements leads to lung hypoplasia, the most critical consequence of which is a reduced surface area for gaseous exchange following birth. Lung function tests in babies born to mothers who have smoked during pregnancy show a relative reduction of 50% in small airway dimension.[8] Maternal smoking in pregnancy almost certainly determines poorer lung function in the child's future adult life and has been linked to a susceptibility to the development of chronic obstructive pulmonary disease (COPD).

It is not difficult for even the most addicted smoker to accept that passive smoking by children is not good for their lungs. Pooled analyses of school-aged children demonstrate a 1.4% reduction in forced expiratory volume in one second (FEV1), a 5% decrease in mid-expiratory flow rates and a 4.3% decrease in end-expiratory flow rate in those children exposed regularly to tobacco smoke.[9] But these analyses failed to demonstrate significant effects when it was only the father that smoked and showed much greater effects in those children whose mothers smoked in pregnancy.

For children of six years or less, wheeze with viral infection is more likely if a member of the household smokes. Smoking does not cause children to develop asthma or allergy but does exacerbate symptoms in those that have the disease. In older children wheeze, cough, phlegm, and breathlessness are 20–40% more common amongst those regularly exposed to tobacco smoke.[10] Symptoms reduce if a parent stops smoking or as the child gets older he or she spends less time in the household.

Systematic reviews have demonstrated a causal relationship between parental smoking and respiratory infections and acute middle ear disease. Chronic middle ear disease is 20–50% more frequent in children exposed to household smoke.[11] More specifically, passive smoking in children is a risk factor for RSV, bronchiolitis, pulmonary tuberculosis and meningococcal disease. The latter is supported by the observation that smokers are more likely to be carriers of meningococci. Passive smoking is also a risk factor for dental caries in children.

There is unequivocal evidence linking maternal smoking with sudden infant death syndrome (SIDS).[12] Even after adjustment for powerful confounders such as sleeping position and socio-economic status, maternal smoking doubles the risk of SIDS. The risk is higher in smoking mothers who share a bed with their infant. Possible explanations for this increased risk include neuro-developmental abnormalities leading to sleep apnoea, a reduced ventilatory response to hypoxia and abnormal pulmonary development. In addition, infantile colic is twice as common.[13]

The usual response of smoking parents when challenged by the GP that their child's health is suffering as a result of their habit is, 'But I always smoke outside the house'. However, hair cotinine (a nicotine metabolite) concentrations in children are similar whether the parent smokes indoors or outdoors.[14] So, cessation is the only reasonable option for a responsible parent. There is such a wealth of evidence indicating the harm smoking does to children that it must be a priority to target smoking cessation advice to parents and those wanting to start a family. Ideally all smoking women should be encouraged and supported to cease their habit before conceiving.

Meningitis vaccines

The spectre of 'meningitis' in children causes anxiety among parents, particularly when their child has a febrile illness. There is a significant workload from the resulting primary care consultations, many of which are out of hours. In the very early stages of disease it may be difficult to differentiate bacterial meningitis from self-limiting febrile illness. But failure to do so can have catastrophic consequences for the child's health and a significant negative impact on a GP's career. Fatality rates for bacterial meningitis are 5–10%. About 20% of survivors have serious neurological sequelae such as hydrocephalus, deafness and seizures.[15] Considerable progress has been made in the primary prevention of childhood meningitis through vaccination. This section describes recent advances and future prospects in meningitis vaccines for children.

Haemophilus influenzae type B (Hib) is an important cause of meningitis in children age six months to two years. In 1992 a vaccine against Hib was introduced into the UK immunisation schedule. Following the successful introduction of the vaccine, the number of UK cases of Hib meningitis in young children fell from 920 in 1992 to 25 in 1994.[16] This was the first of the new class of conjugated meningitis vaccines designed to induce long-term immunological memory. Conjugation of the antigenic bacterial polysaccharide capsule to an immunogenic carrier protein (such as tetanus or diphtheria toxoid) enhances antibody response to the polysaccharide and induces long-term memory.[17] The success of the Hib vaccine has encouraged the recent and ongoing development of other conjugate vaccines to protect against *Neisseria meningitidis*, *Streptococcus pneumoniae* and Group B streptococcus, likewise all important causes of bacterial meningitis in children.

There are five principal serotypes of *Neisseria meningitides* responsible for virtually all invasive meningococcal disease (meningitis and/or septicaemia): A, B, C, W135 and Y. These serogroups are based on the structure of the outer polysaccharide capsule. In Europe most meningococcal disease is caused by groups B and C, in sub-Saharan Africa by group A and in the United States 30% of infections attributed to group Y.[18] Although polysaccharide vaccines to A, C, W135 and Y have been available for the past two decades they have not been effective for children under five years who mount a poor and short-lived antibody response to them. In 1999 a group C conjugate vaccine was introduced into the UK immunisation schedule. Since then the incidence of group C disease in young children has sharply fallen and estimated vaccine effectiveness for age two to three years is 92%.[19]

Figure 5.2 **Lab-confirmed cases of meningitis C**

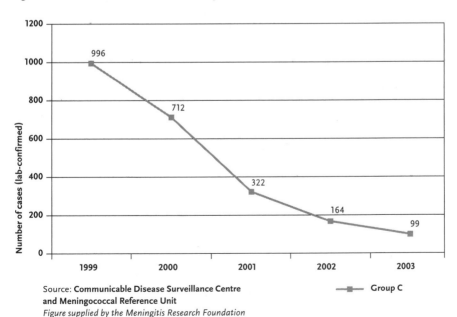

Source: **Communicable Disease Surveillance Centre and Meningococcal Reference Unit**
Figure supplied by the Meningitis Research Foundation

The development of conjugate vaccines to A, W135 and Y is at an advanced stage. Within the next few years there will be a combination conjugated vaccine available, which offers children long-term protection against A, C, W135 and Y meningococcal disease.

The development of a vaccine for group B meningococcal disease has not been straightforward. The main problem is that the polysaccharide capsule of the serogroup B meningococcus is identical to sialic acid polysaccharides found in human embryonic brain tissue. The B capsule is 'seen' by the human immune system as a self-antigen and is poorly immunogenic. Attempts have been made at modifying the capsule and exploring other outer membrane structures as potential vaccine constituents. Pharmaceutical companies are exploring the complete group B meningococcal genome to identify other potential protein candidates for vaccine development. Group B vaccines are unlikely to be in use in the next five years and when they eventually arrive they are likely to be very expensive.

Streptococcus pneumoniae has 90 known serotypes, but just five were responsible for 74% of isolates in children with invasive disease (meningitis and/or septicaemia) in England and Wales between 1993 and 1995. In 2000 a conjugated pneumococcal vaccine was licensed for use in the United States. This vaccine, which induces immunity against seven pneumococcal serotypes, is reported to have prevented 94% of invasive pneumococcal cases.[20] Although there is pressure to introduce this conjugated vaccine into the UK childhood immunisation schedule, the Joint Committee on Vaccination and Immunisation has so far resisted. This is because of the relatively low prevalence of pneumococcal disease in the UK, concern that there may be a shift of invasive bacteria to serotypes not covered by the vaccine and current public concern about childhood vaccines following the MMR debate.

Group B streptococcus is the most common cause of neonatal meningitis. Whilst antenatal prophylactic penicillin is currently the main prevention, conjugate vaccines have been developed in the United States and Japan.[21] One of the problems with these vaccines is who to target to receive them. It is difficult to obtain ethical approval for vaccinating pregnant women and neonatal meningitis often occurs in the first few days of life, before it is feasible to administer a vaccine.

The development of conjugate vaccine technology has heralded a major advance in the quest for a universal vaccination to prevent meningitis in children. The future challenge will be to produce a safe, efficacious and affordable combination meningitis vaccine. Primary care is well placed to deliver such a vaccine which will come as a welcome relief to all parents and professionals for whom this disease results in so much uncertainty.

Health impact of childhood obesity

The developed world faces major health challenges as a result of the current obesity epidemic. The impact on primary care will be considerable as the prevalence in adults of cardiovascular disease, diabetes and orthopaedic problems rise sharply. However, good child health provides a foundation for good adult health and it is worthwhile promoting an understanding in primary care of the health problems associated with childhood obesity. This section aims to provide an update of our current understanding of the short- and long-term consequences of childhood obesity.

The definition of childhood obesity is currently under debate, although most paediatricians accept a working definition of a body mass index (BMI) – (weight in kg)/(height in metres)^2– above the 98th centile.[22] Reference data for BMI centile charts represent a compilation of 11 UK surveys between 1978 and 1990. The validity of this definition of childhood obesity is underscored by the strong relationship BMI has with short- and long-term morbidity for the child. The extent of the problem is staggering. Recent data from English children show 10% of six-year-olds to be obese, rising to 17% of 15-year-olds.[23] There are two principal reasons for this surge in obesity rates: an unbalanced diet and a sedentary lifestyle. It is probably the latter that is of greatest importance. Time spent with televisions and computers reduces physical activity and it is a salutary observation that in 2004 only 5% of children make their own way to school whilst 20 years ago that figure was 90%.

So what are the health consequences of obesity in children? The early programming of an unfavourable cardiovascular risk factor profile is a major concern. The odds ratio of an obese child having a blood pressure above the 95th centile compared with a child of normal weight is 4.5 for systolic and 2.4 for diastolic pressures.[24] Other cardiovascular risk factors in obese children include raised low-density and reduced high-density lipoprotein (HDL) levels, raised triglycerides and high fasting-insulin concentrations. Fifty-eight percent of obese five- to ten-year-olds have at least one of these cardiovascular risk factors and 25% have two or more. The extent of asymptomatic atherosclerotic lesions in childhood is predicted by the number of cardiovascular risk factors. For obese children the odds ratio for atherosclerosis in a child with two risk factors is 9.7 and with three risk factors is 43.5. Moreover there are abnormalities in left ventricular mass and function, endothelial function and C reactive protein levels. Longitudinal studies have demonstrated the persistence of these risk factors in children into adulthood and their association with adult cardiovascular disease. Obese children are at significant risk of developing cardiovascular disease later in life.

The increasing prevalence of obesity in children is leading to an increasing prevalence of diabetes. An increase in abdominal adipose tissue results in insulin resistance and glucose impairment. A recent study reported that 25% of overweight four- to ten-year-olds and 21% of overweight teenagers were glucose intolerant.[25] In addition, obese children have a twofold risk of developing Type 1 diabetes. Life expectancy in children developing Type 1 diabetes before the age of seven years is reduced by an average of 18%.

Studies have described an association between obesity and the risk of developing and the severity of asthma, atopy and wheeze.[26] Polycystic ovary syndrome, foot and knee problems and sleep apnoea may all be associated with childhood obesity. The psychological consequences of being an 'obese' child must not be underestimated. Low self-esteem, depression, bullying and behavioural problems are all more common among obese children. Girls are at greater risk of psychological problems than boys and psychological morbidity increases with age.

The link between child obesity and adult obesity is strong. Sixty-nine percent of obese six- to nine-year-olds and 89% of obese ten- to fourteen-year-olds are obese as adults.[27] Obesity in adulthood is more likely if the child has an obese parent. The problem is compounded with a parallel rise in adult obesity rates. Even after adjustment for powerful confounders such as intelligence quotient there is solid evidence linking childhood obesity with less favourable educational achievement, income and socio-economic status.

Although an obese child with short stature may warrant investigations to exclude an underlying cause, most of the work in primary care should be directed toward childhood obesity prevention and recognition of associated complications. There are a number of strategies that could help. Promotion of prolonged breast-feeding has a consistent protective effect.[28] Recognising excessive weight gain in the first year of life, like weight loss, is important. Possessing BMI charts and demonstrating to children and parents that there is a problem. Encouraging healthy eating and physical activity. Energy expenditure does make a difference. Childhood obesity is a major public health problem. Whilst the responsibility primarily lies with parents, brief pieces of intervention advice from primary care health professionals can be beneficial for the child's health.

References

1. van den Hoogen B G, de Jong J C, Groen J, *et al.* A newly discovered human pneumovirus isolated from young children with respiratory tract disease. *Nat Med* 2001; **7**: 719–24

2. Williams J V, Harris P A, Tollefson S J, *et al.* Human metapneumovirus and lower respiratory tract disease in otherwise healthy infants and children. *N Engl J Med* 2004; **350**: 443–50

3. Jartti T, van den H B, Garofalo R P, Osterhaus A D, Ruuskanen O. Metapneumovirus and acute wheezing in children. *Lancet* 2002; **360**: 1393–4

4. Stockton J, Stephenson I, Fleming D, Zambon M. Human metapneumovirus as a cause of community-acquired respiratory illness. *Emerg Infect Dis* 2002; **8**: 897–901

5. Saraiya M, Berg C J, Kendrick J S, *et al.* Cigarette smoking as a risk factor for ectopic pregnancy. *Am J Obstet Gynecol* 1998; **178**: 493–8

6. Terry R R, Kelly F W, Gauzer C, Jeitler M. Risk factors for maternal colonization with group B beta-hemolytic streptococci. *J Am Osteopath Assoc* 1999; **99**: 571–3

7. Anderson G D, Blidner I N, McClemont S, Sinclair J C. Determinants of size at birth in a Canadian population. *Am J Obstet Gynecol* 1984; **150**: 236–44

8. Hanrahan J P, Tager I B, Segal M R, *et al.* The effect of maternal smoking during pregnancy on early infant lung function. *Am Rev Respir Dis* 1992; **145**: 1129–35

9. Cook D G, Strachan D P, Carey I M. Health effects of passive smoking. Parental smoking and spirometric indices in children. *Thorax* 1998; **53**: 884–93

10. Cook D G, Strachan D P. Health effects of passive smoking. Parental smoking and prevalence of respiratory symptoms and asthma in school age children. *Thorax* 1997; **52**: 1081–94

11. Strachan D P, Cook D G. Health effects of passive smoking. Parental smoking, middle ear disease and adenotonsillectomy in children. *Thorax* 1998; **53**: 50–6

12. Anderson H R, Cook D G. Passive smoking and sudden infant death syndrome: review of the epidemiological evidence. *Thorax* 1997; **52**: 1003–9

13. Reijneveld S A, Brugman E, Hirasing R A. Infantile colic: maternal smoking as potential risk factor. *Arch Dis Child* 2000; **83**: 302–3

14. Nelson R. Smoking outside still causes second-hand smoke exposure to children. *Lancet* 2002; **359**: 1675

15. Segal S, Pollard A J. The future of meningitis vaccines. *Hosp Med* 2003; **64**: 161–7

16. Peltola H. Worldwide Haemophilus influenzae type b disease at the beginning of the 21st century: global analysis of the disease burden 25 years after the use of the polysaccharide vaccine and a decade after the advent of conjugates. *Clin Microbiol Rev* 2000; **13**: 302–17

17. Buttery J P, Moxon E R. Designing meningitis vaccines. *J R Coll Physicians Lond* 2000 **34(2)**: 163–8

18. Bethell D, Pollard A J. Meningococcal vaccines. *Expert Rev Vaccines* 2002; **1**: 75–84

19. Morley S L, Pollard A J. Vaccine prevention of meningococcal disease, coming soon? *Vaccine* 2001; **20**: 666–87

20. Black S, Shinefield H, Fireman B, *et al.* Efficacy, safety and immunogenicity of heptavalent pneumococcal conjugate vaccine in children. Northern California Kaiser Permanente Vaccine Study Center Group. *Pediatr Infect Dis J* 2000; **19**: 187–95

21. Baker C J, Edwards M S. Group B streptococcal conjugate vaccines. *Arch Dis Child* 2003; **88**: 375–8

22. Reilly J J, Wilson M L, Summerbell C D, Wilson D C. Obesity: diagnosis, prevention, and treatment; evidence-based answers to common questions. *Arch Dis Child* 2002; **86**: 392–4

23. Reilly J J, Dorosty A R. Epidemic of obesity in UK children. *Lancet* 1999; **354**: 1874–5

24. Freedman D S, Dietz W H, Srinivasan S R, Berenson G S. The relation of overweight to cardiovascular risk factors among children and adolescents: the Bogalusa Heart Study. *Pediatrics* 1999; **103**: 1175–82

25. Sinha R, Fisch G, Teague B, Tamborlane W V, Banyas B, *et al.* Prevalence of impaired glucose tolerance among children and adolescents with marked obesity. *N Engl J Med* 2002; **346**: 802–10

26. Figueroa-Munoz J I, Chinn S, Rona R J. Association between obesity and asthma in 4–11-year-old children in the UK. *Thorax* 2001; **56**: 133–7

27. Whitaker R C, Wright J A, Pepe M S, Seidel K D, Dietz W H. Predicting obesity in young adulthood from childhood and parental obesity. *N Engl J Med* 1997; **337**: 869–73

28. von Kries R, Koletzko B, Sauerwald T, *et al.* Breast feeding and obesity: cross sectional study. *BMJ* 1999; **319**: 147–50

Acknowledgement

I am grateful to Dick Moyon-White for comments on earlier drafts of this manuscript.

CHAPTER 6

Women's Health

Sarah Jarvis

▶ **KEY MESSAGES**

- Many new surgical techniques of endometrial ablation for the treatment of menorrhagia have been developed in recent years. Their availability varies across the country, but there is little difference in efficacy between the different methods.

- Women must be given all the information they need to make an informed choice of treatment for menorrhagia.

- The metabolic implications of polycystic ovary syndrome (PCOS), including effects on development of diabetes and cardiovascular disease, need to be considered in all women with the diagnosis.

- Changes in prescribing patterns for hormone replacement therapy (HRT) have significant implications for both short-term symptom control and long-term prevention of osteoporosis.

- The shift to liquid-based technology for cervical cytology should improve sensitivity in detection of potentially cancerous lesions, as well as patient satisfaction.

- Anastrozole offers the first real hormonal alternative to tamoxifen for the adjuvant treatment of breast cancer.

Introduction

Recent years have seen a revolution in the management of a wide variety of medical conditions relating to women's health. In some cases, the revolution has been for the good, with development of more effective, better tolerated treatment options and investigations. In other cases, however, changes in thinking have been precipitated by adverse research findings, which have been picked up by the lay media and publicised in an often unbalanced, sensationalist fashion. Presented with this situation most women depend on primary care, as their first port of call, to provide a balanced and objective picture, allowing them to make informed choices.

The issues covered in this chapter include:

▶ advances in the management of menorrhagia, including new surgical options

▶ the changing focus of treatment in PCOS

▶ the facts behind the scare stories relating to long-term use of HRT, and the short and long-term management options this information throws up

▶ new national guidance on liquid-based technology for cervical screening

▶ a new long-term drug option for improved outcomes in breast cancer.

Advances in the management of menorrhagia

While only about 40% of women presenting with symptomatic menorrhagia have a monthly menstrual blood loss exceeding the 80 ml required for a diagnosis of 'objective' menorrhagia,[1] subjective heavy menstrual loss can be both distressing and inconvenient. Flooding – bleeding that cannot be contained by both tampon and sanitary pad – has traditionally been used as an indication of menorrhagia, but there is little to suggest that this method provides an accurate measurement of objective menorrhagia.[1] In recent years, however, evidence has proved that many of the existing licensed medications are relatively ineffective, and at the same time a variety of surgical treatments have been developed.

Medical management of menorrhagia

Tranexamic acid, an antifibrinolytic drug given at a dose of 1–1.5 g, 3–4 times a day during the heaviest 3–4 days of the menstrual cycle, reduces menstrual blood flow by an average of 52 ml.[2] NSAIDs are less effective at reducing menstrual blood loss, but they do also reduce dysmenorrhoea.

Oral progestogens have been licensed for many years for the treatment of menorrhagia, with medroxyprogesterone acetate given at a dose of 2.5–10 mg daily for 5–10 days monthly, beginning on days 16–21 of the menstrual cycle.[3] However, systematic review of the evidence shows little benefit from progestogens given in this regime.[4]

The Mirena Intra-Uterine System (IUS) is now licensed for the treatment of menorrhagia, as well as for contraceptive purposes. Irregular, but usually light, bleeding may persist after insertion of an IUS for up to six months, although bleeding is reduced by up to 90% after 12 months.[5] Up to 20% of women request removal of the IUS within one year of insertion, as a result of side effects including headache, breast tenderness, back pain and abdominal bloating,[6] but the incidence of side effects is not significantly different than for other treatments for menorrhagia of similar efficacy.[7]

For the treatment of menorrhagia, the IUS is more effective than oral cyclical progestogens, NSAIDs or tranexamic acid.[7] Efficacy rates are comparable to those of endometrial ablation, but the IUS has the advantage, compared to surgical options, of allowing the woman the choice of regaining her fertility at a later date, by removal of the device.[8,9]

Surgical options for menorrhagia

Recent years has seen the development of a wide variety of methods of endometrial ablation, which provide relief from menorrhagia with a shorter operating time, lower complication rate and faster recovery than hysterectomy. Methods include transcervical endometrial resection, rollerball, laser, microwave and thermal balloon ablation. Continued bleeding after endometrial resection is usually light, but does affect between 30% and 90% of women undergoing the procedure.[8,9] There is little difference in the relative efficacy of the different methods of endometrial ablation.[8–10] Satisfaction rates, likewise, vary little between methods, and are generally high.[10]

Hysterectomy is the only treatment for menorrhagia guaranteed to bring about a 100% reduction in menstrual blood loss. It does, however, involve major surgery, which carries a 25% risk of complication, including sepsis, blood loss requiring transfusion, anaemia, urinary retention, and haematoma.[11]

Queries have been raised in the past about longer-term complications, including interruption of the pelvic nervous supply and consequent reduction in sexual pleasure. There have also been doubts about the relative likelihood of reduced sexual wellbeing if total hysterectomy (abdominal as well as vaginal) rather than subtotal abdominal hysterectomy, with preservation of the cervix, is carried out.[12] In fact, recent research has shown that not only are satisfaction rates following hysterectomy high (and higher than after endometrial ablation), but that sexual satisfaction actually increases.[12]

Implications for practice

The three major advances in the treatment of menorrhagia in recent years have been the licensing of the IUS for its management, the development of a variety of methods of endometrial ablation, and the finding that sexual satisfaction is not diminished by any form of hysterectomy. Treatment for menorrhagia should not be limited to those women who have evidence of monthly menstrual flow greater than 80 ml, and the choice of treatment should be tailored to the individual woman's circumstances. The implications of the various treatments on fertility should always be discussed.

Polycystic ovary syndrome – new definitions, new treatments

The clinical features of PCOS include oligomenorrhoea, anovulation, infertility, hirsutism, acne and obesity.[13,14] Diagnostic criteria include the presence of multiple small cysts within the ovaries, raised plasma testosterone levels and increased luteinising hormone (LH) levels compared to follicle stimulating hormone (FSH) levels.[13,14] Since the condition was first described by Stein and Leventhal in the early 1930s, there has been much debate about the number of criteria that must be fulfilled for a diagnosis of PCOS to be made, and consequently about the incidence of the condition. Currently accepted criteria suggest that 5–10% of women of reproductive age are affected.[15]

In recent years, the emphasis on management of women with PCOS has moved from regulation of periods and induction of ovulation where appropriate, towards a more holistic approach. For instance, the 50% obesity rate among women with PCOS, and the vicious cycle resulting from increased testosterone production in the adipose tissue, makes the management of cardiovascular risk factors in these women a pressing concern. Likewise, an androgenic lipid profile (high levels of LDL cholesterol and triglycerides) and a hypercoagulation state (with elevated levels of plasminogen activator 1) are all very prevalent in women with PCOS.[14,16]

In addition, it is estimated that approximately 35% of obese women with PCOS have impaired glucose tolerance, and that within five to ten years, 30–50%

of these will go on to develop Type 2 diabetes mellitus (DM). Furthermore, PCOS is associated with gestational diabetes, which is itself a risk factor for later development of Type 2 DM. Overall, it is estimated that 10% of obese women with PCOS will develop diabetes by the age of 40 years.[16]

It is recognised that the mechanism behind development of Type 2 DM in women with PCOS centres around insulin resistance, and the consequent development of hyperinsulinaemia.[15] Insulin resistance modifies reproductive function both by the direct action of insulin on steroidogenesis, and by the disruption of insulin-signalling pathways in the central nervous system. In recent years, then, there has been increasing research into the use of metformin and other insulin sensitising agents to treat both the features of PCOS and the overall diabetes-related health outcomes of women with PCOS.

The results are very encouraging. Systematic review and meta-analysis suggests that as well as reducing fasting insulin concentrations, blood pressure, and LDL-cholesterol levels, metformin increases rates of ovulation in women with PCOS.[15] In addition, it is more effective than Dianette, the cyproterone acetate-containing combined oral contraceptive pill with anti-androgenic properties, in treating hirsutism.[17] No research into the relative efficacy of metformin and Dianette in the treatment of acne in PCOS was found in a literature search, but it is a logical inference from the above findings that metformin might also have a role in the management of this characteristic symptom.

Implications for the future

Looking to the future, it is likely that interest will turn to the role of drugs that can delay the onset of Type 2 DM in the management of women with PCOS, as well as other groups at high risk of developing the condition. For instance, several studies into the use of the angiotensin converting enzyme inhibitor (ACE-I) and angiotensin receptor blocker (ARB) drugs presently used for the management of hypertension have looked at the development of diabetes, as well as the progression of microalbuminuria in patients already diagnosed with Type 2 DM.[18,19] Current indications for ACE-Is and ARBs include the control of hypertension, the management of heart failure, the prevention of recurrence of myocardial infarction and the progression of diabetic renal disease in diabetic patients with microalbuminuria.

Several of these indications are recognised as important enough for specific inclusion in the clinical indicators of the quality and outcomes framework of the new GMS contract.[20] With an estimated increase in the incidence of diabetes worldwide from 130 million to 300 million in the 30 years between 1995 and 2025, and with an estimated 1 million undiagnosed diabetics in the

UK alone, any effective treatment to prevent the development of diabetes and its complications in high-risk patients is likely to prove cost effective in the long term.

HRT – new information on long-term risks

The world of women's health has been largely dominated in the last year by emerging research relating to adverse consequences of long-term HRT. Of particular concern has been the new findings relating to an increased risk of breast cancer in women taking combined (oestrogen/progesterone) preparations of HRT. Interestingly, the increased risk of breast cancer associated with HRT has been known for some years, but previous studies have suggested that the implications for mortality were not significant. For instance, while research five years ago suggested a 35% increased risk in breast cancer associated with taking HRT for more than ten years, the postulation was that these cancers had a lower mortality rate, and that overall mortality from breast cancer was not adversely affected.[21]

In 2002, the results of the Women's Health Initiative study were published. This study, based in the USA, involved 16,000 healthy women randomised to receive placebo or continuous combined HRT, containing 0.625 mg equine oestrogen and 2.5 mg medroxyprogesterone acetate (this regime is most similar to Premique, which is prescribed in the UK and contains 0.625 mg equine oestrogen and 5 mg medroxyprogesterone acetate). The study was terminated early because of an unacceptably high incidence of adverse events among women taking active HRT.[22] The implications for HRT and the prescribing risks connected with taking combined HRT for ten years are outlined in Box 6.1.

Box 6.1 **Implications for prescribing HRT (MHRA, December 2003)** [23]

- For treatment of menopausal symptoms, the benefits of short-term use of HRT outweigh the potential risks in most women.

- For these women, the minimum effective dose should be used for the shortest duration.

- HRT should not be considered first-line therapy for the long-term prevention of osteoporosis in women who are over 50 years of age and at an increased risk of fractures.

- Patients already using or considering using HRT long-term for the prevention of osteoporosis should have their medicine reviewed at their next appointment.

- HRT should not be prescribed for the prevention of heart disease.

In the UK, there was remarkably little national media coverage of the study. Some gynaecologists questioned the relevance of the study to British populations, since the average age of the women studied was 63 years. Nonetheless, the results from the Women's Heath Initiative trial were taken very seriously by the Committee on Safety of Medicines, which, as a consequence of this emerging evidence for long-term risks of HRT, published an update of its guidance on the use of HRT (see Box 6.1).[23]

Far more public anxiety was generated by the publication of the Million Women Study in August 2003.[24] As the title suggests, more than one million women, aged 50–64 years, were followed in the UK between 1996 and 2001. The main findings of the study were as follows:

- Taking combined oestrogen/progestogen HRT for ten years increased the likelihood of developing breast cancer by 19 per 1000 users (absolute increased risk 1.9% over ten years) – a relative risk of 2.0.

- Over ten years, the background risk of a woman of this age developing breast cancer is about 2% – the relative risk of 2.0 means that taking combined HRT would double her risk over this period.

- Taking combined HRT for five years increased risk of developing breast cancer by 6 in 1000 women (0.6% over five years) – a relative risk of 1.3.

- Taking oestrogen-only HRT for ten years increased risk of breast cancer by about 5 in 1000 (0.5% over ten years) – a relative risk of 1.25.

- Use of tibolone was associated with a relative increased risk of developing breast cancer of 1.45.

- There was no significant difference in the risk of breast cancer between oral, transdermal or implanted preparations.

- There was no significant difference between the effects of progestogen given sequentially or continuously on the incidence of breast cancer, although the number of women who had switched preparations was not known.

- The use of oestrogen-only HRT in non-hysterectomised women is associated with an increased risk of developing endometrial cancer. However, the combined increase in risk associated with non-hysterectomised women taking oestrogen-only HRT for ten years is 15–19 extra cancers (five extra breast cancers and 10–14 extra endometrial cancers). This is similar to the figure of 19 extra cancers (all extra breast cancers) associated with ten years' use of combined oestrogen/progestogen HRT.

▶ The increased risk of breast cancer has disappeared by five years after stopping HRT, whether combined oestrogen/progestogen, oestrogen only or tibolone HRT.

Implications for practice

So where does this leave postmenopausal women and the GPs who must advise them? It would appear that there are two main areas of consideration:

1. the management of short-term symptoms related to the menopause, including hot flushes and vaginal dryness, and

2. the management of long-term risks for development of osteoporosis in postmenopausal women.

Short-term management of symptoms of the menopause

Hot flushes are experienced by up to 85% of women at some stage during their menopausal years, and are often the most distressing menopausal complaint. They can lead to sleep disturbance and thence to irritability and lethargy.

As discussed above, the Committee on Safety of Medicines and the MHRA (the Medicines and Healthcare products Regulatory Agency) have published updates of their guidance on the use of HRT (see Box 6.1) in the light of the Women's Health Initiative study and the Million Women Study.

In the past, the effectiveness of HRT in reducing or preventing menopausal symptoms such as hot flushes has been such that relatively little research has been carried out on alternative therapies in women in whom use of HRT was not contra-indicated. However, hot flushes are a significant problem in women receiving cytotoxic and hormonal therapies as part of their treatment for breast cancer, as these treatment modalities are commonly associated with accelerated menopause and short-term menopausal symptoms. Consequently, there has been a growing body of research into the use of alternative treatments of menopausal hot flushes in patients. Table 6.1 details some alternatives to consider.

Table 6.1 **Alternative treatments of menopausal hot flushes**

Treatment	Dosage	Result
Red clover isoflavane	40 mg daily	20–25% reduction in hot flushes (not significantly different from placebo) [25]
Red clover isoflavane	80 mg daily	44% reduction in hot flushes compared with placebo after 12 weeks, as well as improvement in the Greene Climacteric Scale Score[26]

Treatment	Dosage	Result
Red clover isoflavone	57 mg and 82 mg total isoflavone daily	No significant difference in reduction of hot flushes between 82 mg isoflavone, 57 mg isoflavone and placebo group. Subjects in 82 mg isoflavone group experienced significantly more rapid reduction in hot flushes than 57 mg or placebo groups[27]
Phytoestrogens in soya supplements	90 mg isoflavines	No significant difference in reduction of hot flushes compared to placebo[28]
Topical progesterone cream		83% reduction in hot flushes compared with 19% reduction in placebo group[29]
Paroxetine	12.5 or 25 mg daily over 6 weeks	Median reductions in hot flushes of 62.2% (12.5 mg daily) and 64.6% (25 mg daily) group, compared with 37.8% in the placebo group[30]
Venlafaxine	75 mg daily	60% reduction in hot flushes compared with 27% reduction in placebo group[31]

Prevention of osteoporosis in postmenopausal women

The Royal College of Physicians of London (RCP) has issued guidelines on the identification of patients at high risk of osteoporosis, and their management.[32] These can be used in conjunction with the guidelines published in the MeReC Bulletin on prevention of osteoporosis-related fractures in the elderly[33] to identify women in need of preventive treatment for osteoporosis on the basis of dual energy X-ray absorptiometry (DEXA) scanning. In addition, new guidelines have just been produced on the management of glucocorticosteroid-induced osteoporosis.[34]

The National Institute for Clinical Excellence (NICE) is undertaking consultation on the cost effectiveness of alternatives to HRT for the prevention of osteoporosis-related fractures for both secondary and primary prevention. Its initial draft consultation document, produced in December 2003, recommended that no woman be given osteoporosis-preventive treatment without a history of fragility fracture, and that even with a history of fragility fracture, women under the age of 65 should not be given osteoporosis-preventive treatment in the absence of other risk factors (severe osteoporosis on DEXA scanning or maternal history of hip fracture). Such was the outcry from professional and patient bodies at this guidance that NICE has set up working parties to look at factors that might identify women at particularly high risk for primary prevention. The resulting guidance of these working parties is awaited.

Interestingly, the RCP guidelines accept that DEXA scanning has a relatively poor predictive power for future osteoporotic fractures. Given the size of the problem – the annual cost of osteoporotic fractures in a single UK Primary Care Organisation of 100,000 is estimated at £2,800,600[35] – some GPs may feel that there is an argument for treating all women with risk factors for osteoporosis, regardless of DEXA scanning results.

However, the lessons of HRT should remind us all that long-term therapies carry potential risks as well as benefits. These risks must be weighed up carefully against the benefits in terms of reduced admissions, reduced mortality and improved quality of life for many patients. In addition, the cost of long-term preventive therapy needs to be borne in mind. Having said this, one must not let anxieties over risks, such as those relating to long-term HRT usage, prevent us from adequately treating women who are at risk. There is evidence that even after hospitalisation for osteoporosis-related fracture, and despite the recommendation that all patients having suffered such a fracture should be treated with osteoporosis-preventing medication,[32] many high-risk patients are not receiving adequate preventive therapy.[36]

_& Raloxifene.

Selective Estrogen Receptor Modulators (SERMs)

SERMs are licensed for the prevention and treatment of postmenopausal osteoporosis. They increase bone mineral density and reduce the risk of vertebral fracture,[37] although they have not, as yet, been proven to protect against non-vertebral fractures. Osteoporotic vertebral fractures are an important cause of chronic back pain, with up to 40,000 vertebral fractures diagnosed in the UK annually.[38] In fact, the lifetime risk of a vertebral fracture is significantly higher than that of a hip fracture.[39] In addition, in contrast to HRT, SERMs actually reduce the risk of invasive breast cancer by up to 72%.[40] Side effects include hot flushes and leg cramps.

Bisphosphanates
Bisphosphanates are effective at reducing osteoporotic fractures and increasing bone mineral density. They need to be used with caution in patients with moderate renal impairment, and are contraindicated in patients with severe renal impairment. In addition, they are associated with a significant incidence of upper gastrointestinal disturbance, resulting in caveats on prescribing information. Despite this, research suggests that a high proportion of patients

receiving this medication have both insufficiencies of creatinine clearance and pre-existing upper gastrointestinal disease, both of which are common in the elderly patients most at risk of osteoporosis.[41]

Calcium and vitamin D

Both the RCP guidelines and the MeReC Bulletin guidelines stress that while calcium and vitamin D supplements do not have as great an effect on osteoporosis as SERMs or bisphosphanates, they are cheap and well tolerated. They can therefore be recommended both as an adjunctive therapy in women with osteoporosis on DEXA scanning, and as an adjunct to lifestyle advice for women with osteopenia on DEXA scanning.[33]

Liquid-based cytology for cervical screening

The national cervical screening programme for detecting early changes linked to cervical cancer has been a standard part of mainstream primary care for decades. Before 1990, payment for cervical smears was made on the basis of item-of-service payments for each procedure. Under the GP contract of 1990, a system of targets for cervical smears was introduced, with payments at a lower level made for achieving a target of 50% among eligible women, and a higher payment for achieving a target of 80%. Under the new GMS contract, which came into effect on 1st April 2004, payment for cervical screening will form part of Additional Services.[20]

As primary care has shifted from a GP-led to a team-based service, and as the proportion of practices employing practice nurses has increased, the task of carrying out cervical smears has increasingly fallen to the practice nurse. For over 50 years, the Papanicolaou or 'Pap' smear test has been the gold standard tool for carrying out cervical smears in the NHS, as well as in most other countries.

This method, however, has significant shortcomings. Overall, about 10% of Pap smears are reported as inadequate on staining and examination by a cytologist. Potential causes of inadequate smears include problems with sample collection, suboptimal preparation, blood, inflammatory exudate or mucus obscuring the smear, or insufficient cervical cells for adequate interpretation.

With liquid-based cytology (LBC), a plastic broom rather than a spatula is used. Instead of wiping the spatula onto a slide, which risks the loss of a large proportion of cervical cells removed by the spatula but not transferred onto the slide, the whole broom is snapped off and rinsed immediately into a vial of preservative fluid. All the cervical cells are thus transferred to the laboratory, where they can be separated from blood and other debris before examination. This makes LBC up to 12% more sensitive than Pap smears.[42]

All these factors have been considered by the advisory members of the NICE guidance board, which has just reported on its recommendations for the future of cervical screening.[42] The report uses a meta-analysis of data derived from 14 studies, comparing the efficacy, cost effectiveness and other comparators between LBC and Pap smears.

It concludes that while moving to an LBC-based system for the national NHS cervical screening programme will involve a start-up cost of about £10.3 million, there will be cost savings from a reduction in the present 250,000–300,000 inadequate cervical smears that must, under the present system, be retaken each year. The cost of these repeat smears is significant, not only in terms of workforce implications in primary care and in the laboratory, but also in terms of patient anxiety and non-compliance with follow-up.

Other advantages of the LBC system taken into account by the NICE guidance include:

▶ reduction in smear taking and consultation time of about five minutes per patient

▶ capacity for carrying out tests for chlamydia and human papilloma virus (HPV) on the same LBC sample

▶ overall preference for LBC over Pap smears on the part of patients and health care professionals

▶ increased sensitivity in detecting high-grade lesions with features of severe dyskaryosis.

Implications for practice

The NICE guidance on liquid-based cytology for cervical screening recommends a move from a Pap smear-based system to an LBC-based system for cervical screening. The initial cost is likely to be offset by savings in time and reductions in workload secondary to inadequate smears. In addition, the increased sensitivity of the method, and the likely improved compliance that will result from patient preference of LBC over Pap smears, give this advance the potential both to improve quality of care and to save lives.

Anastrozole for breast cancer

For many years, tamoxifen has been the drug of choice for the longer-term adjuvant management of breast cancer. However, 2001 saw the preliminary results of trials on the first real alternative, anastrozole. Tamoxifen works by partially blocking oestrogen receptors within each cancer cell, thereby preventing circulating oestrogen from stimulating the growth of breast cancer cells. In contrast, anastrozole blocks production of oestrogen and therefore reduces circulating levels.

The preliminary results of the trial suggest that in comparison to tamoxifen, anastrozole:

- significantly increases time to recurrence and improves disease-free interval, defined as local, contralateral or distant breast cancer recurrence or death (14% reduction compared to tamoxifen at four years)

- reduces the incidence of endometrial cancer (0.1% vs. 0.7%)

- reduces the incidence of vaginal bleeding (3% vs. 12.2%)

- is associated with a lower incidence of thromboembolic events and DVT (2.2% vs. 3.8%)

- increases the incidence of musculoskeletal disorders such as joint pain (30.3% vs. 23.7%)

- is associated with a higher incidence of fractures (7.1% vs. 4.4%).[43]

At present, research is ongoing, but as a result of preliminary analysis anastrozole is now licensed for adjuvant treatment of postmenopausal women with oestrogen receptor-positive, early invasive breast cancer who are unable to take tamoxifen therapy because of a high risk of thromboembolism or endometrial abnormalities, as well as for the treatment of hormone receptor-positive or -unknown, advanced breast cancer in postmenopausal women.

Implications for practice

Breast cancer is the most common form of cancer in women, with an incidence of 2% in the ten years after the menopause.[24] The preliminary results of the ATAC trial on anastrozole must be interpreted with caution, in view of its relatively recent development. Nonetheless, there are hopeful signs that this new advance will revolutionise both the quality of life and the longevity of future generations of women with breast cancer.

References

1. Rees M, McPherson A. Menstrual Problems. In: McPherson A (editor). *Women's problems in general practice*. Oxford: Oxford Medical Publications, 1993. p 171–97.

2. Cooke I, Lethaby A, Farquhar C. Antifibrinolytics for heavy menstrual bleeding. Cochrane Database Syst Rev. 2000; **(2)**: CD000249. Oxford: Update Software.

3. British Medical Association and the Royal Pharmaceutical Society of Great Britain. British National Formulary, March 2003

4. Coulter A, Kelland J, Peto V, *et al.* Treating menorrhagia in primary care. An overview of drug trials and a survey of prescribing practice. *Int J Technol Assess Health Care* 1995; **11**: 456–71

5. Lethaby A E, Cooke I, Rees M. Progesterone/progestogen releasing intrauterine system versus placebo or any other medication for heavy menstrual bleeding. Cochrane Database Syst Rev 2000; **(2)**: CD002126

6. Stewart A. The effectiveness of the levonorgestrol-releasing intrauterine system in menorrhagia: a systematic review. *Br J Obstet Gynae* 2001; **108**: 74–86

7. Levonorgestrol intrauterine system for menorrhagia. *Drug Ther Bull* 2001; **39**: 85–7

8. Barrington J W, Arunkalaivanan A S, Abdel-Fattah M. Comparison between the levonorgestrol intrauterine system (LNG-IUS) and thermal balloon ablation in the treatment of menorrhagia. *Eur J Obstet Gynecol Reprod Biol* 2003; **108(1)**: 72–8

9. Henshaw R, Coyle C, Low S, Barry C. A retrospective cohort study comparing microwave enometrial ablation with levonorgestrol-releasing intrauterine device in management of heavy menstrual bleeding. *Aust NZ J Obstet Gyenae* 2002; **42(2)**: 205–9

10. Consumers Association. Which operation for menorrhagia? *Drug Ther Bull* 2000; **38**: 7–80

11. Dicker R C, Greenspan J R, Strausss L T, *et al.* Complications of abdominal and vaginal hysterectomy among women of reproductive age in the United States – the Collaborative Review of Sterilization. *Am J Obstet Gynaecol* 1982; **144**: 841–8

12. Roovers J-P, van der Bom J, van der Haart C H, *et al.* Hysterectomy and sexual wellbeing: prospective observational study of vaginal hysterectomy, subtotal abdominal hysterectomy and total abdominal hysterectomy. *BMJ* 2003; **327**: 774–7

13. Hull M G. Epidemiology of infertility and polycystic ovarian disease: endocrinological and demographic studies. *Gyn Endocrinol* 1987; **1**: 235–45

14. Polson D W, Adams J, Wadsworth J, Franks S. Polycystic ovaries and associated clinical and biochemical features in young women. *Clin Endocrinol* Oxford: 1999; **51**: 779–86

15. Lord J M, Flight I H, Norman R J. Metformin in polycystic ovary syndrome: systematic review and meta-analysis. *BMJ* 2003; **327**: 951–5

16. Legro R. Diabetes prevalence and risk factors in polycystic ovary syndrome. *Obstet Gynaecol Clin North Am* 2001; **28**: 99–109

17. Harborne L, Fleming R, Lyall H, *et al.* Metformin or antiandrogen in the treatment of hirsutism in polycystic ovary syndrome. *J Clin Endocrinol Metab* 2003; **88(9)**: 4116–23

18. Mogensen C E, Neldam S, Tikkeanen I, *et al.* Randomised controlled trial of dual blockade of rennin-angiotensin system in patients with hypertension, microalbuminuria, and non-insulin dependent diabetes: the candesartan and lisinopril microalbuminuria (CALM) study. *BMJ* 2000; **321**: 1440–4

19. Yusuf S, Pfeffer M A, Swedberg K, *et al.* CHARM Investigators and Committees. Effects of candesartan in patients with chronic heart failure and preserved left-ventricular ejection fraction: the CHARM-Preserved Trial. *Lancet* 2003; **362(9386)**: 777–81

20. DoH. *Investing in General Practice: The New General Medical Services Contract.* London: Department of Health, 2003

21. Faiz O, Fentiman I S. Hormone Replacement therapy and breast cancer. *IJCP* 1998; **52**: 98–101

22. Writing Group for the Women's Health Initiative Investigators. Risks and benefits from estrogen plus progestin in healthy postmenopausal women: principal results from the Women's Health Initiative randomised controlled trial. *JAMA* 2002; **288**: 321–33

23. Safety update on long-term HRT. *Current Problems in Pharmacovigilance.* Oct 2002; **28**: 11–12. See Medicines and Healthcare Products Regulatory Agency website: www.mhra.gov

24. Million Women Study Collaborators. Breast cancer and hormone-replacement therapy in the Million Women Study. *Lancet* 2003; **362**: 419–427

25. Baber R J, Templeman C, Morton T, Kelly G E, West L. Randomized placebo-controlled trial of an isoflavone supplement and menopausal symptoms in women. *Climacteric* 1999 Jun; **2(2)**: 85–92

26. van de Weijer P H, Barentsen R. Isoflavones from red clover (Promensil) significantly reduce menopausal hot flush symptoms compared with placebo. *Maturitas* 2002; **42**: 287–93

27. Tice J A, Ettinger B, Ensrud K, Wallace R, Blackwell T, Cummings S R. Phytoestrogen supplements for the treatment of hot flashes: the Isoflavone Clover Extract (ICE) Study: a randomized controlled trial. *JAMA* 2003 Jul 9; **290(2)**: 207–14

28. Van Patten C L, Olivotto G, Chambers K. Effects of soy phytoestrogens on hot flashes in postmenopausal women with breast cancer: a randomised controlled clinical trial. *Am Soc Clin Oncol* 2002; **20(6)**: 1449–55

29. Leonetti H B, Lonog S, Anasti J N. Transdermal progesterone cream for vasomotor symptoms and postmenopausal bone loss. *Obst Gynaecol* 1999; **94(2)**: 225–8

30. Stearns V, Beebe K L, Iyengar M, Dube E. Paroxetine controlled release in the treatment of menopausal hot flashes: a randomized controlled trial. *JAMA* 2003 Jun 4; **289(21)**: 2827–34

31. Loprinzi C L, Pisansky T M, Fonseca R, *et al.* Pilot evaluation of venlafazine hydrochloride for the therapy of hot flashes in cancer survivors. *J Clin Oncol* 1998; **16**: 2377–81

32. Royal College of Physicians. *Osteoporosis – clinical guidelines: summary and recommendations.* London: RCP, 1994. See: www.rcplondon.ac.uk\files\osteosummary.pdf

33. Common issues in osteoporosis. *MeRec Bulletin* 2001; **12(2)**

34. National Osteoporosis Society. *Primary Care Strategy for Osteoporosis and Falls.* Bath: NOS, 2002

35. Bone and Tooth Society of Great Britain, Royal College of Physicians, National Osteoporosis Society. *Guidelines on the prevention and treatment of glucocorticosteroid-induced osteoporosis.* June 2003

36. Panneman M J, Lips P, Sen S S, Herings R M. Undertreatment with anti-osteoporotic drugs after hospitalisation for fracture. *Osteoprosis Int* 2004; **15**: 120–4

37. Ettinger B, *et al.* Reduction of vertebral fracture risk in postmenopausal women with osteoporosis treated with raloxefine. *JAMA* 1999; **282(7)**: 637–45

38. National Osteoporosis Society. *What is osteoporosis?* See: www.nos.org.uk/osteo.asp

39. Cummings S R, Black D M, Rubin S M. Lifetime risk of hip, Colles' or vertebral fracture and coronary heart disease among white postmenopausal women. *Ann Int Med* 1998; **128**: 793–800

40. Cauley J A, Norton L, Lippman M E, Eckert S, *et al*. Continued breast cancer risk reduction in postmenopausal women treated with raloxefine: 4-year results from the MORE trial. *Breast Cancer Res Treatment* 2001; **65(2)**: 125–34

41. Bernett G B, Feldman S, Martin H, *et al*. An opportunity for medication risk reduction, health care provider collaboration, and improved patient care: a retrospective analysis of osteoporosis management. *J Am Med Dir Assoc* 2003; **4(6)**: 329–36

42. National Institute for Clinical Excellence. Final appraisal determination – guidance on the use of liquid-based cytology for cervical screening. Review of existing guidance, number 5. London: NICE, August 2003

43. The ATAC (Arimidex, Tamoxifen, Alone or in Combination) Trialists' Group. Anastrozole alone or in combination with tamoxifen versus tamoxifen alone for adjuvant treatment of postmenopausal women with early breast cancer: first results of the ATAC randomised trial. *Lancet* 2002; **359**: 2131–9

CHAPTER 7

Sexual Health

Dr Anna Graham

▶ **KEY MESSAGES**
- The key to providing appropriate sexual health advice is to first take a sexual history.
- Taking a sexual history needs to be done confidentially and non-judgementally.
- Practices need to undertake confidentiality training and require all staff to sign confidentiality statements.
- Partner notification can be done in a variety of settings including general practice.

RECENT ADVANCES ▼

- Surveys suggest that an increasing number of people have more sexual partners than ever before.
- Screening for chlamydia is becoming more widespread in the UK.
- New treatments for patients with HIV have been highly successful at reducing progression to AIDS.
- The government produced the first ever *National Strategy for Sexual Health and HIV* in 2001 – it called for a broader role for general practice in the promotion of better sexual health.
- A new course for those working in primary care has been devised aiming to equip participants with the basic knowledge, skills and attitudes for the effective management of sexually transmitted infections.

Introduction

Essential elements of good sexual health are defined as 'equitable relationships and sexual fulfilment with access to information and services to avoid the risk of unintended pregnancy, illness or disease' in the government's *National Strategy for Sexual Health and HIV*.[1]

The key to the provision of appropriate sexual health advice to an individual patient is assessment of risk, by taking a sexual history. In order to obtain a sexual history confidentiality must be ensured. It is recommended that the whole practice be involved in an update of confidentiality training and explanation on how to take a sexual history is provided in this chapter. A summary is provided of recent advances in key areas of sexual health: contraception, sexually transmitted infection management, abortion and sexual problems. In addition, an overview is provided of the *National Strategy for Sexual Health and HIV* as it relates to those working in general practice. Finally, details on training opportunities in sexual health are given.

Confidentiality in general practice

This is a thorny but crucial issue for those involved in providing sexual health care in a general practice setting. It is well known that young people especially, but this applies to all patients, are keen to be reassured about confidentiality. If, in a consultation with an individual patient, reassurance on this issue is made we must know exactly what we mean by this reassurance. The whole team must be made aware of the issues involved. This includes reception and domestic, as well as clinical, staff. The reason for this is particularly obvious in parts of the country where staff are drawn from the same community as their patients, but applies to all working in any health care setting, where remarks such as 'I saw your son/daughter at the practice last week' can be disastrous.

The Royal College of General Practitioners has produced, in collaboration with others, a toolkit on *Confidentiality and Young People*.[2] The materials for a training session in the practice are provided as well as a recommendation that all staff sign confidentiality agreements. Examples of these are included. The toolkit is a valuable resource for individual practices and for sexual health promotion specialists supporting primary care.

Risk assessment and sexual history taking

In order to provide appropriate sexual health advice it is essential to take an accurate sexual history. This has been a compulsory element of history taking in genitourinary medicine (GUM) clinics for a long time but many working in general practice have shied away from the exercise. The key challenge is to do so confidentially and non-judgmentally. Matthews and Fletcher[3] point out that health professionals working in primary care consult patients from across the risk spectrum for sexual ill health, including many at no risk.

There are a number of types of consultation where taking a sexual history can be useful, including contraceptive counselling, targeting sexual health promotion advice, for example when providing travel advice or doing a smear, and when deciding whether testing for a sexually transmitted infection (STI) is appropriate. Symptoms cannot be relied upon as they may be diverse and ambiguous and much infection is asymptomatic. Taking a sexual history requires confidence, sensitivity and confidentiality (Box 7.1).

Doctors and nurses may at first find taking a sexual history difficult for two reasons:

▶ lack of experience

▶ embarrassment for the patient and the practitioner.

Box 7.1 **Principles of taking a sexual history**[4]

If possible the patient should be seen alone. If a partner or relative is present some people will be reluctant to reveal personal information.

▶ Ask permission and explain why you are asking these questions – that the answers help you to assess the risk for STIs.
▶ Check with the patient their history if you are unclear what they mean. Avoid the temptation to reassure the person prematurely.
▶ Don't make assumptions about sexual orientation. Use terms such as 'partner'.
▶ Use the right terminology avoiding terms such as 'gay' because men who have sex with men may not identify themselves as such.
▶ Only ask what you need to – know don't ask unnecessary or intrusive questions.

A full sexual history could include questions about:[5]

▶ duration and severity of symptoms (Box 7.2)
▶ most recent episode of sexual intercourse
  ▷ timing (in relation to symptoms)
  ▷ type and duration of relationship (regular or casual)
  ▷ type of sexual intercourse (possible sites of infection)
  ▷ use of condom and contraception
  ▷ gender of partner (sexual orientation)

A full sexual history could include questions about:[5] *continued*

> ▶ details of previous sexual partners (these should be obtained in relation to duration of symptoms – to find out about new partners and who needs to be contact traced – but are also needed to assess risk in those without symptoms, given the burden of asymptomatic infection)
> ▶ sexual intercourse abroad or with partners from other countries (risk of antibiotic resistant gonorrhoea, tropical STIs or HIV risk)
> ▶ previous STIs, tests for STIs including HIV, hepatitis B
> ▶ contraceptive choice and actual use (risk of unplanned pregnancy and infection)
> ▶ menstrual, cervical cytology and obstetric history in women
> ▶ drug history, including allergies, self treatment, non-prescribed drugs and injection drug use

Box 7.2 **Clinical symptoms and signs of some sexually transmitted infections (potential causes in brackets)**[5]

> ▶ *Urethritis* (in men: chlamydia, gonorrhoea, rarely trichomonas, genital herpes, warts)
> Urethral discomfort or itching on micturition
> Urethral discharge: purulent (typically gonorrhoea), mucopurulent or clear (typically non-specific urethritis including chlamydia)

> ▶ *Urethritis* (in women: chlamydia, gonorrhoea)
> Urinary frequency or urethral discomfort, 'cystitis'

> ▶ *Cervicitis* (chlamydia, gonorrhoea)
> Intermenstrual bleeding
> Post-coital bleeding
> Cervical mucopurulent discharge

> ▶ *Vaginitis* (trichomoniasis and non-sexually transmitted candida and bacterial vaginosis)
> Vaginal soreness or irritation (trichomoniasis or candida)
> Vaginal discharge: lumpy (typically candida), smelly, thin and homogeneous (typically bacterial vaginosis)

> ▶ *Proctitis* (gonorrhoea, chlamydia, herpes simplex, warts, rarely amoebiasis in homosexual men)
> Rectal discomfort, discharge, lumps or ulceration

> ▶ *Conjunctivitis* (chlamydia, gonorrhoea)

> ▶ *Upper genital tract infection* (chlamydia, gonorrhoea, anaerobic infections)
> Women (pelvic inflammatory disease): Dyspareunia, lower abdominal pain, adnexal tenderness and/or mass, fever +/– symptoms of cervicitis
> Men (epididymo-orchitis): Testicular swelling and pain, fever

---

> ▶ *Genital ulceration* (herpes simplex, syphilis, rarely chancroid, donovanosis, lymphogranuloma venereum)

> ▶ *Genital lumps* (genital warts, molluscum contagiosum, scabies)

> ▶ *Complicated infections*
> Chlamydia: Reiter's syndrome (urethritis, seronegative arthritis, iritis)
> Gonorrhoea: Disseminated infection (arthritis, endocarditis, meningitis), Bartholin's cyst
> Primary herpes simplex: urinary retention, constipation, radiculomyelopathy, systemic viraemia

The author has never found a patient surprised or unwilling to answer questions of this nature in a general practice setting. It is more often the case that that the author has trepidation in bringing up the topic. The patient may be at very low risk of a sexually transmitted infection and the clinician may decide with the patient not to pursue this line. Occasionally the patient may be at very high risk such as those who have travelled in parts of the world with a high prevalence of HIV, or work in the sex industry; in both of these examples full infection screens are to be encouraged, with the patient's consent.

Contraception

Patterns of use of contraception and family planning services
The majority of contraceptive advice is provided in general practice. Over the last quarter century there has been an overall decrease in the use of family planning clinics with increases in attendance at these services seen only in the under 20s.[6] Between 1975 and 1998–99 the proportion of girls under 16 visiting family planning clinics increased from 1–8%. For girls aged 16–19 the proportion increased from a minimum of 12% in 1988–89 to 22% in 1998–99. The majority of contraceptive advice given to the over 20s is in general practice.

There is a need to encourage women to use non-user dependent methods with lower failure rates, such as injectables and implants as well as condoms to avoid infection.

New methods of contraception
Cerazette®
This is the first third-generation progestogen only pill (POP) containing desogestrel (75µg daily). POPs are used by only 5% of women in the UK. This new pill reliably inhibits ovulation in 97% of cycles. In a direct head-to-head comparison study Cerazette® was compared to a 30µg levonorgestrel POP. The levonorgestel-only POP inhibited ovulation in 71% of cycles. Pregnancy rates are expressed by calculating the Pearl Index (PI) (number of pregnancies per 100 women years):

Desogestrel	PI = 0.41 (95% CI: 0.085 to 1.204)
Levonorgestrel	PI = 1.55 (95% CI: 0.422 to 3.963)

It appears that desogestrel prevents more pregnancies but the confidence intervals overlap and the difference is not statistically significant. The bleeding pattern of those taking desogestrel is more variable than that of levonorgestrel users. The desogestrel containing POP costs £8.85 for a three-month supply compared to £3.31 for the most expensive alternative POP.[7,8]

Yasmin®

This new combined oral contraceptive does appear to have similar contraceptive efficacy to other similar pills but is a lot more expensive (£14.70 for three-months supply compared to, for example, £2.58 for the same quantity of Microgynon 30®). Each Yasmin® pill contains 30 µg ethinylestradiol plus 3 mg drospirenone (a derivative of spironolactone).

At the launch of this combined oral contraceptive, company advertising suggested that it was 'the pill for well-being', with 'no associated weight gain' and a 'demonstrable positive effect' on premenstrual symptoms and skin condition. The evidence for these claims is based on two unblinded randomised trials. The well-being claim is based on a survey of 237 women (a 10% sample) from one of the trials. It is unclear how the sample was chosen and the respondents were aware of which drug they were taking and so the results may be biased. The weight claim is based on self-reported weight from women measured at home which again could be biased. The weight change was very small (less than 1 kg).[9]

Cerazette® and Yasmin® are not recommended as first choice contraceptives. It is possible that their use in selected patients may be appropriate.

Evra®

This is a transdermal patch delivering 150 µg norelgestromin and 20 µg ethinylestradiol daily into the systemic circulation. The patch is applied weekly for three weeks followed by a patch-free week. The method of action and efficacy of the patch was similar to a triphasic oral preparation in a comparative study. A Cochrane systematic review compared the efficacy, cycle control, compliance and safety for the contraceptive patch and for the combined oral contraceptive.[10] The review concluded that self-reported compliance was better with the patch but, overall, the efficacy data are similar for both methods. The cost of a month's supply of Evra® is £7.74 compared to 86p for a month of Microgynon 30®.

Levonelle-2®

A new licence was granted in the autumn of 2003 to allow both doses to be given at the same time. Evidence suggests that this is as effective as separating doses by 12 hours. It is possible this change will lead to the full dose being taken more often.

Sexually transmitted infections

Sexual behaviour in Britain

The second National Survey of Sexual Attitudes and Lifestyles 2000 (Natsal 2000) was undertaken in 1999–2001 and provides the most reliable and recent data on sexual risk practices in the UK. A stratified sample of addresses was selected from the small-user postcode address file for Britain. At each selected address residents aged 16–44 years were enumerated and one randomly selected and invited to participate by the interviewer. The unadjusted response rate was 63.1% (11,161 respondents). A computer-assisted self-interview component allowed respondents to key in their responses to sensitive questions into a laptop computer. The main findings were:[11]

- ▶ mean numbers of heterosexual partners in the past five years were 3.8 (SD 8.2) for men and 2.4 (SD 4.6) for women

- ▶ homosexual partnerships were reported by 2.6% (95% CI: 2.2–3.1) of both men and women

- ▶ mean number of new partners in the past year varied from 2.04 (SD 8.4) for single men aged 25–34 years to 0.05 (SD 0.3) for married women aged 35–44 years

- ▶ 4.3% (95% CI: 3.7–5.0) of men reported paying for sex

- ▶ 14.6% (95% CI: 13.4–16.0) of men and 9.0% (95% CI: 8.2–10.0) of women had concurrent partnerships in the past year. Concurrent (or simultaneous) partnerships occur where individuals are engaged in more than one sexual partnership during the same time period. These relationships increase the opportunity for transmission of STIs.

A comparison of Natsal 2000 with the results of the same survey undertaken in 1990–91 showed that all of the above risk behaviours had increased significantly. The largest increases were seen in the under-25s and those not cohabiting or married. This helps to explain the doubling of diagnoses of chlamydia, gonorrhoea and syphilis over the past five years.[12]

Screening for chlamydia trachomatis infection

Chlamydia is the commonest bacterial STI in the UK – 80% of women and 50% of men who have this infection have no symptoms. In order for there to be a case for implementing a screening programme, results from good quality randomised trials, demonstrating a reduction in mortality or morbidity, should be available. This is not, and is unlikely ever, to exist. Three studies have or are assessing the utility of screening for this infection in the UK:

1. The Wirral and Portsmouth Department of Health pilots

2. National Survey of Sexual Attitudes and Lifestyles 2000 (Natsal 2000)

3. Chlamydia screening studies (ClaSS).

In The Wirral and Portsmouth the aim was to assess the feasibility and acceptability of opportunistic screening at a variety of health care settings. The focus was on sexually active 16–24-year-old women. From September 1999 to August 2000 urine tests for chlamydia were offered to women in general practice and specialist settings. A central office sent out results; on The Wirral this was a Community Hospital and in Portsmouth the GUM clinic. Positives were referred to GUM clinics for partner notification and treatment, or this was undertaken by the test site, or at the central office. One-third of patients were recruited at a consultation for contraceptive advice and one-third reported symptoms at the time the test was offered. The prevalence of infection was 9.8% (95% CI: 9.3 to 10.3) in Portsmouth and 11.2% (95% CI: 10.3 to 12.1) on The Wirral.

This pilot was acceptable and feasible with a higher than expected prevalence found. It was an opportunistic screening programme with a significant minority of patients reporting symptoms at testing. This pilot included a broad range of clinical settings but did not include men in a systematic way.[13]

In contrast to this pilot the National Survey of Sexual Attitudes and Lifestyles 2000 was a population-based sample where half of all sexually experienced respondents were invited to provide a urine sample for testing for chlamydia. From this, 2.2% (95% CI: 1.5–3.2%) men and 1.5% (95% CI: 1.1–2.1%) women were found to have chlamydia. The highest prevalence was found in 18–24-year-old women (3.0%) and 25–34-year-old men (3.0%). Non-married status, age, partner concurrency, and increasing numbers of sexual partners were associated with prevalent infection. These findings are very similar to Dutch and Danish population-based screening studies.[14]

The chlamydia screening studies are based in Bristol and Birmingham general practices. Men and women aged 16–39 years are invited to provide a urine sample by postal request. A randomised trial comparing partner notification undertaken by practice nurses with health advisers in GUM clinics is included. The results of this study will be available at the end of 2004.

Chlamydia screening has now been rolled out by the Department of Health to ten further pilot sites in England in non-general practice settings. The reason given for not rolling out to general practice in the invitation to tender was of 'logistical issues that need to be addressed'. Other important unanswered questions include the assessment of the costs and benefits of who should be screened, whether screening should also be offered to men and what the long-term benefits of screening might be. The natural history of untreated asymptomatic infection is unlikely to ever be known. It has been assumed that the sequelae of untreated symptomatic infection can be prevented by treatment and that this can be extrapolated to those with asymptomatic infection.

What does this mean for clinicians working in general practice now? The most sensible approach is to test for chlamydia when the symptoms reasonably suggest this could be the cause (for example when a woman presents with intermenstrual bleeding)[15] and to screen when a patient is at risk, as assessed by taking a sexual history.

The next issue is how best to test or screen. In men, collection of a first void urine in a plain urine sample bottle is appropriate. The test most likely to be performed on this specimen is a nucleic acid amplification test which has high specificity and sensitivity. This may not be available to general practice based samples in your area – it is worth checking with your local laboratory. The government is currently making funds available to support its introduction countrywide. In many parts of the country the best way to take a sample from women remains an endocervical swab taken with a swab specifically designed for this purpose. One can ensure that the sample taken will include endocervical cells, as chlamydia is an intracellular organism, by rotating the swab several times within the endocervical canal whilst taking the sample. It is likely that the taking of a urethral swab at the same time enhances the sensitivity of the tests. Urine samples, in both men and women, and vulvo-vaginal swabs may become the preferred specimens in years to come.

It is not necessary to perform a test of cure except when the case is a pregnant woman and/or erythromycin is used to treat the infection.

Gonorrhoea

Eighty-five per cent of men will be symptomatic in the first ten days of infection with gonorrhoea, whereas 70% of women are asymptomatic. If a man presents with urethral discharge in general practice it is not uncommon to refer them to the local GUM clinic. However, it is possible to manage them initially in general practice and this obviates the need for the patient to wait for an appointment (and possibly not bother).

What tests should we do in general practice? If a man has an obvious discharge I would ask his permission to take samples for chlamydia (first void urine in plain urine specimen pot) and gonorrhoea (charcoal swab). It is not necessary to place the swab inside the urethra if there is obvious discharge as the discharge can be milked onto the swab (by the patient if preferred).

Treating gonorrhoea requires knowledge of local resistance to antibiotics. It is necessary to call the local laboratory for recommendations. Follow-up needs to include a test of cure as well as partner notification – this may best be done in a GUM clinic.

HIV

HIV remains a rare infection in the UK (47,000 infected individuals identified since 1982, 0.1% prevalence 15–49 years).[4] It is primarily associated with identifiable risk factors:

- ▶ men who have sex with men

- ▶ injecting drug users

- ▶ those living in countries of high prevalence

- ▶ those have received medical treatment or a blood transfusion in countries of high prevalence

- ▶ men and women who have sex with any of the above.

Since 1999 the most frequent route of acquisition of newly reported HIV infection in the UK has been through heterosexual sex. Most homosexually acquired infections are in white males (89%), but 57% of heterosexually acquired and 60% of vertically acquired infections are in people of black African origin, mainly acquired in sub-Saharan Africa. The impact of more recent HIV epidemics in sub-Saharan Africa is now being seen, primarily in London where over 70% of black Africans in the UK live.[5]

Impact of HIV treatments on survival

In 1996 'highly active antiretroviral therapy' or 'HAART' was introduced to treat HIV positive patients. Since the introduction of these drugs the risk of progression to AIDS has fallen substantially.[16] For this reason patients at high risk of acquiring HIV need to be made aware of these therapeutic advances and their availability in the UK when deciding whether to be tested for HIV.

Antenatal HIV

During pregnancy the risk of vertical transmission of HIV from mother to infant without treatment is 15–30%. This is reduced to 1–2% with the use of antiretroviral drugs, delivery by caesarean section, careful obstetric management and avoidance of breast feeding. It is therefore important to identify previously undiagnosed pregnant women with HIV early in pregnancy. For this reason a national policy was introduced in 1999 to offer and recommend testing to all pregnant women in England. This has been introduced inconsistently across the country.

Anonymous testing for HIV provides the most reliable surveillance data. In 2001 this was undertaken in 72% of live births. Among women giving birth in London the prevalence was one in 286. Elsewhere in England prevalence is low but increasing (one in 2256 in 2001). The rate is highest in women born in Central and East Africa. Of all HIV infected women giving birth in 2001 for whom country of birth was known 77% (239 of 309) were born in sub-Saharan Africa.[17]

HIV pre-test discussion

Testing for HIV is now considered part of the repertoire of tasks in sexual health that all general practice teams should consider doing.[1] The pre-test discussion needs to be a non-judgemental process enabling the patient to make a decision whether or not to test.[3] If doing HIV testing you must have arrangements for dealing with a positive diagnosis and onward referral. A sexual history needs to be taken first to assess an individual's risk of HIV. Patients need to be informed of the availability of new treatments for HIV. The standard HIV test detects HIV antibodies. It may take up to three months for antibodies to be detected after acquisition of HIV. This may affect when the test is done and whether it needs to be repeated.

It is essential to explain how and when you plan to give the result to the patient prior to taking the test. If the result is negative you need to consider if a re-test is necessary. If the test is positive the patient is likely to be shocked so keep information to a minimum focusing on how they will cope over the next few days. A confirmatory HIV test is usually undertaken involving referral to the GUM clinic.[4]

Partner notification

The management of STIs includes the notification and treatment of sexual partners. Re-infection by an untreated sexual partner can lead to suppression of partially treated symptoms, delayed diagnosis of ascending infection and continued transmission. Partner notification is a difficult issue for those working in general practice without the back-up from health advisers on site. One answer is to refer all those with a STI to the GUM clinic. However, GUM clinics are unable to cope with demand and often suffer from long waiting times. In England, in 2002, the median time to first appointment at a GUM clinic was 12 days for men and 14 days for women.[12] The Brook Advisory Centres in London showed that very few of its referrals to GUM clinics were seen there.[18]

In some parts of the UK health advisers based in GUM clinics undertake partner notification for patients identified in general practice settings as a matter of routine. Patients give permission to be contacted when the original test sample is taken.

Another solution is to undertake partner notification in general practice. The clinician would do so by taking a sexual history and explaining to the patient the importance of telling their contacts to seek medical help from their GP or GUM clinic. It is probably reasonable to ask patients to inform all sexual partners in the previous three months (longer if none). This would be extended for HIV as this infection often has a long asymptomatic period.

Any patient treated for a sexually transmitted infection must be advised not to have sexual intercourse, even with a condom, until they and their partner(s) are fully treated so as to avoid re-infection.

Problems with sexual function

A recent survey of patients attending general practices in London shows that problems with sexual function are common – 97 of 447 (22%) men and 422 of 1065 (40%) women received a diagnosis according to international classification of diseases. Erectile failure and loss of sexual desire were the most common diagnoses in men, the only independent predictor was being bisexual. Lack of sexual desire and failure of orgasmic response were the most common in women. Independent predictors of such diagnoses in women were increasing age, poorer physical health, increasing psychological distress and sexual dissatisfaction. Up to 30% of this sample reported seeking sexual advice from their doctor. However, only 3–4% had an entry relating to sexual difficulties in their practice records. This suggests that doctors may be reluctant to record sensitive data.[19]

As part of Natsal 2000 (see p. 116) persistent sexual problems – lasting at least six months – in people who had at least one heterosexual partner in the previous year were investigated and shown to be less prevalent – 6.2% men and 15.6% women reported problems related to sexual function.[20]

Authors of both of these recently published papers suggest that labelling 'lack of sexual desire' as a disease is questionable as this is reported by such a large proportion of the populations studied.

Abortion

There are widespread variations in access to abortion services. Long waits have especially serious implications for younger women who may present later in their pregnancy. This is acknowledged in *The National Strategy for Sexual Health and HIV* which states that:

> 'From 2005...women who meet the legal requirements have access to an abortion within three weeks of the first appointment with the GP or other referring doctor.'[1]

Policy

There is no National Service Framework (NSF) for sexual health to date although this has been called for by a government select committee. *The National Strategy for Sexual Health and HIV*, published in 2001, was the first of its kind.[1] It called for 'a broader role for those working in primary care settings'. The strategy outlines three different 'levels' of service provision (Box 7.3). Level one has a number of elements of sexual health care, which the strategy suggests should ideally be available in all general practice settings. It is acknowledged in the strategy that in order for these elements to be available in every general practice setting there are training needs that need to be fulfilled.

Level two services will be made available in community settings, for example, primary care teams with a special interest in sexual health, family planning and GUM clinics.

Specialist clinical teams will deliver the more specialist aspects of care across more than one PCT. These elements of sexual health care are listed as Level three responsibilities.

Box 7.3 **Levels of service provision**

Level one	▶ Sexual history and risk assessment ▶ STI testing for women ▶ HIV testing and counselling ▶ Pregnancy testing and referral ▶ Contraceptive information and services ▶ Assessment and referral of men with STI symptoms ▶ Cervical cytology screening and referral ▶ Hepatitis B immunisation
Level two	▶ Intrauterine device insertion ▶ Testing and treating STIs ▶ Vasectomy ▶ Contraceptive implant insertion ▶ Partner notification ▶ Invasive STI testing in men

Level three	▶ Sexual health services needs assessment
	▶ Support provider quality, clinical governance at all levels
	▶ Provide specialist services:
	  ▷ Outreach for STI prevention
	  ▷ Outreach contraception services
	  ▷ Specialised infections management, including co-ordination of partner notification
	  ▷ Highly specialised contraception
	  ▷ Specialised HIV treatment and care

Training in sexual health

Sexual health often affords little time in the undergraduate curriculum and is not part of core general practice training. Courses have been developed in order to provide clinicians providing sexual health care, especially in general practice settings, with the skills needed to do so. The two most commonly held qualifications are the DFFP (Diploma in the Faculty of Family Planning) and the recently devised Sexually Transmitted Infection Foundation (STIF) Course. The former has been around for many years and is run by the Faculty of Family Planning and Reproductive Health Care, part of the Royal College of Obstetricians and Gynaecologists. This qualification has recently been updated, and now includes some STI teaching. Faculty courses (both basic training and updating) are listed on the Faculty website (see Resources).

The Faculty journal includes Faculty guidance and new product reviews produced by their Clinical Effectiveness Unit initiated in 1997. This guidance is available to all on the Faculty web site (see Resources).

The STIF course was devised by the Medical Society for the Study of Venereal Diseases (now renamed British Association for Sexual Health and HIV (BASHH)) in response to *The National Strategy for Sexual health and HIV* in order to support providers of level one and two services. The aim of the course is to equip participants with the basic knowledge, skills and attitudes for the effective management of STIs. It is a workshop-based two-day course with role-playing activities to rehearse sexual history taking using scenarios commonly found in everyday general practice. GUM consultants in some parts of the country run the course.

BASHH has a Clinical Effectiveness Group that has, to-date, produced 24 evidence-based guidelines in the area of sexually transmitted infections since its foundation in 1997. These and listings of local STIF courses are available from the BASHH website (see Resouces).

It is unfortunate that there is not a qualification in 'sexual health' which includes all facets of this subject. It is possible in time that this will be developed nationally and there are some local initiatives to do so such as the 'Postgraduate Award for Sexual Health in Primary Care' for GPs and practice nurses initially piloted in the West Midlands Deanery,[21] and now an accredited six-month modular course at Warwick University (see Resouces).

References

1. Department of Health. *The national strategy for sexual health and HIV.* London: Department of Health, 2001. www.dh.gov.uk/assetRoot/04/05/89/45/04058945.pdf (accessed 09/09/2004)

2. Royal College of General Practitioners and Brook. *Confidentiality and young people. Improving teenagers' uptake of sexual and other health advice.* London: Royal College of General Practitioners and Brook, 2000. [Available from the Department of Health. Email: DOH@prolog.uk.com, for free ref: 31451]

3. Matthews P, Fletcher J. Sexually transmitted infections in primary care: a need for education. *Br J Gen Prac* 2001; **51**: 52–56

4. British Association for Sexual Health and HIV. Sexually Transmitted Infections Foundation Course. Course Manual. London: British Association for Sexual Health and HIV, August 2003

5. Low N. Sexual health. In: Kai J (ed) *Ethnicity, health and primary care.* Oxford: Oxford University Press, 2003. pp. 161–72

6. Botting B, Dunnell K. Trends in fertility and contraception in the last quarter of the 20th century. *Population Trends* 2000; summer (**100**): 32–9

7. Cerazette New product review. www.ffprhc.org.uk

8. Collaborative study group on the desogestrel-containing progestogen-only pill. A double blind study comparing the contraceptive efficacy, acceptability and safety of two progestogen-only pills containing desogestrel 75 μg/day or levonorgestrel 30 μg/day. *Eur J Contracept Reprod Health Care* 1998; **3**: 169–78

9. Is Yasmin a 'truly different' pill? *Drug Ther Bull* 2002; **40(8)**: 57–9

10. Gallo M F, Grimes D A, Schulz K F. Skin patch and vaginal ring versus combined oral contracetives for contraception. In: *Cochrane Database of Systematic Reviews*. Oxford: 2003; 1

11. Johnson A M, Mercer C H, Erens B, *et al*. Sexual behaviour in Britain: partnerships, practices and HIV risk behaviours. *Lancet* 2001; **358**: 1835–42

12. Sexual Health in Britain: Recent changes in high-risk sexual behaviours and the epidemiology of sexually transmitted infections including HIV. London: HIV/STI Division. Health Protection Agency, 2002 www.hpa.org.uk/infections/topics_az/hiv_and_sti/publications/sexual_health.pdf (accessed 9/09/2004)

13. Department of Health. A pilot study of opportunistic screening for genital chlamydia trachomatis infection in England (1999–2000). Summary Report. www.dh.gov.uk/assetRoot/04/07/44/99/04074499.pdf (accessed 9/09/2004)

14. Fenton K A, Korovessis C, Johnson A M, McCadden A, McManus S, Wellings K, Mercer C H, Carder C, Copas A, Nanchahal K, Macdowall W, Ridgway G, Field J, Erens B. Sexual behaviour in Britain: reported sexually transmitted infections and prevalent genital chlamydia trachomatis infection. *Lancet* 2001; **358**: 1851–54

15. Sellors J W, Pickard L, Gafni A, *et al*. Effectiveness and efficiency of selective vs universal screening for chlamydial infection in sexually active young women. *Arch Intern Med* 1992; **152**: 1837–44

16. CASCADE Collaboration. Determinants of survival following HIV-1 seroconversion after the introduction of HAART. *Lancet* 2003; **362**: 1267–74

17. Department of Health. Prevalence of HIV and hepatitis infections in the UK. Annual report of the unlinked anonymous prevalence monitoring program. London: HMSO, December 2002. See: www.hpa.org.uk

18. Vanehegan G, Wedgewood A. Young peoples' understanding of safer sex and their attitude to referral for STI screening – two audits from London Brook Advisory Centres. *J Fam Plann Reprod Health Care* 1999; **25**: 22–4

19. Nazareth I, Boynton P, King M. Problems with sexual function in people attending London general practitioners: cross sectional study. *BMJ* 2003; **327**: 423–6

20. Mercer C H, Fenton K A, Johnson A M, Wellings K, Macdowall W, McManus S, Nanchahal K, Erens B. Sexual function problems and help seeking behaviour in Britain: national probability sample survey. *BMJ* 2003; **327**: 226–7

21. Smallcombe J. Improving GPs' skills and services in sexual health and HIV. *The New Generalist* 2003; **1(2)**: 45–6

Useful Resources

Useful web addresses

Faculty of Family Planning and Reproductive Health Care:
www.ffprhc.org.uk

British Association for Sexual Health and HIV (formally the Medical Society for the Study of Venereal Diseases and Association of Genitourinary Medicine):
www.BASHH.org

Postgraduate Award for Sexual Health in Primary Care:
www2.warwick.ac.uk/fac/med/healthcom/primary_care/courses_intro/courses/sexhealth/ (accessed 14/10/04)

CHAPTER 8

Diabetes Mellitus

A M Farooqi, L S Levene

▶ **KEY MESSAGES**

- The prevalence of Type 2 diabetes is increasing dramatically, with significant implications for primary care's workload.

- An oral glucose tolerance test (OGTT) is less likely to miss early Type 2 diabetes than a fasting blood glucose test, but further guidance is awaited about optimal population screening.

- Tight glycaemic control and aggressive reduction of cardiovascular risk are at the core of reducing morbidity and mortality in people with diabetes.

- Although newer oral hypoglycaemic drugs and insulin formulations may have the potential to improve glycaemic control in some patients, their precise role in diabetic care is subject to debate. The National Institute for Clinical Excellence (NICE) offers evidence-based guidance for practitioners on this. Good diet, increased physical activity and regular monitoring are still important in all people with diabetes.

- Optimal management of diabetic complications should follow evidence-based management pathways.

- Effective health education is important in prevention, in improving outcomes and in empowering patients to take a greater role in the management of their disease.

- The delivery of the standards outlined in the National Service Framework (NSF) for diabetes and of the quality indicators listed in new GMS contract will increase both the role and workload of primary care in diabetes care.

RECENT ADVANCES ▼

- The onset of Type 2 diabetes can be prevented or delayed in high-risk individuals by modification of lifestyle to improve adverse risk factors (weight loss, better diet, greater physical activity).

- Tight glycaemic control reduces micro- and macro-vascular complications in people with diabetes. New oral agents and insulin formulations may have a role in improving glycaemic control.

- Vigorous effective correction of adverse cardiovascular risk factors, such as raised blood pressure and dyslipidaemia, has been shown to reduce morbidity and mortality in people with diabetes.

- Health education has evolved from a didactic to a more patient-centred approach, using a variety of innovative techniques. However, further research is needed to evaluate effectiveness.

- The NSF for diabetes outlines the improvements in diabetic care that need to be achieved over the next decade, to be delivered both by primary and secondary care.

The management of diabetes mellitus has become increasingly important in primary care's workload and to government health policy. This is a brief overview of the many recent advances in knowledge, such as the UK Prospective Diabetes Study (UKPDS) and the MRC/BHF study, of the important statements of government policy (NSFs) and of the authoritative clinical guidelines published by NICE, SIGN and the ADA. This chapter focuses on the most important points for general practitioners involved in managing people with diabetes. A list of abbreviations and sources of further information can be found at the end of the chapter.

Epidemiology and diagnosis

We are currently witnessing a worldwide explosion in the prevalence of Type 2 diabetes, projected to rise to 300 million individuals by 2010.[1] This increase

is modelled from the observed increase worldwide in recent years and anticipated changes in risk factors such as ageing, obesity and lower activity levels.
Even though Western European Caucasians seem to have a comparatively low
genetic predisposition to developing Type 2 diabetes, the UK is likely to see a
50% increase in numbers of sufferers from an estimated 2 million (3.6% prevalence) in 2000 to 3 million (4.5% prevalence) in 2010. General practitioners
whose lists contain a high proportion of ethnic populations (e.g. Indo-Asians,
Afro-Caribbeans) will see a significantly greater increase in prevalence of diabetes in their practice populations. Such populations have a greater pre-dispo-
sition to Type 2 diabetes and this will find greater expression due to increased
obesity and lack of physical activity related to Western lifestyles.

The diagnosis of diabetes

Diagnosis is based upon whether the plasma glucose level is above an agreed
threshold (criteria). International consensus has been reached over the criteria
proposed by the ADA (see Table 8.1) in 1997; however, there has been a vigorous international debate over which diagnostic test to use for diagnosis. The
ADA has a strong preference for using fasting plasma glucose levels. However,
the Decode Study[2] in Europe demonstrated that a fasting glucose result, as
opposed to a two-hour post-load glucose level, would miss about one-third (33%)
of people with diabetes. Undertaking large numbers of OGTTs would have
major logistical and workload implications. A pragmatic approach for general
practice is to carry out an OGTT on those patients with an initial impaired
fasting glucose (6.1–6.9 mmol/l). This strategy would detect more than 80%
of undiagnosed people with diabetes.

Table 8.1 **Interpretation of blood glucose results**

	Fasting plasma glucose	2 hours post 75g glucose load
Normal glucose homeostasis	≤6.0 mmol/l	≤7.7 mmol/l
Impaired fasting glucose (IFG)	6.1–6.9 mmol/l	Not applicable
Impaired glucose tolerance (IGT)	Not applicable	7.8–11 mmol/l
Diabetes mellitus	≥7.0 mmol/l*	>11.1 mmol/l*/**

*On two occasions, or on a single occasion if symptoms (thrush, polyuria, weight loss) are present.
**Also random plasma glucose.

Screening for diabetes

On the face of it, Type 2 diabetes fulfils many of the criteria for screening. It is an important health problem that can be effectively treated and acceptable diagnostic tests are available. However, there are no current national recommendations for screening, due to a number of unanswered questions.

Who to screen?

There is no data on the cost-effectiveness of population screening or on the screening of high-risk groups. However, simulation modelling suggests high-risk screening may be more cost effective with 50% detection of all possible cases from 18% of the population.[3] Whilst national guidance is awaited it would seem sensible to screen high-risk cases (see Box 8.1).

How to screen?

Screening by random glucose has sensitivity of about 70% and specificity of 65–80% in a number of studies. Screening by glucosuria has a low sensitivity (as low as 16% in some studies) and the specificity of a positive test ranges from 11% to 37%. HbA$_1$c has poor sensitivity (about 60%) but with high specificity (97%).[4-5]

The most sensible current consensus is to use fasting glucose with an OGTT (still the gold standard for diagnosis) for those with impaired fasting glucose (IFG).

How often to screen?

There is no current recommendation or authoritative guidance on how often to screen even with high-risk groups.

Further authoritative guidance on screening for diabetes is awaited from the National Screening Committee (NSC), itself dependent on the results of current trials such as Diabetes Heart Disease and Stroke Screening Study (DHDS) and ADDITION, a randomised trial of the cost-effectiveness of screening and intensive multi-factorial intervention for Type 2 diabetes. These studies are expected to report their findings in the next two to three years.

The prevention of diabetes

There is increasing evidence that the early detection of pre-diabetic conditions (IFG and IGT) is important, because it is now known that such individuals are at increased risk of developing Type 2 diabetes and/or vascular disease, for which there are potentially effective interventions to prevent or delay onset.

Lifestyle modification, for example based upon reducing obesity (defined as a body mass index (BMI) greater than 30 kg / m²) and increasing physical activity, have been shown to delay the onset of Type 2 diabetes in higher risk individuals. Trials from the USA,[6] Finland[7] and China[8] have demonstrated that programmes aimed at bringing lifestyle changes (dietary change, weight reduction and increased physical activity) can reduce the progression of IGT to overt diabetes by 40–60%. The interventions involved intensive patient education and support. Less intensive advice is less successful.

Another approach to prevention may include the use of drugs, such as metformin[6] or inhibitors of the renin-angiotensin system,[9–10] which show some experimental promise as agents that can delay the onset of Type 2 diabetes.

The importance of early effective interventions to prevent diabetes are recognised in standard one (prevention) of the NSF. However, any system for providing education and support needs to be effective, sustainable and universally accessible. By these criteria, the United Kingdom has some way to go. The role of the NHS would need to be supported and complimented by government policy (e.g. taxation, advertising, school curriculum), and would require considerable resources if applied to large populations.

The metabolic syndrome

Metabolic syndrome is present when any three of the following occur in an individual: hypertension, central obesity, hyperglycaemia, dyslipidaemia and insulin resistance.[11] This syndrome is increasingly recognised as being important in people at risk of, or with, diabetes. Its presence indicates a high risk of developing cardiovascular disease and requires aggressive correction of the relevant risk factors. Metabolic syndrome is more common in Indo-Asians to the extent that a BMI greater than 23 in Indo-Asians, as compared to 25 in Caucasians, indicates increased risk.[12]

Box 8.1 **Major risk factors for Type 2 diabetes**[13]

Age >40 years
1st degree relative with Type 2 diabetes
BMI >30 Kg/m²
Non-white racial group
History of gestational diabetes, IGT or IFG

	Sensitivity	Specificity
Random bld gluc	70%	65-80%
Glucosuria	16%	11-37%
Hb A₁C	60%	97%

Blood glucose management

Optimal glycaemic control has been shown to reduce morbidity and mortality in people with diabetes.[14-15] To achieve and maintain good glycaemic control, the 'empowered and enabled' patient, acting upon the results of self-monitoring, needs to carefully balance lifestyle (diet, physical activity) and blood glucose-lowering medication.

Self-monitoring

This is essential for self-care and for optimal control. Urinalysis provides only an approximate and delayed estimation of blood glucose levels; therefore, it has a limited role, mainly in some stable Type 2 diabetics. Blood glucose monitoring (BGM) provides accurate information, enabling more precise glycaemic control. BGM is now recommended for all Type 1 and gestational diabetics, and for many people with Type 2 diabetes. The aim is for pre-meal/fasting blood glucose levels of 4–7 mmol/l. A wide range of monitors are available (not available on prescription at NHS expense), but each requires its own brand of test strip (which can be prescribed at NHS expense). Details are available in the current issue of Monthly Index of Medical Specialities (MIMS). Whichever method is used, it must be accompanied by suitable patient education to enable improved self management of glycaemia. Diabetes UK recently issued a position statement recommending that people with diabetes be given information, choice and support in self-monitoring, using either a blood or urine method that is most appropriate for them 'without restrictions on the type and numbers of testing strips'.[16] July 2003

Diet

Diabetes UK has recently issued a comprehensive list of consensus-based recommendations for people with diabetes.[17] Nutritional advice should try to achieve and maintain:

▶ the reduction of risk of microvascular disease by achieving near normal glycaemia without undue risk of hypoglycaemia

▶ the reduction of risk of macrovascular disease, including management of body weight, dyslipidaemia and hypertension.

The main differences from previous UK recommendations are:

▶ greater flexibility in proportions of energy derived from carbohydrate and monosaturated fats, the latter now promoted as the main source of dietary fat

▶ further liberalisation in the consumption of sucrose

▶ more active promotion of carbohydrate foods with a low glycaemic index

▶ greater emphasis on the benefits of regular exercise (see *p. 134*).

The latest recommendations for the composition of a suitable diet are summarised in Table 8.2.

The content and delivery of advice should respect patients' personal, religious and cultural circumstances; take into account willingness to change; and enable appropriate choices to be made – better compliance is more likely. Primary care professionals with appropriate knowledge and training should provide relevant advice. Referral to a qualified dietician is helpful, either where this level of knowledge is unavailable or in dealing with more complex issues.

Table 8.2 **Summary of recommendations for the composition of a diet for people with diabetes** [17]

Component	Comments
Protein	Not > 1 g per kg body weight (different for nephropathy and children)
Total fat	<35% of energy intake
Saturated + transunsaturated fat	<10% of energy intake
n-6 polyunsaturated fat	<10% of energy intake
n-3 polyunsaturated fat	Eat fish, especially oily fish 1–2 times weekly Fish oil supplements not recommended
cis- monounsaturated fat*	10–20%
Total carbohydrate*	45–60%
Sucrose	Up to 10% of daily energy, eaten within the context of a healthy diet Consider using non-nutritive sweeteners where appropriate if overweight and/or hypertriglyceridaemic
Fibre	No quantitative recommendation *Soluble fibre* has beneficial effects on glycaemic and lipid metabolism *'Insoluble' fibre* has no direct effects on glycaemic and lipid metabolism, but its high satiety content may help weight loss and is advantageous to gastrointestinal health

continued overleaf

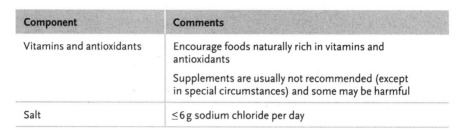

Component	Comments
Vitamins and antioxidants	Encourage foods naturally rich in vitamins and antioxidants
	Supplements are usually not recommended (except in special circumstances) and some may be harmful
Salt	≤6 g sodium chloride per day

*combined should total 60–70% of energy intake

Physical activity[18]

An appropriately increased level of physical activity improves insulin resistance and lipid profiles (reduced triglycerides and increased high-density lipoprotein (HDL) cholesterol); thus improving glycaemic control, reducing vascular risk and protecting against the development of Type 2 diabetes. Ideally, individuals should aim to undertake 30 minutes of moderately intense physical activity at least five days per week, although any increased physical activity in sedentary individuals is likely to be beneficial. Exercise programmes are now increasingly available and many accept referrals from primary care (called 'exercise on prescription'). Any programme must be tailored to the individual, and should take account of current health, aims and preferences. Any advice provided needs to pay attention to glycaemic levels, fluid balance and foot care. However, physical activity need not always involve a formal exercise regime. Regular walking and other home-based activities will increase strength, mobility and cardiovascular fitness.

Oral drug therapy

An overview

In people with Type 2 diabetes, there is a progressive deterioration of pancreatic beta cell function, combined with insulin resistance. Both mechanisms need to be tackled in order to achieve and maintain good glycaemic control. The main classes of medications act by improving either insulin secretion (secretagogues) or insulin action. NICE has published guidelines for the management of blood glucose,[19] supplemented by technology appraisals of some of the important newer drugs (see discussion of glitazones opposite). New classes of oral agents that improve either insulin secretion or action may become available in the future.

Drug therapy is likely to involve 'stepping up' oral therapy by increasing dosages and using combinations of different drug classes, with the introduction of insulin an eventual step for many patients. If a trial of improved diet either fails or is unsuitable to achieve normoglycaemia, then introduction of either metformin or a sulphonylurea is the recommended first line, followed by a combination of both (subject to contraindications and tolerance).

Drug details are available in chapter 6, section 1.2 of the latest edition of the British National Formulary.

Insulin secretagogues

The well-established sulphonylurea class is one of NICE's drug classes of choice. There are many sulphonylureas available. NICE recommends a generic preparation of a once-daily drug. The older long-acting preparations, gliben-clamide and chlorpropamide, are best avoided because of increased weight gain and a greater risk of hypoglycaemia.

Two agents (repaglinide and nateglinide) belonging to a new class, meglitinide analogues (or post-prandial glucose regulators), are now available in the UK. Due to their quicker onset and shorter duration of action, they may have a role in obese or fasting patients not ideally suited to sulphonylureas. The benefit that these agents may have in reducing long-term complications by specifically acting upon post-prandial hyperglycaemia is currently debatable.

Drugs that improve insulin action

The biguanide metformin is the first-line choice in obese Type 2 diabetics, and can be combined with insulin secretagogues, glitazones or insulin. A stepped approach to increasing dose reduces gastrointestinal side effects. Metformin reduces cardiovascular risk and, despite several contraindications, it is quite safe if used in accordance with recently published guidelines,[20] particularly if avoided in patients with raised serum creatinine (greater than $150\,\mu mol/l$), tissue hypoxia (such as myocardial infarction and sepsis), for three days after administration of contrast medium containing iodine (creatinine must return to normal), or two days before general anaesthesia.

Two agents in the glitazones drug class (rosiglitazone and pioglitazone) were launched in the UK in 2000. They do not increase secretion of insulin, but promote peripheral glucose utilisation (reducing insulin resistance). Although their current UK licence is for both monotherapy and in combination with either metformin or sulphonylureas (but not in triple therapy or with meglitinide analogues or insulin), NICE currently only recommends their use in those unable to take metformin and a sulphonylurea in combination because of lack of tolerance or a contraindication to one of these drugs.[21] When prescribing glitazones, liver function needs to be monitored.

Insulin

Overview

There is a bewildering array of insulin preparations available. Animal-based insulins are being used progressively less and developments are based upon human-sequence insulins. The main recent advances have been:

▶ new categories of insulin: the rapid-acting and prolonged-acting insulins

▶ new delivery systems: pens, infusion devices

▶ new regimens: in particular, basal–bolus.

However, the most important developments in primary care are the increased readiness and role of the primary health care team to convert Type 2 patients onto insulin.

Preparations

Two new rapid-acting preparations, lispro and aspart, are now available. Their onset is within five to ten minutes, with a peak of action at one hour, and duration of action of three to five hours.

The prolonged-acting insulin glargine has a duration of action of 24 hours and a prolonged plateau of concentration rather than a peak, with an apparently reduced risk of hypoglycaemia when compared to older intermediate- or prolonged-acting insulins. A recent NICE technology appraisal[22] recommends the use of glargine as a treatment option in patients with Type 1 diabetes and in some patients with Type 2 diabetes.

Delivery systems

In addition to the new pens and infusion devices now available, alternative methods of insulin delivery are being explored for future use. These include different routes of administration (via nasal mucous membranes or inhalers). Although some may become available within the next two to three years, inflexible dosage and reduced bio-availability may limit their usefulness.

Regimens

In addition to the well-established twice daily regimen, two newer regimens are being used more frequently.

The first, basal–bolus, makes use of the above-mentioned rapid- and prolonged-acting insulins and is becoming increasingly popular. Rapid-acting insulin is administered with each meal, with a single evening dose of prolonged-acting insulin acting as the basal insulin. This regimen requires more frequent

BGM, but allows much greater flexibility.

Another regimen is the combination of a single injection of prolonged-acting insulin (as before) with an oral agent, such as metformin. This may be suitable for elderly and other groups of people with diabetes.

Other and future developments

In the UK about 50 Type 1 patients per year receive pancreatic transplants, often combined with renal transplants for those in renal failure. However, these patients must take life-long anti-rejection medication. Other Type 1 patients are being given islet cell transplants in specialist centres.

These techniques could eventually become redundant if a promising treatment, announced by US researchers in November 2003, involving the administration of a protein (TNF-alpha) to reverse auto-immune destruction of islet cells is found to work in humans, as well as in mice.

Cardiovascular risk and diabetes

Cardiovascular disease (CVD) is a very significant cause of morbidity and mortality in people with diabetes, especially Type 2, whose overall risk is of an equivalent magnitude to non-diabetics with a history of established coronary heart disease (CHD).[23] The traditional risk factors for cardiovascular disease have been shown to be of special importance for people with diabetes, who have at least double the risk of developing it compared to non-diabetics.[24] Therefore, the effective correction of these risk factors is crucial in managing diabetes, a disease whose adverse impact is predominately vascular.

Evaluating cardiovascular risk

The overall risk usually arises from the combined impact of multiple cardiovascular risk factors. Several calculators, based upon data from Framingham (with few diabetics and non-whites), are readily available to calculate the risk of cardiovascular outcomes over a ten-year period for given combinations of clinical and demographic variables and to assess the impact of relevant interventions.[25] However, all of these calculators suffer from two main drawbacks:

1. they risk under-estimation in certain ethnic groups (Indo-Asians and Afro-Caribbeans) and in individuals with a positive family history of CVD

2. they are less helpful in younger diabetics whose 'impending' event is likely to occur more than ten years into the future, but who are, nonetheless, at greater risk than the non-diabetic population over their lifetime.

The UKPDS has been looking to develop diabetes-specific models based upon its data; it has already produced one for evaluating stroke risk.[26]

Targets

Reducing vascular risk is one of the key aims of diabetic management, but the interventions are to alter risk factors, which are surrogate, not real disease, endpoints. The targets set out by the Diabetes NSF and NICE may not always be achievable, a point recognised by the less stringent targets attracting maximum quality points in the new GMS contract. Targets should be set at a realistic and achievable level for the individual patient.[27] All treatable risk factors should be addressed in patients identified as high risk,[28] with any improvement likely to be of benefit.[29]

Blood pressure

The current consensus for target blood pressure for people with diabetes is 140/80, with the lower 130/75 for those with evidence of renal disease (e.g. microalbuminuria).

Such targets are based upon evidence from studies such as UKPDS 36,[30] which demonstrated significant reduction in cardiovascular complications from a 10 mmHg reduction in systolic blood pressure and the Hypertension Optimal Treatment (HOT)[31] study which showed a 50% reduction in major cardiovascular risk events comparing 80 mmHg to 90 mmHg diastolic blood pressure.

To achieve the required target levels for blood pressure is difficult and often requires several anti-hypertensive agents (30% of the 'tight control' group in UKPDS required three or more drugs). The latest British Hypertension Society Guidelines offer a practical guide for prescribing combinations of agents.[51]

In view of the strong link between microvascular renal damage and hypertension, blockade of the renin-angiotensin system with ACE inhibitors or angiotensin receptor-blocking agents are the drugs of choice. The benefits of these drugs[32-3] may be related to anti-hypertensive and other effects, such as endothelial protection. The relative merits and risks of other drug classes continue to be vigorously debated, but ultimately the actual level of blood pressure achieved should be of prime importance.

Dyslipidaemia

The 4S,[34] CARE[35] and LIPID[36] studies have all shown the benefits of lipid lowering of cardiovascular risk in secondary prevention. Although the percentage of diabetics in these studies was not high, benefits were equivalent to, or greater than, the non-diabetic cohort.

The current National Clinical Guidelines recommend the following targets for lipids: [37]

1. total cholesterol less than 5.0 mmol/l, or low-density lipoprotein cholesterol (LDL-C) less than 3.0 mmol/l

2. triglycerides less than 2.3 mmol/l.

More recently, the landmark MRC/BHS study[29] showed a significant reduction in cardiovascular complications for people with diabetes, with and without prior CHD, treated with high-dose simvastatin, although detailed breakdown of the data is still awaited. The Collaborative Atorvastatin Diabetes Study (CARDS) (reported at the American Diabetes Association (2004) conference) was terminated early as it showed a significant reduction in major cardiovascular events in diabetics treated with 10 mg atorvastatin – regardless of whether their initial cholesterol level is raised or not. Any improvement in dyslipidaemia therefore appears to be beneficial and statins remain the treatment of choice. Further primary prevention studies with both statins and fibrates are ongoing. The eventual recommendation that all people with diabetes should be treated with lipid-lowering agents is a distinct, if expensive, possibility.

The first of a new generation of statins, rosuvastatin, which is claimed to be more potent, was recently launched in the UK but has been reported recently to be associated with myopathy at higher doses. Other classes are cholesterol absorption inhibitors (e.g. ezetimibe) and extended-release nicotinic acid (e.g. sustained-release niacin). Drugs that act in novel ways are currently still in the developmental stages. It is likely that many of these newer agents will require further trials or a technology appraisal by NICE to determine their precise role in cholesterol management.

Obesity

In people with Type 2 diabetes, obesity (as discussed in the section above on prevention), especially truncal, results in increased insulin resistance and, thus, increased cardiovascular risk. The anti-obesity agents, orlistat and sibutramine, have a role in weight loss, but should be prescribed in combination with education and support for lifestyle modification as the main approach. Both drugs are expensive and have been appraised by NICE.[38-9]

Aspirin

Aspirin at a daily dose of 75–150 mg should be used as secondary prevention for cardiovascular disease in people with diabetes unless contraindicated.

Recently it has been suggested that, for primary prevention, aspirin is safe for those with a ten-year risk of cardiovascular disease greater than 15%, but unsafe at a risk at or less than 5%. On this basis, most diabetics over the age of 30 would qualify for aspirin prophylaxis based on the use of a cardiovascular risk prediction chart. In order to minimise the risk of a cerebrovascular event, it is recommended that aspirin is commenced only when blood pressure is controlled.

Diabetic complications

Three of the Diabetes NSF's 13 standards relate to the early detection and optimal management of long-term complications. Cardiovascular disease is discussed elsewhere. The main target organs remaining to be discussed here are eyes, kidneys, feet and neuropathy.

Eyes

The main developments relevant to primary care are related to screening:

▶ increased use of the 'gold-standard' mydriatic retinal photography, requiring organisation and collaboration across trusts [40]

▶ the Diabetes NSF's stated aim of offering retinal screening to 80% of all diabetics by March 2006, rising to 100% by the end of 2007. [41]

The management pathways following assessment are set out in Table 8.3.

Table 8.3 **Management pathways following eye assessment** [40]

Care Pathway	Visual Acuity	Lens	Retina	Other Factors
Routine review (1 year)	Unchanged	Clear OR Minimal opacities	No changes OR Minimal/low risk background	
Early review (3 to 6 months)			New or worsening lesions OR Exudates >1 dd* from fovea	Renal disease OR Rapid improvement of blood glucose

Care Pathway	Visual Acuity	Lens	Retina	Other Factors
Routine referral to ophthalmologist		Cataracts interfering with vision	View is obscured (but beware of possibility of significant retinopathy)	
Rapid referral (within 4 weeks) to ophthalmologist	Unexplained drop		Hard exudates <1 dd from fovea OR Macular oedema OR Unexplained findings OR Pre-proliferative retinopathy OR More advanced (severe) retinopathy	
Urgent referral (within 1 week) to ophthalmologist			New vessels	Pre-retinal and/or vitreous haemorrhage OR Rubeosis iridis
Emergency referral (same day) to ophthalmologist	Sudden loss		Retinal detachment	

*dd = disc diameter

Kidneys[42]

The presence of albumin in urine in people with diabetes may indicate early nephropathy and also acts as a marker for diabetic retinal disease and increased cardiovascular risk. Annual screening for microalbuminuria (urinary albumin excretion between 30 and 300 mg / day, undetectable by standard test strips) in both Type 1 and 2 diabetics is now being recommended. The preferred and practical method is to estimate the albumin : creatinine ratio on an early morning sample, with ratios equal to or greater than 2.5 mg / mmol in males and 3.5 mg / mmol in females taken to indicate microalbuminuria. Positive tests need repeating within a month for confirmation. The community prevalence of microalbuminuria in diabetics is likely to be in the region of 20%.[43]

If albuminuria is found, then the following may prevent or delay deterioration in renal function:

- ▶ tight blood pressure control (< 135 / 75) with drugs that inhibit the rennin-angiotensin system (ACE or ARA) as the preferred first line

- ▶ optimal glycaemic control

- ▶ smoking cessation

- ▶ correction of abnormal lipid profile.

Referral to a nephrologist is advised if renal impairment develops (raised serum creatinine greater than 150 mmol / l).

Feet

The main role for primary care is the early detection of high-risk individuals (with neuropathy and/or vascular disease) and of those with complications, such as foot ulcers or gangrene, followed by prompt optimal management (summarised in Table 8.4). Current guidance is based upon RCGP guidelines published in 2000,[44] due to be updated shortly by NICE.

Table 8.4 **Summary of assessment and indicated management pathways for diabetic feet**[45]

Level of risk	Assessment findings	Interventions
Low risk	Normal sensation AND ▶ Good pulses ▶ No previous ulcer ▶ No foot deformity ▶ Normal vision	▶ No specific podiatrist input ▶ Trained patient undertakes own nail care ▶ Review in 12 months
Moderate risk	▶ Loss of sensation OR ▶ Absent pulses (or previous vascular surgery) OR ▶ Significant visual impairment OR ▶ Physical disability (e.g. cerebrovascular accident (CVA), gross obesity)	▶ Regular podiatry (at 4–12 week intervals) ▶ Interim review at 2–6 months

Level of risk	Assessment findings	Interventions
High risk	▶ Previous ulcer due to neuropathy/ ischaemia OR ▶ Absent pulses and neuropathy OR ▶ Callus with risk factor (neuropathy, absent pulse, foot deformity) OR ▶ Previous amputation	▶ Refer to podiatrist with special interest in diabetes OR ▶ Refer to local hospital-based specialist diabetes team
Active foot disease	▶ Active foot ulceration OR ▶ Painful neuropathy difficult to control	Contact local hospital-based specialist diabetes team for urgent appointment
Emergency foot problem	▶ Critical ischaemia, as characterised by: ▷ Rest or night pain OR ▷ Pale/mottled foot OR ▷ Dependent rubor OR ▷ Ischaemic ulceration OR ▷ Gangrene ▶ Severe infection, as characterised by: ▷ Abscess OR ▷ Cellulitis	Emergency referral to hospital

Neuropathy

Diabetic neuropathy is common. Pain management has been improved by the use of newer agents such as gabapentin, as opposed to conventional painkillers. The management of erectile dysfunction has been transformed by the introduction of oral sildenafil in 1999. Other similar agents include tadalafil and vardenafil.

Health education

Effective health education is now recognised to be much more than a didactic transfer of knowledge from professional to patient; rather, it is centred on producing appropriate behaviour change in the patient's lifestyle. The experiences of other health care professionals, such as psychologists and dieticians, have demonstrated the benefits of incorporating various techniques and concepts within the consultation and of the imaginative use of group work. The use of effective consultation techniques, an awareness of the trans-theoretical model [46] of change, together with the application of cognitive behaviour therapy and

Cycle delany
1992

motivational interviewing techniques are within the capabilities of most primary health care professionals. Although the evidence supporting the use of these various techniques remains largely unproven in diabetic health education, such a patient-centred approach aims to encourage and enable patients to take a more active role in their care, which is at the heart of NSF Standard 3, *Empowering people with diabetes.*

In the UK two health education programmes are worth mentioning:

1. The Dose Adjustment Programme for Normal Eating (DAFNE) for patients on insulin is an intensive group education programme designed to 'empower' patients to adjust insulin dosages based upon blood glucose levels.[47]

2. The Diabetes Education for Self-Management: Ongoing and Newly Diagnosed (DESMOND) is a national initiative, developing and evaluating group self-management education programmes for people with type 2 diabetes. This is currently for those who are newly diagnosed, but the project seeks to develop an ongoing structured education programme that can form the basis of systematic continuous care for people with diabetes. This programme is at the pilot stage in 14 UK centres and is being co-ordinated by the Diabetes Centre, University Hospitals of Leicester.

Organisation of diabetes care in the NHS

Diabetes is now an important part of government health policy. The recent publication of the NSF for Diabetes (Standards in 2001, Delivery Strategy in 2002); NICE guidelines – based on clinical and cost-effectiveness based evidence; and the quality and outcomes indicators in the new GMS contract, provide the framework for delivering high-quality care to people with diabetes throughout the NHS, including an important role for primary care.

The key elements and inter-relationship of these publications are summarised in Table 8.5 opposite. Relevant NICE guidance, which has a direct impact on general practitioners, is indicated in the middle column.

Table 8.5 **How NSF standards link to NICE guidance and the new GMS contract**

NSF Standards[48]	NICE Guidance[49]	GMS 2 contract[50]
Standard 1 The NHS will develop, implement and monitor strategies to reduce the risk of developing Type 2 diabetes in the population as a whole and to reduce the inequalities in the risk of developing Type 2 diabetes	Orlistat for the treatment of obesity in adults (March 2001) Sibutramine for obesity in adults (October 2001)	Quality outcomes framework
Standard 2 The NHS will develop, implement and monitor strategies to identify people who do not know they have diabetes	No NICE guidelines	The practice can produce a register of all patients with diabetes mellitus
Standard 3 All children, young people, and adults with diabetes will receive a service which encourages partnership in decision making, supports them in managing their diabetes and helps them to adopt and maintain a healthy lifestyle. This will be reflected in an agreed and shared care plan in an appropriate format and language. Where appropriate, parents and carers should be fully engaged in this process	Patient education models for diabetes (April 2003)	
Standard 4 All adults with diabetes will receive high-quality care throughout their lifetime, including support to optimise the control of their blood glucose, blood pressure and other risk factors for developing the complications of diabetes	Pioglitazone for Type 2 diabetes (March 2001) Rosiglitazone for Type 2 diabetes (August 2000) Insulin analogues for the treatment of diabetes – insulin glargine (December 2002) Management of Type 2 diabetes – blood glucose (September 2002)	The percentage of patients with diabetes whose notes record BMI in the previous 15 months The percentage of patients with diabetes in whom there is a record of smoking status in the previous 15 months, except those who have never smoked where smoking status should be recorded once

continued overleaf

NSF Standards[48]	NICE Guidance[49]	GMS 2 contract[50]
Standard 4 *continued*	Glitazones for the treatment of Type 2 diabetes (August 2003)	The percentage of patients with diabetes, who smoke and whose notes contain a record that smoking cessation advice or referral to a specialist service, where available, has been offered in the last 15 months
		The percentage of diabetic patients who have a record of HbA1c or equivalent in the previous 15 months
		The percentage of patients with diabetes in whom the last HbA1c is 7.4 or less (or equivalent test/reference range depending on local laboratory) in last 15 months
		The percentage of patients with diabetes in whom the last HbA1c is 10 or less (or equivalent test/reference range depending on local laboratory) in last 15 months
		The percentage of patients with diabetes who have had influenza immunisation in the preceding 1 September to 31 March
Standard 6 All young people with diabetes will experience a smooth transition of care from paediatric diabetes services to adult diabetes services, whether hospital or community-based, either directly or via a young people's clinic. The transition will be organised in partnership with each individual and at an age appropriate to and agreed with them	No NICE guidance	

NSF Standards[48]	NICE Guidance[49]	GMS 2 contract[50]
Standard 7 The NHS will develop, implement and monitor agreed protocols for rapid and effective treatment of diabetic emergencies by appropriately trained health care professionals. Protocols will include the management of acute complications and procedures to minimise the risk of recurrence	No NICE guidance	
Standard 8 All children, young people and adults with diabetes admitted to hospital, for whatever reason, will receive effective care of their diabetes. Wherever possible, they will continue to be involved in decisions concerning the management of their diabetes	No NICE guidance	
Standard 9 The NHS will develop, implement and monitor policies that seek to empower and support women with pre-existing diabetes and those who develop diabetes during pregnancy to optimise the outcomes of their pregnancy	Antenatal care; routine care of healthy pregnant women (October 2003)	
Standard 10 All young people and adults with diabetes will receive regular surveillance for the long-term complications of diabetes	Management of Type 2 diabetes; retinopathy- early management and screening (February 2002) Renal disease – prevention and management (February 2002)	The percentage of patients with diabetes who have a record of retinal screening in the previous 15 months The percentage of patients with diabetes with a record of the presence or absence of peripheral pulses, in the previous 15 months The percentage of patients with diabetes with a record of neuropathy testing in the previous 15 months

continued overleaf

NSF Standards[48]	NICE Guidance[49]	GMS 2 contract[50]
Standard 10 *continued*		The percentage of patients with diabetes who have a record of the blood pressure in the last 15 months
		The percentage of patients with diabetes in whom the blood pressure is 145 / 85 or less
		The percentage of patients with diabetes who have a record of microalbuminuria testing in the previous 15 months (exception reporting for patients with Proteinuria)
		The percentage of patients with diabetes who have a record of serum creatinine testing in the previous 15 months
		The percentage of patients with diabetes with Proteinuria or microalbuminuria who are treated with ACE inhibitors (or A2 antagonists)
		The percentage of patients with diabetes who have a record of total cholesterol in the previous 15 months
		The percentage of patients with diabetes whose last measured total cholesterol within the previous 15 months is 5 mmol / or less
Standard 12 All people with diabetes requiring multi-agency support will receive integrated health and social care	No NICE guidance	

References

1. Amos A F, McCarty D J and Zimmet P. The rising global burden of diabetes and its complications: estimates and projections to the year 2010. *Diabet Med* 1997; **14**: S7–S85.

2. DECODE Study. Is fasting glucose sufficient to define diabetes: Epidemiological data from 20 European studies. *Diabetologia* 1999; **42**: 647–54

3. Hofer T P, Vijan S and Hayward R A. Estimating the microvascular benefits of screening for type 2 diabetes. *Int J Technol Assess Health Care* 2000; **16**: 822–33

4. Rolifling C C, White R R, Wiedmeyer H, *et al*. Use of glycated haemoglobin (HbA1c) is more sensitive than fasting blood glucose as a screening test for diabetes. *Diabetes Care* 2000; **23**: 187–91

5. Davidson M B, Schriger D L, Peters A L and Lorder B. Relationship between fasting plasma glucose and glycated haemoglobin: potential for false positive diagnosis of Type 2 diabetes using new diagnostic criteria. *JAMA* 1999; **281(13)**: 1203–210

6. Knowler W C, Barrett-Connor E, Fowler S E, *et al*. for the Diabetes Prevention Programme Research Group. Reduction in the incidence of Type 2 diabetes with lifestyle intervention or metformin. *N Engl J Med* 2002; **346**: 393–403

7. Tuomilehro, Lidstrom J, Erikson J G, *et al*. Prevention of Type 2 diabetes mellitus by changes in lifestyle amongst subjects with impaired glucose tolerance. *N Engl J Med* 2001; **333**: 1343–50

8. Pan X, Li G, Hu Y, *et al*. Effects of diet and exercise in preventing NIDDM in people with impaired glucose tolerance. The Da Qing IGT and Diabetes Study. *Diabetes Care* 1997; **20**: 537–544

9. Dählof B, Devereux R B, Kjeldsen S E, *et al*. for the LIFE study group. Cardiovascular morbidity and mortality in the Losartan Intervention For Endpoint reduction in hypertension study (LIFE): a randomised trial against atenolol. *Lancet* 2002; **359**: 995–1003

10. Yusuf S, Gerstein H, Hoogwerf B, *et al*. (for the HOPE Study Investigators). Ramipril and the development of diabetes. *JAMA* 2001; **286**: 1882–5

11. Reavon G M. The role of insulin resistance and disease. *Diabetes* 1988; **37**: 1595–607

12. Hanif M W, *et al*. Obesity is highly prevalent in Indo-Asians with metabolic syndrome. *Diabetes* 2002; **19(S2)**: 33

13. Wareham N J, Griffin S J. Should we screen for Type 2 diabetes. Evaluation against National Screening Committee criteria. *BMJ* 2001; **322**: 986–9

14. The Diabetes Control and Complications Trial Research Group. The effect of intensive treatment of diabetes on the development and progression of long-term complications in insulin-dependent diabetes mellitus. *N Engl J Med* 1993; **329**: 977–86

15. Stratton I M, Adler A I, Neil H A W, *et al*. Association of glycaemia with macrovascular and microvascular complications of Type 2 diabetes (UKPDS 35): prospective observational study. *BMJ* 2000; **321**: 405–12

16. Diabetes UK Position Statement. Home monitoring of blood glucose levels. July 2003. See: www.diabetes.org.uk/infocentre/state/monitoring.htm (accessed 10/09/2004)

17. Connor H, Annan F, Bunn E, *et al*. for the Nutritional Subcommittee of the Diabetes Care Advisory Committee of Diabetes UK. The implementation of nutritional advice for people with diabetes. *Diabet Med* 2003; **20**: 786–807

18. Diabetes UK Care recommendation. Physical activity and diabetes. March 2003. See: www.diabetes.org.uk

19. NICE Guideline Development Group and Recommendations Panel. Inherited Clinical Guideline G. Management of Type 2 diabetes: Management of blood glucose. London: National Institute for Clinical Excellence, September 2002. See: www.nice.org.uk

20. Jones G C, Macklin J P, Alexander W D. Contraindications to the use of metformin (Editorial). *BMJ* 2003; **326**: 4–5

21. NICE Appraisal Committee. Technology Appraisal Guidance No. 63: Guidance on the use of glitazones for the treatment of Type 2 diabetes. London: National Institute for Clinical Excellence, August 2003. See: www.nice.org.uk

22 NICE Appraisal Committee. Technology Appraisal Guidance No. 53. Guidance on the use of long-acting insulin analogues for the treatment of diabetes – insulin glargine. London: National Institute for Clinical Excellence, December 2002. See: www.nice.org.uk

23. Haffner S M. Coronary heart disease in patients with diabetes. *N Engl J Med* 2000; **342(14)**: 989–97

24. Stamler J, Vaccaro O, Neaton J D, *et al.* Diabetes, other risk factors, and 12-yr cardiovascular mortality for men screened in the Multiple Risk Factor Intervention Trial. *Diabetes Care* 1993; **16(2)**: 434–44

25. British Hypertension Society. See: www.hyp.ac.uk/bhs/Cardiovascular_Risk_Charts_and_ Calculators.htm (accessed 10/09/2004)

26. Kothari V, Stevens R J, Adler A I, *et al.* Risk of Stroke in Type 2 Diabetes Estimated by the UK Prospective Diabetes Study Risk Engine (UKPDS 60). *Stroke* 2002; **33**: 1776–81

27. Winocour P H. Effective diabetes care: a need for realistic targets. *BMJ* 2002; **324**: 1577–80

28. Law M R, Wald N J. Risk factor thresholds: their existence under scrutiny. *BMJ* 2002; **324**: 1370–6

29. Collins R, Armitage J, Parish S, *et al.* for the Heart Protection Study Collaborative Group. MRC/BHF Heart Protection Study of cholesterol lowering with simvastatin in 20,536 high-risk individuals: a randomised placebo-controlled trial. *Lancet* 2002; **360(9326)**: 7–22

30. Adler A I, Stratton I M, Neil H A W, *et al.* Association of systolic blood pressure with macrovascular and microvascular complications of type 2 diabetes (UKPDS 36): prospective observational study. *BMJ* 2000; **321**: 412–19

31. Hannsen C, Zanchetti A, Carruthers S G, *et al.* Effects of blood pressure lowering and low dose aspirin in hypertension: principal results of the Hypertension Optimal Treatment (HOT) randomised trial. *Lancet* 1998; **351**: 1755–62

32. The Heart Outcomes Prevention Evaluation Study Investigators. Effects of an angiotensin-converting-enzyme inhibitor, ramipril, on death from cardiovascular causes, myocardial infarction, and stroke in high-risk patients. *N Engl J Med* 2000; **342**: 145–53

33. Fox K M; EURopean trial on reduction of cardiac events with Perindopril in stable coronary artery disease Investigators. Efficacy of perindopril in reduction of cardiovascular events among patients with stable coronary artery disease: randomised, double-blind, placebo-controlled, multicentre trial (the EUROPA study). *Lancet* 2003; **362(9386)**: 782–8

34. Scandinavian Simvastatin Survival Study. Randomised trial of cholesterol lowering in 4444 patients with coronary heart disease: the Scandinavian Simvastatin Survival Study. *Lancet* 1994; **344**: 1383–9

35. Goldberg R B, Mellies M J, Sacks F M, *et al.* Cardiovascular events and their reduction with pravastatin in diabetic and glucose-intolerant myocardial infarction survivors with average cholesterol levels: subgroup analyses in the cholesterol and recurrent events (CARE) trial. The Care Investigators. *Circulation* 1998; **98**: 2513–9

36. Long-Term Intervention with Pravastatin in Ischaemic Disease (LIPID) Study Group. Prevention of cardiovascular events and death with pravastatin in patients with coronary heart disease and a broad range of initial cholesterol levels. *N Engl J Med* 1998; **339**: 1349–57

37. McIntosh A, Hutchinson A, Feder G, *et al. Clinical guidelines and evidence review for Type 2 diabetes. Lipids management.* Sheffield: ScHARR, University of Sheffield, 2002. See: http://shef.ac.uk/guidelines

38. NICE Appraisal Committee. *Technology Appraisal Guidance No. 22: Guidance on the use of orlistat for the treatment of obesity in adults.* London: National Institute for Clinical Excellence, March 2001. See www.nice.org.uk

39. NICE Appraisal Committee. *Technology Appraisal Guidance No. 31: Guidance on the use of sibutramine for the treatment of obesity in adults.* London: National Institute for Clinical Excellence, October 2001. See: www.nice.org.uk

40. NICE Guideline Development Group and Recommendations Panel. *Inherited Clinical Guideline E. Management of Type 2 diabetes: Retinopathy – screening and early management.* London: National Institute for Clinical Excellence, February 2002. See: www.nice.org.uk

41. Department of Health. *National Service Framework for Diabetes: Delivery Strategy.* London: HMSO, December 2002

42. NICE Guideline Development Group and Recommendations Panel. *Inherited Clinical Guideline F. Management of Type 2 diabetes: Renal disease – prevention – and early management.* London: National Institute for Clinical Excellence, February 2002. See: www.nice.org.uk

43. Levene L S, McNally P G, Fraser R C, *et al.* What characteristics are associated with screening positive for microalbuminuria in patients with diabetes in the community? Abstract presented to Diabetes UK 2002 professional conference, accepted for publication in *Practical Diabetes International*

44. Hutchinson A, McIntosh A, Feder G, *et al. Clinical guidelines for Type 2 diabetes: prevention and management of foot problems.* London: Royal College of General Practitioners, 2000

45. Adapted from the Tayside foot risk assessment protocol quoted in: *Scottish Intercollegiate Guidelines Network. Management of Diabetes: A national clinical guideline (number 55).* Edinburgh: SIGN Executive, Royal College of Physicians, November 2001. See: www.sign.ac.uk

46. Prochaska J O, DiClemente C C. Stages of change in the modification of problem behaviors. *Prog Behav Modif* 1992; **28**: 183–218

47. DAFNE Study Group. Training in flexible, intensive insulin management to enable dietary freedom in people with type 1 diabetes: dose adjustment for normal eating (DAFNE) randomised controlled trial. *BMJ* 2002; **325**: 746–9

48. Department of Health. *National Service Framework for Diabetes: Standards.* London: HMSO, 2001

49. NICE. *Compilation: Summary of Guidance issued in England and Wales.* Issue 7. London: National Institute for Clinical Excellence, 2003

50. General Practice Committee. *The New GP Contract.* London: GPC, 2003

51. Williams B, Poulter N R, Brown M J, *et al.* British Hypertension Society. Guidelines for hypertension management 2004. (BHS-IV): Summary. *BMJ* 2004; **328**: 634–40

List of abbreviations

4S • Scandinavian Simvastatin Survival Study

ADA • American Diabetes Association

ADDITION • Anglo-Danish-Dutch Study of Intensive Treatment in People With Screen Detected Diabetes in Primary Care

BHF • British Heart Foundation

BMI • body mass index

CARDS • Collaborative Atorvastatin Diabetes Study

CARE • Cholesterol And Recurrent Events trial

CHD • coronary heart disease

CVA • cerebrovascular accident

DAFNE • dose adjustment for normal eating randomised controlled trial

DCCT • Diabetes Control and Complications Trial

DECODE • Diabetes Epidemiology: Collaborative Analysis of Diagnostic Criteria in Europe

DESMOND • Diabetes Education for Self-Management: Ongoing and Newly Diagnosed

DHDS • Diabetes Heart Disease and Stroke Screening Study

EUROPA • EURopean trial On reduction of cardiac events with Perindopril in stable coronary Artery disease

GMS • General Medical Services

HbA1c • Haemoglobin A1c (glycosylated haemoglobin)

HOPE • Heart Outcomes Prevention Evaluation Study

HOT • Hypertension Optimal Treatment

IFG • impaired fasting glucose

IGT • impaired glucose tolerance

LIFE • Losartan Intervention For Endpoint reduction in hypertension study

LIPID • Long-Term Intervention with Pravastatin in Ischaemic Disease Study

MRC • Medical Research Council

NICE • National Institute for Clinical Excellence

NSF • National Service Framework

OGTT • oral glucose tolerance test

PMS • Personal Medical Services

SIGN • Scottish Intercollegiate Guidelines Network

UKPDS • United Kingdom Prospective Diabetes Study

Further information sources

In a rapidly changing field, keeping up-to-date is likely to involve regular perusal of suitable internet sites and journals. The authors recommend the following as starting points for those wishing to keep abreast of developments in diabetes:

Electronic

1. National Electronic Library of Health (NeLH) is available free to NHS staff via the NHSNet online: www.nelh.nhs.uk/. In addition to having excellent links to NSFs, NICE, PubMed and a host of 'goodies', those with a personal ATHENS (Access To Higher Education via NISS authentication System, obtainable from the local postgraduate medical library) username and password, will be able to access remotely many electronic resources, such as the Cochrane Library.

2. Diabetes UK, formerly the British Diabetic Association, caters not only for health care professionals, but also for patients and other interested lay people, at 10 Parkway, London NW1 7AA, telephone (020) 7424 1000 (GPs and practice nurses can join the Primary Care section). Available at: www.diabetes.org.uk. Diabetes UK also publishes various papers and journals, available to its members.

3. The American Diabetes Association (ADA) publishes comprehensive and referenced clinical practice recommendations that are updated annually, available at: www.diabetes.org.

Journals

1. There are a number of free journals that focus on diabetes and cardiovascular disease, which often have useful articles aimed at the generalist, such as *Practical Diabetes International*, which is published every two months and is excellent. PMH Publications, PO BOX 100, Chichester, West Sussex, PO18 8HD, mail it free on request to health care professionals.

2. Important research and reviews about diabetes may be published in eminent peer-reviewed journals with wide circulation, such as the *British Medical Journal*, the *Lancet*, or *The New England Journal of Medicine*, or those with specialist interest, such as *Diabetes Care*, *Diabetic Medicine*, or *Diabetologia*. These are either available on subscription or are held in many hospital postgraduate libraries.

Books

1. Levene LS. *Management of Type 2 Diabetes Mellitus in Primary Care: A Practical Guide.* Edinburgh: Butterworth Heinemann, 2003

2. Krentz AJ, Bailey CJ. *Type 2 Diabetes in Practice.* London: Royal Society of Medicine Press, 2001

CHAPTER 9

Cardiology

Tom Fahey, Knut Schroeder

▶ KEY MESSAGES
- Hormone replacement therapy (HRT) should no longer be used for the prevention of cardiovascular disease.
- Cardiovascular risk estimation should always be the starting point for primary prevention of cardiovascular disease.
- Shared decision-making is important in the management of cardiovascular disease.
- Exercise-based cardiac rehabilitation can reduce cardiac death.

RECENT ADVANCES ▼
- Ambulatory blood pressure monitoring is better at predicting cardiovascular outcomes than conventional blood pressure measurements.
- Clopidogrel is an effective alternative to aspirin for preventing ischaemic events in people with stable cerebrovascular, cardiovascular and peripheral vascular disease.
- Direct thrombin inhibitors appear to be equivalent to warfarin in terms of effectiveness.
- A number of electronic devices are now available to treat atrial fibrillation.
- Percutaneous transluminal coronary angioplasty (PTCA) may be superior to thrombolysis in the short term in patients who are prone to occlusion or re-occlusion of the artery responsible for an infarction.
- Implantable cardioverter defibrillators are effective for secondary and primary prevention of cardiac arrest.

Primary Prevention

Pharmacological interventions, drug interactions and drugs that are likely to cause harm

Key messages

- HRT can no longer be recommended for the prevention of cardiovascular disease.

- There is potential for an antagonistic interaction between aspirin and ibuprofen; caution concerning co-prescribing of these drugs is required.

The effect of HRT on cardiovascular disease has become much clearer in recent years. Combined therapy, oestrogen and progestogen increase the risk of breast cancer, coronary heart disease, stroke and venous thromboembolism.[1-2] These risks are counter-balanced by reducing the risk of hip fracture and colon cancer. In terms of the overall balance of risks and benefits, HRT results in two serious adverse events per 1000 women treated for one year. After five years the risk of one serious adverse risk increases to one per 100 women treated.[1]

The currently agreed recommendation is that HRT is effective for reducing vasomotor symptoms at the time of the menopause. It does not have any effect on quality of life in older women without menopausal symptoms.[1,3] In addition, it does not have any effect on symptoms of depression, insomnia, sexual functioning or cognition.[1] HRT can no longer be recommended for prevention of cardiovascular disease, indeed current evidence suggests that there is a small but significant increase in cardiovascular risk.[4]

There is some evidence from laboratory studies that ibuprofen, a non-aspirin non-steroidal anti-inflammatory drug (NSAID), can inhibit the antiplatelet effect of aspirin. Such an interaction is of significant public health importance because of the widespread use of NSAIDs.[5] Pharmaco-epidemiology studies have neither fully confirmed nor refuted such an interaction. One recent study using a dispensed prescribing database, found that the rates of all-cause mortality and cardiovascular mortality were higher amongst patients with cardiovascular disease who were taking ibuprofen and aspirin compared with those taking aspirin alone.[6] These findings, however, have not been confirmed in a different study that examined prescription data for aspirin or ibuprofen after discharge from hospital.[7] At present the current level of evidence is not sufficient to make definitive recommendations for or against the concomitant use of ibuprofen with aspirin. Further studies to clarify this issue are ongoing but until then relative caution should be given to the co-prescribing of these drugs and alternative NSAIDs or analgesics used if possible.[5]

Cardiovascular risk estimation

Key messages

- Combining overall cardiovascular risk is the starting point for primary prevention of cardiovascular disease.

- Risk scoring tools are by no means perfect at predicting true cardiovascular risk.

- Newer methods including modifications of current risk scoring tools are being developed and evaluated.

Estimation of cardiovascular risk is now seen as the starting point when discussing the risks and benefits of pharmacological and non-pharmacological therapy for cardiovascular disease prevention with patients. All current UK guidelines, including the joint risk tables and Sheffield risk score,[8-9] require calculation of absolute risk by means of confirming and combining cardiovascular risk factors – age, sex, blood pressure, total/HDL cholesterol ratio, smoking status and presence of diabetes. Nearly all risk scores have been based on the Framingham risk equation. However, there is growing unease that risk assessment in general and the Framingham risk equation in particular do not provide an accurate assessment of an individual's cardiovascular risk.[10] In the British Regional Heart Study cohort (a representative sample from 24 UK general practices), Framingham overestimates risk of fatal or non-fatal coronary heart disease (CHD) by 57%. Furthermore, there is regional variation in the extent of overestimation, with overestimation greatest in areas of the UK where the mortality rate from CHD is lowest, for example the South of England (overestimation by 71%), and lowest in areas of the UK where the mortality rate from CHD is highest, for example Scotland (overestimation 28%).[11]

There are several reasons why risk scoring is not as accurate as might be hoped:

▶ variation in cardiovascular mortality between and within countries

▶ a secular decline in the rate of CHD

▶ use of risk factors that have been only measured on one occasion only

▶ the 'risk-paradox' of risk-reducing treatments such as blood pressure lowering drugs and statin therapy

▶ the fact that some ethnic groups, at higher cardiovascular risk, are not represented in the cohorts of patients upon which cardiovascular risk scores are based.[10]

The most important reason for inaccuracy relates to basing primary prevention of cardiovascular disease and drug treatment on 'thresholds' of risk. For example, a recent study examined the predictive ability of the Framingham risk equation in a representative sample of 24 general practices selected to represent the range of cardiovascular disease mortality in the UK – the British Regional Heart Study. In this prospective study 7735 men, aged 40–59 years at entry (1978–80), were randomly selected from the age–sex registers in each of the 24 participating general practices.[11] The Framingham risk equation was applied to all these individuals when they entered the study and they were followed up over a 20-year period and their cardiovascular outcome was ascertained. When the threshold of ≥ 30% over ten-year risk of coronary heart disease risk was assessed (consistent with the recommended threshold from the joint risk tables and the National Service Framework for CHD),[12] around 84% of the disease events occurred in the 'low risk' group – people who might potentially be reassured by the decision that treatment was not indicated for their level of risk.[11] When the threshold was lowered to ≥ 15%, this false negative rate fell to 25%, however the number identified as being at high risk, but who did not have a cardiac event, rose from 6% to 45%.[11]

The reason why risk scoring appears to perform so poorly as a screening tool is due to the fact that individual risk factors have a continuous relationship with cardiovascular disease; the best predictors of cardiovascular risk are those risk factors that cannot be altered, for example age and sex.[13] This has led some commentators to suggest that age alone may be the best way to identify 'high risk' individuals who are at greater risk of cardiovascular disease.[13] Alternative solutions have been proposed to enable risk scores to function more accurately. Recalibration of the Framingham risk function to reflect regional rates or the different rates of cardiovascular disease in different ethnic groups has been proposed, and appears to work well in UK and North American populations.[11,14]

An alternative to recalibration has been the approach adopted by the SCORE (Systemic Coronary Risk Evaluation) investigators who pooled data from twelve European cohorts, and have provided risk-assessment charts for high and low risk countries.[15] Unfortunately the SCORE approach is limited by the use of cardiovascular death as its endpoint and it does not include a variable that takes into account treatment effects.[10] Additionally, the SCORE algorithm cannot be used in many inner city general practices, where the majority of the patients live in areas of socio-economic deprivation or are from black and minority ethnic groups.[10] Thus, both approaches, re-calibration and the SCORE approach, represent valuable modifications but do not alter the underlying challenge of using risk scoring as a screening tool for primary prevention.

Shared decision making in cardiovascular disease

Key messages

- Shared decision making is important in cardiovascular disease, particularly in primary prevention where the risks and benefits of treatment may be quite similar.

- Decision aids improve knowledge and decisional conflict; they are being developed for a wide variety of cardiovascular conditions.

Eliciting patients' preferences should be viewed as an essential element in cardiovascular risk assessment when deciding on whether cardiovascular treatments are necessary. It is important to elicit patient's preferences, as they are likely to differ from a clinician's. For example, patients with high blood pressure often disagree with guidelines and health professionals over the level of cardiovascular risk they are prepared to accept as either safe or hazardous.[16] In patients with atrial fibrillation, willingness to accept treatment with warfarin or aspirin has been shown to be difficult to predict on an individual basis and varies in direction and magnitude in terms of willingness to take preventative treatment and risk aversion to the side effects of treatment.[17]

In order that shared decision making can be facilitated between patients and health professionals, several decision aids have been developed in conditions such as atrial fibrillation and hypertension.[18-19] These decision aids have been shown to increase patients' knowledge about their condition, improve their decisional conflict (a composite measure of how uncertain, unclear, uninformed, and unsupported a patient feels about the decision they have to make), whilst not adversely affecting their anxiety levels.[18-19] It is likely that more of these types of decision aids will become available in the future, possibly over the Internet.

24-hour ambulatory blood pressure monitoring

Key messages

- Ambulatory blood pressure is a better predictor of cardiovascular outcomes than conventional blood pressure measurements.

- Ambulatory blood pressure measurement should be considered if there is a discrepancy between home blood pressure readings and readings taken in primary care.

- An effective alternative to ambulatory monitoring is self-measurement at home which can be used in both diagnosis and management of hypertension.

There is new evidence from a recent prospective cohort study that cardiovascular outcomes in treated patients with high blood pressure are better predicted by ambulatory blood pressure than by conventional blood pressure measurements in general practice.[20] The most striking finding of this study was that individuals on blood pressure lowering medication whose mean 24-hour systolic blood pressure was 135 mmHg or higher were almost twice as likely to suffer a cardiovascular event than those with a mean 24-hour systolic blood pressure of less than 135 mmHg. This finding was regardless of their blood pressure readings taken by a health professional. There is good evidence that 'white coat' hypertension in general practice is more widespread than previously assumed. A comparison of different blood pressure measurements in primary care – readings made by general practitioners, nurses, technicians and self-measurement by patients – showed that readings made by doctors were higher, demonstrating that 'white coat' hypertension is common, occurring in up to one-fifth of patients.

If ambulatory blood pressure measurements are not possible, repeated measurements by a nurse or by the patient themselves will result in much less unnecessary treatment or change in drug treatment.[21] In terms of patient acceptability, there is a trade-off between getting the most accurate readings and patient acceptability – patients are least tolerant of ambulatory blood pressure monitoring when compared to other measurement methods.[22] It seems that self-measurements by patients appear the best tolerated method and provide accurate measurements when obtaining an accurate blood pressure record.[22]

The role of ambulatory blood pressure monitoring in primary care is changing with increasing numbers of patients using self-monitoring devices to record their readings so that drug treatment can be optimised. Self-monitoring of blood pressure at home can help to discover discrepancies between surgery and home measurements.[21] Ambulatory monitoring should be considered in situations where hypertension appears resistant to blood pressure lowering drugs. A raised ambulatory blood pressure of more than 130/80 mmHg would support an increase or change in blood pressure lowering medication, whereas readings below this threshold would back continuation with current therapy and follow-up with ambulatory blood pressure readings every one to two years. Evidence concerning the role of self monitoring as a means by which patients can manage and titrate their own hypertension drugs is not fully established, though some randomised trials have shown that this is a promising development.[23]

Secondary prevention

New models of care, including nurse-led care

Key messages

- Patients are satisfied with nurse-led care.

- There is some evidence on the effectiveness of nurse-led care on secondary prevention clinics for cardiovascular but more evidence is needed for hypertension treatment and management.

The increase in the availability of nurse practitioners in general practice may lead to higher levels of patient satisfaction and quality of care. A recent systematic review by Horrocks and colleagues, of whether nurse practitioners working in primary care can provide equivalent care to doctors, included 11 trials and 23 observational studies.[24] This review showed that patients were more satisfied with the care by a nurse practitioner, although the effect size was relatively small. Nurse practitioners were found to have longer consultations and they requested more investigations. This study found no differences in prescriptions, return consultations, or referrals.

Although nurse-led care appears to be effective in many areas of primary care, there is little evidence to suggest that nurse-led care is effective in the management of hypertension. Oakeshott and colleagues reviewed ten studies of nurse-led management of high blood pressure, which were all of generally high methodological quality in terms of randomisation, blinding, and reports of losses to follow-up.[25] This review found that nurse-led hypertension management and cardiovascular health promotion without a change in prescribing had little or no effect on blood pressure. Only one of the included trials, in which patients with blood pressure levels above certain cut-off points were referred to their GPs for drug treatment, showed an important difference.[26] This review concluded that the most important advantages of nurse-led care included improved anti-hypertensive prescribing, better adherence to treatment and better follow-up due to rigorous application of national guidelines. The authors identified a need for randomised controlled trials, based in primary care, to further evaluate the effectiveness of nurse-led care by specially trained practice nurses in improving blood pressure control.

In terms of secondary prevention of cardiovascular disease, effective implementation can be achieved through nurse-led clinics. Improvements have been demonstrated in terms of the process of care – the prescribing of effective drug therapies and risk factor modification – as well as improvement in health status and quality of life.[27] Furthermore, these changes translate into improved lifestyle and medical change at five-year follow up, with associated improvements in all-cause mortality and coronary events.[28]

New drugs in the treatment of angina and myocardial infarction

Key messages

- Aspirin continues to be the main standard antiplatelet drug.
- Clopidogrel is similarly effective alternative to aspirin for preventing ischaemic events in people with stable cerebrovascular, cardiovascular and peripheral vascular disease.
- Adding clopidogrel to aspirin in people with non-ST segment elevation acute coronary syndrome can reduce further ischaemic events.
- There is some evidence that each drug has 'additive' effects on reducing the risk of cardiovascular disease.

Aspirin continues to be the standard antiplatelet drug therapy but provides only partial protection in people with stable cardiovascular disease, as it affects only one of many pathways leading to platelet activation, with up to 45% of the population being 'resistant' to aspirin. Clopidogrel (Plavix) has replaced its predecessor ticlopidine, due to a better safety profile, with no significant risk of haematological toxicity and infrequent gastrointestinal adverse effects. A number of large randomised trials (for example, the CAPRIE[29] and CURE[30] trials) have provided good evidence for the effectiveness of clopidogrel. This is now indicated as an alternative antiplatelet agent for secondary prevention in individuals who do not tolerate aspirin or for use in acute non-ST elevation acute coronary syndromes. There is some evidence to suggest that one year of clopidogrel therapy following percutaneous coronary intervention is more effective than one month of clopidogrel therapy.[31]

In a systematic review of five randomised trials of secondary prevention it has been shown that combinations of pravastatin and aspirin have additive effects on cardiovascular mortality. Taking both drugs produced a relative reduction in fatal and non-fatal myocardial infarction of about a quarter to a third when compared to taking either of these drugs alone.[32] These findings emphasise that secondary prevention of coronary heart disease requires combination drug therapy to produce the greatest benefits for patients.

Ambulatory electrocardiography for the diagnosis of arrhythmias in primary care

Key messages

- Ambulatory electrocardiography (ECG) can be useful for linking ECG findings to patient symptoms.

- Interpretation can be difficult and should be performed by a trained health professional.

Ambulatory ECG can be useful to detect and classify episodes of abnormal electrical activity of the heart in daily life. Because some abnormalities may only occur while a patient is asleep or under emotional or physical stress, recording an ECG over a longer period of time can be useful. These recordings can be continuous (typically 24 or 48 hours) or intermittent, with some intermittent recorders incorporating a memory loop that allows the capture of fleeting symptoms, the onset of a cardiac arrhythmia, or infrequent syncopes.[33] Based on results from a recent randomised trial, loop recorders have a higher diagnostic yield for patients with syncope or presyncope compared to continuous monitors, but their use may be limited because some patients find them more difficult to operate.[34] Loop devices are particularly useful in the diagnosis of symptomatic arrhythmias and for monitoring the effectiveness and safety of anti-arrhythmic medications.[35]

The most recent recommendations on the use of ambulatory ECG were provided by the American College of Cardiology and the American Heart Association in collaboration with the North American Society for Pacing and Electrophysiology, which published their guidelines in 1999.[36] These guidelines give advice on how to evaluate symptoms of cardiac arrhythmias, assess risk in patients with a previous myocardial infarction, evaluate anti-arrhythmic therapy, assess pacemaker/implantable cardioverter-defibrillator function, or evaluate possible myocardial ischaemia.

The main indication for ambulatory ECG is to determine the association of a patient's symptoms with cardiac arrhythmias, where an ECG recording is needed at exactly the time when the symptoms occur. Clinicians who have received the appropriate training and have gained the necessary skills should perform the assessment of recordings from ambulatory ECG.[33]

Other currently available technologies such as home monitoring systems that allow transmission of patient ECG data as well as information on blood pressure and pulse oximetry via telephone or a wireless approach are not yet widely used but may facilitate the ambulatory titration of anti-arrhythmic medication or the management of heart failure in the future.[35]

Treatment of atrial fibrillation – direct thrombin inhibitors and implantable devices

Key messages

- Patients with atrial fibrillation and no other risk factors who take aspirin do not benefit from oral anticoagulation therapy.

- Rate control with effective oral anticoagulation is the priority over rhythm control with cardioversion.

- Direct thrombin inhibitors appear to have equivalent effectiveness as warfarin, a better safety profile and do not require blood monitoring.

- Devices used to treat atrial fibrillation include: atrial defibrillator; overdrive atrial pacing; atrial pacing; dual site pacing; ventricular pacing.

Atrial fibrillation commonly causes symptoms such as palpitations and short-ness of breath, but is also associated with stroke, heart failure, increased hospital admissions and death.[37] Proper risk stratification is an essential pre-requisite for rational management of atrial fibrillation. Recent evidence shows that, irrespective of age, patients with atrial fibrillation and no additional risk factors (no previous history of stroke or transient ischaemic attack, no treated hypertension or systolic blood pressure 140 mmHg, no symptomatic coronary artery disease or no diabetes) who take aspirin have stroke rates similar to those of age-matched individuals. Therefore the risks of oral anticoagulation therapy outweigh the benefits.[38]

Management of atrial fibrillation most commonly consists of strategies to control rate or rhythm. Two recent randomised trials compared these two strat-egies of rate control: allowing atrial fibrillation to persist but giving patients oral anticoagulant drugs and anti-arrhythmic agents, or rhythm control-giving serial cardioversion so as to try to convert back to sinus rhythm, as well as oral anticoagulants and anti-arrhythmic agents.[39–40] Both studies showed that attempts at cardioversion to produce sinus rhythm did not produce any benefit in terms of quality of life, risk of stroke and overall mortality. These studies show that rate control allied to effective oral anticoagulation is the over-riding priority in the management of patients with atrial fibrillation.[41]

Oral anticoagulants, usually used in the form of warfarin, block the vitamin-K-dependent liver production of clotting factors II (prothrombin), VII, IX and X. However, warfarin has a narrow therapeutic window and requires close monitoring of the international normalised ratio. Recently, direct oral thrombin inhibitors have been introduced and compared to warfarin in terms of effectiveness when treating non-valvular atrial fibrillation. Randomised trials have shown that direct thrombin inhibitors such as ximelagatran, are equivalent in terms of preventing stroke whilst the side effect profile was marginally better in the ximelagatran group, with major bleeding being the same but minor bleeding occurring more often in the warfarin group.[42] As direct thrombin inhibitors do not require regular blood monitoring and have a better safety profile than warfarin, treatment of atrial fibrillation may well change. Ongoing studies of clopidogrel are due to report shortly. The other outstanding issue relates to the longer-term safety of ximelagatran, which is associated with abnormalities in liver enzyme function.[43] _Lancet 2003_

Implantable devices have also been developed to provide an additional therapeutic option in patients with atrial fibrillation.[44] Ventricular pacing during atrial fibrillation is ineffective, but dual chamber pacing has been shown in some studies to be superior to ventricular pacing in reducing both the incidence of atrial fibrillation as well as the progression to chronic atrial fibrillation, although this effect was not seen until two years after the pacemakers had been implanted.[45] Implantable pacemakers and defibrillators are undergoing further development. Their use may become more frequent in the future for decreasing the incidence of atrial fibrillation and to improve patients' quality of life, particularly in combination with other treatments.

Tertiary prevention

Recent developments in cardiac rehabilitation

Key messages

- Exercise-based cardiac rehabilitation can reduce cardiac deaths.
- Cardiac rehabilitation should involve a multidisciplinary team.

There is good evidence to suggest that exercise-based cardiac rehabilitation is effective in reducing deaths from heart disease (total cardiac mortality reduced by 31% (95% C I: 49% to 6%), although it remains unclear whether exercise alone or a more comprehensive intervention of cardiac rehabilitation is better.[46] _— Cochrane review 2004._

Cardiac rehabilitation is indicated in patients who suffered a myocardial infarction, suffer from unstable angina, or who underwent coronary revascularisation.[47] It aims to maintain optimal physical and psychosocial health in patients with heart disease by a multidisciplinary team. Health professionals from different backgrounds are encouraged to work together to provide comprehensive cardiac rehabilitation consisting of:

- ▶ exercise training

- ▶ change in health-related behaviour

- ▶ patient education and psychological support

- ▶ helping patients to return to their normal daily activities and

- ▶ reducing the risk of future cardiac events.

Patients with co-morbidity such as diabetes require particular attention and a more aggressive approach to risk-factor management, since these individuals tend to have a greater adverse risk profile in terms of body mass index (BMI), hypertension, lipid profile, and fitness levels.[48]

The Scottish Intercollegiate Guidelines Network (SIGN) promotes an approach in four phases. After a full evaluation and patient education in hospital (phase 1), many patients may still feel isolated and insecure in the early discharge period and may require psychological and emotional support through home visiting or telephone follow-up (phase 2). The role of the primary health care team consists of a tailored approach to encourage structured exercise training together with providing educational and psychological support (phase 3) along with encouraging long-term maintenance of physical activity and lifestyle change (phase 4).

Specific educational and behavioural goals should include the reduction of misconceptions around heart disease, smoking cessation advice, weight reduction and help with returning to work, which might involve different health professionals including psychologists, cardiologists, or exercise physiologists. Due to the often individually-tailored approach to cardiac rehabilitation, patients will receive care according to their need. There is limited information about the cost-effectiveness of these interventions within different patient groups.

Recent evidence concerning revascularisation

Key messages

- Percutaneous transluminal coronary angioplasty (PTCA) may be superior to thrombolysis in the short term in patients who are prone to occlusion or re-occlusion of the artery responsible for an infarction.

- Routine angiography followed by revascularisation is more effective than a purely conservative approach in unstable coronary artery disease.

There continues to be a dilemma as to how to treat patients with multi-vessel disease who are suitable for treatment using coronary artery bypass grafting (CABG) or percutaneous coronary intervention (PCI), since both procedures are similar in terms of rates of death and other cardiovascular morbidity.[49] However, the risk of repeat revascularisation is lower for CABG, but PCI is not as invasive and less costly, and patients' views, as well as local facilities, are therefore important factors in the decision-making process. In patients with severe left main stem disease, CABG is often more appropriate, whereas single vessel coronary artery disease will mostly be treated with PCI.

Intravenous thrombolysis is used for most patients presenting with myocardial infarction, since it is widely available and reduces mortality, as demonstrated in randomised controlled trials. Mortality is reduced by 30 per 1000 presenting within 0–6 hours and by about 20 per 1000 for those presenting within 7–12 hours from onset of symptoms. To be effective, it is important that thrombolysis is given quickly. The NSF Standard Six states that thrombolysis should be given within 60 minutes of calling for professional help (Call to Needle time). The care delivered for the heart attacks is independently audited by the Myocardial Infarction National Audit Project (MINAP). Since the inception of MINAP in 2000, the percentage of heart attack patients in England receiving thrombolysis within 30 minutes of arrival at hospital has doubled (from 40 to 81%). A recent Cochrane Review suggests that, for patients in whom thrombolysis is contraindicated or who are prone to occlusion or re-occlusion of the artery responsible for the infarct, primary PTCA may be superior to thrombolysis in the short term but may not be sustained.[50] PTCA may be preferred if it is available in experienced centres, but optimal thrombolytic therapy is still an excellent approach. There has been much debate about whether patients with unstable angina or non-ST elevation myocardial infarction should be treated with an invasive or conservative approach.

A recent trial by the British Heart Foundation found that an interventional strategy (routine angiography followed by revascularisation) was more effective than a conservative approach for unstable coronary artery disease. This is because it halves the number of angina episodes requiring hospital admission and the need for revascularisation or repeated revascularisation without an increase in risk of death or myocardial infarction.[51] It is likely that in the future drug eluting stents will be more commonly used despite their high initial cost, since these devices reduce the need for revascularisation.[52]

Only a proportion of patients undergoing revascularisation, however, will be free from angina in the longer term. A Swedish study showed that fewer than half of all women and two thirds of men who undergo revascularisation would be free from angina after four years.[53] At four years, three fifths of patients with chronic stable angina did not suffer from angina and had a similar quality of life compared with the general Swedish population. These findings may help practitioners in counselling patients who undergo revascularisation to form realistic expectations about the effects of the procedure.

Implantable defibrillators

Key messages

- Implantable cardioverter defibrillators are effective for secondary and primary prevention of cardiac arrest.
- Careful clinical decision making should precede their use.

Despite advances in emergency treatment and resuscitation techniques, sudden death due to cardiac arrest continues to be a public health problem. Implantable cardioverter-defibrillator therapy has been shown to prevent sudden cardiac deaths and increase survival in high-risk patients.[54] There is now good evidence that automatic implantable cardioverter defibrillators reduce mortality in high-risk patients with a history of myocardial infarction more than 30 days earlier and left ventricular dysfunction with an ejection fraction of less than 30%.[55] The National Institute for Clinical Excellence (NICE) recommends the use of implantable cardioverter defibrillators for secondary and primary prevention of cardiac arrest.

Secondary prevention is indicated in patients who had:

- ▶ either a cardiac arrest due to ventricular tachycardia or ventricular fibrillation
- ▶ spontaneous sustained ventricular fibrillation leading to syncope or significant haemodynamic compromise
- ▶ sustained ventricular tachycardia without syncope or cardiac arrest but with a reduced ejection fraction of less than 35% and no significant heart failure.

Primary prevention is indicated in patients with:

- ▶ a history of myocardial infarction in addition to non-sustained ventricular tachycardia on 24-hour ECG monitoring
- ▶ inducible ventricular tachycardia on electrophysiological testing or
- ▶ left ventricular dysfunction with an ejection fraction of less than 35% and no worse than class III heart failure.

In cases where spontaneous sustained ventricular tachycardia is associated with minimal symptoms and good cardiac function, or those with syncope of unknown cause with no previous history of myocardial infarction, implantable cardioverter defibrillators should not be routinely considered. These devices are expensive and not without complications, and careful decision making by patients and clinicians is important.[54]

Conclusions

There have been quite a number of developments in the primary, secondary and tertiary management of cardiovascular disease. Primary prevention should be focussed on estimation of cardiovascular risk enabling an informed discussion about the risks and benefits of preventative treatments with patients. New drugs and interventions have altered the immediate longer-term management of post-myocardial infarction patients.

References

1. Grady D. Postmenopausal hormones – therapy for symptoms only. *N Engl J Med* 2003; **348**: 1835–7

2. McPherson K. Where are we now with hormone replacement therapy? *BMJ* 2004; **328**: 357–8.

3. Hays J, Ockene J K, Brunner R L, *et al.* Effects of estrogen plus progestin on health-related quality of life. *N Engl J Med* 2003; **348**: 1839–54

4. Petitti D B. Hormone replacement therapy for prevention. *JAMA* 2002; **288**: 99–101.

5. Kimmel S E, Strom B L. Giving aspirin and ibuprofen after myocardial infarction. *BMJ* 2003; **327**: 1298–9

6. MacDonald T M, Wei L. Effect of ibuprofen on cardioprotective effect of aspirin. *Lancet* 2003; **361**: 573–4

7. Curtis J P, Wang Y, Portnay E L, *et al.* Aspirin, ibuprofen, and mortality after myocardial infarction: retrospective cohort study. *BMJ* 2003; **327**: 1322–3

8. Ramsay L E, Haq I, Jackson P R, *et al.* Targeting lipid-lowering drug therapy for primary prevention of coronary disease: an updated Sheffield table. *Lancet* 1996; **348**: 387–8

9. Ramsay L E, Williams B, Johnston G, *et al.* Guidelines for the management of hypertension: report of the third working party of the British Hypertension Society. *J Hum Hypertens* 1999; **13**: 569–92

10. Brindle P, Holt T. Cardiovascular risk assessment – time to look beyond cohort studies. *Int J Epidemiol* 2004; **33**: 614–15

11. Brindle P, Emberson J, Lampe F, *et al.* Predictive accuracy of the Framingham coronary risk score in British men: prospective cohort study. *BMJ* 2003; **327**: 1267–70

12. Department of Health. *National Service Framework for coronary heart disease*. London: HMSO, 2000

13. Law M R, Wald N J. Risk factor thresholds: their existence under scrutiny. *BMJ* 2002; **324**: 1570–6

14. D'Agostino R B, Grundy S, Sullivan L M, *et al.* Validation of the Framingham coronary heart disease prediction scores: results of a multiple ethnic groups investigation. *JAMA* 2001; **286**: 180–7

15. Conroy R, Pyorala K, Fitzgerald A, *et al.* Estimation of ten-year risk of fatal cardiovascular disease in Europe: the SCORE project. *Eur Heart J* 2003; **24**: 987–1003

16. Steel N. Thresholds for taking antihypertensive drugs in different professional and lay groups: questionnaire survey. *BMJ* 2000; **320**: 1446–7

17. Devereaux P, Anderson D, Gardner M J, *et al.* Differences between perspective of physicians and patients on anticoagulation in patients with atrial fibrillation: observational study. *BMJ* 2002; **323**: 1218–22

18. Man-Son-Hing M, Laupacis A, O'Connor A M, *et al.* A patient decision aid regarding antithrombotic therapy for stroke prevention in atrial fibrillation. *JAMA* 1999; **282**: 737–43

19. Montgomery A A, Fahey T, Peters T J. A factorial randomised controlled trial of decision analysis and an information video plus leaflet for newly diagnosed hypertensive patients. *Br J Gen Pract* 2003; **53**: 446–53

20. Clement D L, De Buyzere M L, De Bacquer D A, *et al.* Prognostic value of ambulatory blood pressure recordings in patients with treated hypertension. *New Engl J Med* 2003; **348**: 2407–15

21. Little P, Gould C, Barnett J, *et al.* Comparison of agreement between different measures of blood pressure in primary care and daytime ambulatory blood pressure. *BMJ* 2002; **325**: 254–9

22. Little P, Barnett J, Barnsley L, *et al.* Comparison of acceptability of and preferences for different methods of measuring blood pressure in primary care. *BMJ* 2002; **325**: 258–9

23. Fahey T, Schroeder K, Ebrahim S. Interventions for improving adherence to treatment in patients with high blood pressure in ambulatory settings. In: Cochrane Collaboration. *Cochrane Library* Issue 4. Chichester: John Wiley & Sons Ltd, 2004

24. Horrocks S, Anderson E, Salisbury C. Systematic review of whether nurse practitioners working in primary care can provide equivalent care to doctors. *BMJ* 2002; **324**: 819–23

25. Oakeshott P, Kerry S, Austin A, *et al.* Is there a role for nurse-led blood pressure management in primary care? *Fam Pract* 2003; **20**: 496–73

26. McHugh F, Lindsay F, Hanlon P. Nurse-led care shared care for patients on the waiting list for coronary artery bypass surgery: a randomised controlled trial. *Heart* 2001; **86**: 317–23

27. Campbell N C, Thain J, Deans H G, *et al.* Secondary prevention clinics for coronary heart disease: randomised trial of effect on health. *BMJ* 1998; **316**: 1434–7

28. Murchie P, Campbell N C, Ritchie L D, *et al.* Secondary prevention clinics for coronary heart disease: four-year follow up of a randomised controlled trial in primary care. *BMJ* 2003; **326**: 84

29. CAPRIE Steering Committee. A randomised, blinded, trial of clopidogrel versus aspirin in patients at risk of ischaemic events (CAPRIE). *Lancet* 1996; **348**: 1329–39

30. Yusuf S, Zhao Mehta S R, *et al.* Clopidogrel in unstable angina to prevent recurrent events trial investigators. Effects of clopidogrel in addition to aspirin in patients with acute coronary syndromes without ST segment elevation. *N Engl J Med* 2001; **345**: 494–502

31. Steinhubl S R, Berger P B, Mann J T. Early and sustained dual oral antiplatelet therapy following percutaneous coronary intervention: a randomized controlled trial. C R E D O investigators. Clopidogrel for the reduction of events during observation. *JAMA* 2002; **288**: 2411–20

32. Hennekens C H, Sacks F M, Tonkin A, *et al.* Additive benefits of pravstatin and aspirin to decrease risks of cardiovascular disease. *Arch Intern Med* 2003; **164**: 40–4

33. Kadish A H, Mason J W, Buxton A E, *et al.* ACC/AHA Clinical competence statement on electrocardiography and ambulatory electrocardiography. *J Am Coll Cardiol* 2001; **38**: 2091–100

34. Sivakumaran S, Krahn A D, Klein G J, *et al.* A prospective randomised comparison of loop recorders versus Holter monitors in patients with syncope or presyncope. *Am J Med* 2003; **115**: 1–5

35. Zimetbaum P J, Josephson M E. The evolving role of ambulatory arrhythmia monitoring in general clinical practice. *Ann Intern Med* 1999; **130**: 848–56

36. Crawford M H, Bernstein S J, Deedwania P C, *et al.* ACC/AHA guidelines for ambulatory electrocardiography: a report of the American College of Cardiology/American Heart Association Task Force on Practice Guidelines (Committee to Revise the Guidelines for Ambulatory Electrocardiography). Developed in collaboration with the North American Society for Pacing and Electrophysiology. *J Am Coll Cardiol* 1999; **34**: 912–48

37. Benjamin E J, Wolf Pa, D'Agostino R B, Silbershatz H, Kannel W B, Levy D. Impact of atrial fibrillation on the risk of death: the Framingham Heart Study. *Circulation* 1998; **98**: 946–52

38. van Walraven C, Hart R G, Wells G A, *et al.* A clinical prediction rule to identify patients with atrial fibrillation and a low risk for stroke while taking Aspirin. *Arch Intern Med* 2003; **163**: 936–43

39. Wyse D G, Waldo A L, DiMarco J P, *et al.* Atrial Fibrillation Follow-up Investigation of Rhythm Management (AFFIRM) Investigators. A Comparison of Rate Control and Rhythm Control in Patients with Atrial Fibrillation. *N Engl J Med* 2002; **347**: 1825–33

40. Van Gelder I C, Hagens V E, Bosker H A, *et al.* A comparison of rate control and rhythm control in patients with recurrent persistent atrial fibrillation. *N Engl J Med* 2002; **347**: 1834–40

41. Falk R H. Management of atrial fibrillation – radical reform or modest modification? *N Engl J Med* 2002; **347**: 1883–4

42. SPORTIF III investigators. Stroke prevention with the oral direct thrombin inhibitor Ximelagatran compared with warfarin in patients with non-valvular atrial fibrillation (SPORTIF III): a randomised controlled trial. *Lancet* 2003; **362**: 1691–8

43. Verheugt F. Can we pull the plug on warfarin in atrial fibrillation? *Lancet* 2003; **362**: 1686–7

44. Cooper J M, Katcher M S, Orlov M V. Implantable devices for the treatment of atrial fibrillation. *N Engl J Med* 2002; **346**: 2062–8

45. Skanes A C, Krahn A D, Yee R. Progression to chronic atrial fibrillation after pacing: the Canadian Trial of Physiologic Pacing. *J Am Coll Cardiol* 2001; **38**: 167–72

46. Jolliffe J A, Rees K, Taylor R S, Thompson D, Oldridge N, Ebrahim S. Exercise-based rehabilitation for coronary heart disease (Cochrane Review). In: *The Cochrane Library*, Issue 3. Chichester: John Wiley & Sons Ltd, 2004

47. Ades P A. Cardiac rehabilitation and secondary prevention of coronary heart disease. *N Engl Med* 2001; **345**: 892–902

48. Banzer J A, Maguire T E, Kennedy C M, *et al.* Results of cardiac rehabilitation in patients with diabetes mellitus. *Am J Cardiol* 2004; **93**: 81–4

49. Schofield P M. Indications for percutaneous and surgical revascularisation: how far does the evidence base guide us? *Heart* 2004; **89**: 565–70

50. Steinbrüchel D, Hughes P. Primary Percutaneous interventions versus fibrinolytic therapy for acute myocardial infarction (Cochrane Review). In: *The Cochrane Library*, Issue 3. Chichester: John Wiley & Sons Ltd, 2004

51. Fox K A, Poole-Wilson P A, Henderson R A. Interventional versus conservative treatment for patients with unstable angina or non-ST-elevation myocardial infarction: the British Heart Foundation RITA 3 randomised trial. Randomised Intervention Trial of unstable Angina (RITA) Investigators. *Lancet* 2002; **360**: 743–51

52. Bhargava B, Karthikeyan G, Abizaid A S, *et al.* New approaches to preventing restenosis. *BMJ* 2003; **327**: 274–9

53. Brorsson B, Bernstein S J, Brook R H, *et al.* Quality of life of patients with chronic stable angina before and four years after coronary revascularisation compared with a normal population. *Heart* 2002; **87**: 140–5

54. DiMarco J P. Medical progress: implantable cardioverter-defibrillators. *N Engl J Med* 2003; **349**: 1836–47

55. Moss A S, Zareba W, Hall W J. Prophylactic implantation of a defibrillator in patients with myocardial infarction and reduced ejection fraction. Multicenter automatic defibrillator implantation trial II investigators. *N Engl J Med* 2002; **346**: 877–83

Further reading/contact organisations/websites

Cardiac Rehabilitation • www.cardiacrehabilitation.org.uk

Scottish Intercollegiate Guidelines Network • www.sign.ac.uk

American College of Cardiology • www.acc.org

American Heart Association • www.americanheart.org

British Heart Foundation • www.bhf.org.uk

British Hypertension Society • www.bhsoc.org

National Institute for Clinical Excellence • www.nice.org.uk

CHAPTER 10

Respiratory Medicine

Hilary Pinnock

▶ **KEY MESSAGES**
- Diagnosis: Objective diagnosis and assessment of patients with asthma or chronic obstructive pulmonary disease (COPD) is a prerequisite of appropriate management.

- Monitoring: Structured care involving regular review improves asthma morbidity and may enable the provision of holistic care for COPD.

- Management: Guidelines define strategies for the management of asthma and COPD – their application will be influenced by the individual clinical circumstances and the patient's preference.

- Self-management: Written, personalised asthma action plans improve health outcomes and should be offered to all people with asthma. The role of self-management for people with COPD has not yet been clarified.

- Delivery of care: General Practitioners with a Special Interest (GPwSIs) have the potential to support recent initiatives designed to improve the delivery of care to people with respiratory disease.

The General Medical Services (GMS) contract[1] focuses attention on the provision of high-quality routine care for patients with chronic disease. The quality markers defined by the contract endorse the need for objective diagnosis and structured care recommended by the British Thoracic Society/Scottish Intercollegiate Guideline Network (BTS-SIGN) British Guideline for the Management of Asthma[2] and the National Institute for Clinical Excellence (NICE) guideline on the management of COPD in adults in primary and secondary care.[3] This chapter will discuss the key recommendations of these guidelines, and their implementation in the pragmatic world of general practice.

Diagnosis of asthma and COPD

Recent advances

- Objective tests should be used to confirm a diagnosis of asthma before long-term therapy is started.

- Spirometry should be undertaken on all patients with suspected COPD both to confirm the diagnosis and assess severity.

- The GMS contract sets targets for both these parameters.

Objective diagnosis of asthma

The key diagnostic feature of asthma is the variability of the symptoms, signs, and lung function. Diagnosis can be considered as a three-stage process.

1. **Typical history:** Variable symptoms of wheeze, shortness of breath, chest tightness, and cough suggest a diagnosis of asthma, although some of the patients with mild asthma seen in primary care may have intermittent symptoms occurring only after exposure to an allergen or after a viral infection. Audible wheeze may only be present during exacerbations. A personal or family history of atopy adds weight to the diagnosis.

2. **Objective tests:** A peak flow is the most convenient test of lung function for the diagnosis of asthma. The demonstration of variability requires multiple readings recorded over a period of time to demonstrate diurnal variation, deterioration on exposure to a trigger or reversibility after treatment. An isolated normal peak flow carried out in the surgery does not exclude the diagnosis of asthma. Peak flow charting involves the patient in the diagnostic process and has the advantage of capturing objective evidence of variability at the time the patient has symptoms, allowing an assessment of the severity and frequency of symptoms. In addition, the best peak flow can be established as a baseline for future management plans. Significant variability is defined as 20% or more, with a minimum change of 60 l/min. Spirometry may also be used to demonstrate reversibility (significance is defined as 15% or more, with a minimum change of 200 ml) but, because of the variable nature of asthma, normal spirometry does not exclude the diagnosis.

3. **Response to treatment:** Failure to respond to a trial of asthma treatment, such as inhaled steroids, should prompt reconsideration of the diagnosis.[2] The differential diagnosis of adults with symptoms of cough and wheeze includes COPD, heart failure, bronchiectasis and hyperventilation.

Structured recording of these three diagnostic steps is important, both clinically and to facilitate the auditing of quality indicators for the GMS contract. Suitable templates can be designed for computer systems to ensure accurate coding. Some practical hints for peak flow charting and recording a diagnosis of asthma are included in Box 10.1.

Box 10.1 **Ensuring an objective diagnosis of asthma: some practical hints**

- Provision of simple written instructions may facilitate teaching during the course of a busy surgery or patients can be referred to an asthma-trained practice nurse.

- Patients should be asked to record the best of three peak flow readings each morning and evening and at times when they are symptomatic and when they feel well. For patients experiencing regular symptoms it should be possible to obtain sufficient readings over the course of a week to support or question a diagnosis.

- Variability of more than 20% is highly suggestive of asthma.

- Many of the patients with mild asthma in general practice will only demonstrate peak flow variability during times of exacerbations so that lack of 20% variability does not exclude the diagnosis. It should, however, lead to consideration of alternative diagnoses, especially if the patient was symptomatic at the time.

- The diagnostic process should be recorded in the patient's records. These stickers may be downloaded from the GPIAG website http://gpiag.org and printed onto Avery labels to facilitate recording in paper records.

Asthma diagnosis: (three ticks confirms a diagnosis of asthma)

Yes ☐	**A typical history**	Variable symptoms of wheeze, cough, shortness of breath, chest tightness. PMH or FH of atopy
Yes ☐	**20% variability**	Peak flow diary showing: 20% diurnal variation 20% reduction after trigger 20% response to treatment
Yes ☐	**Response to treatment**	Symptomatic response to β-agonist, oral or inhaled steroid

Asthma: diagnosed / not diagnosed / suspected

Source: **General Practice Airways Group (GPIAG)**

Objective diagnosis of asthma in infants

Making a diagnosis in young children is more complex, both because objective tests of lung function are not feasible in routine practice and because of a growing awareness of the different phenotypes of asthma in infancy. Viral associated wheeze is common in infancy: many will outgrow their symptoms by school age, some will have asthma throughout childhood, a few will have lifelong asthma and, 'occasionally' children will have other more serious pathology.[4]

The three components of the diagnostic process, an appropriate history, objective evidence and a response to treatment, need to be modified for infants:

1. Persistent symptoms of cough and wheeze, especially in the presence of atopy, suggest asthma.

2. Wheeze, heard by a health care professional, should be noted in the patient's records as objective confirmation of the parent's description.

3. A trial of treatment may be a useful strategy.[5] A clear response to bronchodilation is helpful, but for more chronic symptoms a course of inhaled steroids may be more appropriate. Paradoxically, the 'reasonable starting dose' of inhaled steroids suggested for children may have to be increased for infants because of the practical problems of delivering adequate doses to the lung – some authors have suggested up to 400 µg beclomethasone twice daily for two months.[6] A good symptomatic response supports a diagnosis of asthma, but it is important to withdraw treatment to exclude spontaneous resolution. A poor response suggests that asthma is unlikely and should prompt consideration of alternative causes for the child's symptoms. Clear documentation of the response to treatment and follow-up to establish the lowest effective maintenance dose of inhaled steroids are crucial.

Objective diagnosis of COPD

COPD is a chronic, slowly progressive disorder in which the airflow obstruction is fixed or only minimally reversible.[3] In contrast with asthma, symptoms and signs develop insidiously and lung function deteriorates slowly over years. Other causes of productive cough and breathlessness, such as bronchiectasis, need to be considered in the differential diagnosis of chronic symptoms, while a rapid deterioration should prompt a search for other pathology such as lung cancer or heart failure. Co-morbidity is common, with other smoking-related and age-related diseases occurring in 40% of COPD patients investigated after an acute exacerbation.[7] For the primary care clinician the key distinction is often between asthma and COPD; a distinction that is made more complex as some patients with asthma develop irreversible remodelling, and patients with COPD may have 'some reversibility'.[3] The diagnosis is suggested by the history and clarified with spirometry.

▶ **Typical history:** A smoker, presenting with a history of slowly progressive, productive cough, wheeze and shortness of breath, with an onset of troublesome symptoms after the age of 35 years suggests a diagnosis of COPD.

▶ **Spirometry:** A consistently low peak flow with no variability in a smoker with typical symptoms may suggest COPD but the objective diagnosis and assessment of severity requires spirometry.[3] An FEV_1 (forced expiratory volume in 1 second) less than 80% of predicted and an FEV_1 / FVC (forced expiratory volume in 1 second / forced vital capacity) ratio less than 70% confirms obstruction. Some patients with COPD will show significant reversibility (>15% and 200 ml increase in FEV_1), but a substantial increase in FEV_1 (more than 400 ml) suggests a diagnosis of asthma.[3] Some key points for the provision of a spirometry service are given in Box 10.2.

Box 10.2 **Spirometry: some practical points**

- A range of reasonably priced spirometers ideal for use in primary care are readily available. They all require regular servicing and manufacturers' instructions for calibration should be followed.

- Adequate training, whether of respiratory nurses or health care assistants, is essential to ensure that the satisfactory readings are obtained. Technical training on the use of specific instruments is available from the manufacturers, and a range of suitable courses are available from respiratory training centres (see Resources).

- Patients should be prepared for the procedure. They should be clinically stable and should not have used a short-acting bronchodilator for six hours, a long-acting bronchodilator for 12 hours or theophyllines for 24 hours.

- Spirometry takes time, particularly in older patients with severe COPD who may need to rest for some minutes between blows.

A fact sheet on spirometry, with a brief guide to interpretation is available from the GPIAG website (www.gpiag.org). '*Spirometry in Practice*' a practical booklet on spirometry in primary care is available from the BTS consortium: copd@imc-group.co.uk.

The recent NICE guideline recommends classification into mild, moderate and severe COPD as FEV_1 falls below 80%, 50% or 30% of predicted, bringing

UK practice into line with international guidelines.[3,8] Although lung function is a good indicator of prognosis, it does not accurately reflect disability and may underestimate the impact of the disease in some patients while overestimating it in others. The GMS contract has adopted a 70% threshold for the implementation of quality markers for COPD on the basis that symptoms are relatively unlikely at higher levels of lung function.[1]

There is growing evidence that reversibility testing with bronchodilators and oral steroids do not predict the therapeutic value of bronchodilators or inhaled steroids, which should be judged on the basis of clinical benefit.[9] Demonstration of poor reversibility, however, is important for diagnostic purposes, principally to exclude the diagnosis of asthma.

Screening for COPD

The accelerated decline in lung function can be prevented if the patient can be encouraged to stop smoking.[10] It is therefore suggested that identifying patients with mild COPD combined with intensive smoking cessation advice could reduce the burden of COPD by preventing progression to severe, disabling disease.[3] The practicability, effectiveness, and cost-effectiveness of screening for COPD needs to be evaluated in UK primary care before widespread adoption of this theoretical benefit can be recommended.[11–12] Case-finding has been explored as a practical approach to identifying patients at risk of COPD.[13–14] The presence of a cough in a smoker is emerging as a useful marker, correlating better with the diagnosis of COPD than wheeze or shortness of breath.

An additional problem for detecting mild COPD is that a single reading cannot indicate the rate of decline of lung function.[12] A normal FEV_1 of 80% of predicted may represent a considerable loss of lung function if that patient's baseline was 120% of predicted.

Monitoring of asthma and COPD in general practice

Recent advances

- Proactive, structured review of asthma is associated with favourable clinical outcomes.

- COPD is a disabling condition and regular review is recommended to ensure increasing support is provided as the condition deteriorates.

- The GMS contract sets targets for both these parameters.

Regular review of people with asthma

Regular review of people with asthma is associated with a reduced exacerbation rate and improved symptom control[15] and is a recommendation of the BTS-SIGN asthma guideline[2] endorsed by the GMS contract.[1]

The content of a review will vary according to the needs of the individual patient but a key component is the standardised recording of asthma control. Because of the variable nature of asthma, a peak flow undertaken in the clinic is of limited value in assessing asthma status. The simple morbidity score, promoted by the Royal College of Physicians,[16] (see Figure 10.1) consists of three questions that could be used at every asthma review to monitor progress. Tools incorporating similar questions have been used successfully to screen for those with more severe problems.[17] Refinements to improve sensitivity to change are currently being evaluated and may include replacing the 'yes/no' answers with a '0–7' score to reflect the number of days affected in the previous week.

Figure 10.1 **Royal College of Physicians' three questions.**[16]

In the last week / month	Yes	No
Have you had difficulty sleeping because of your asthma symptoms (including cough)?	☐	☐
Have you had your usual asthma symptoms during the day (cough, wheeze, chest tightness or breathlessness)?	☐	☐
Has your asthma interfered with your usual activities (e.g. housework, work, school etc)?	☐	☐

It is recommended that the answers to these three morbidity questions should be recorded at every routine review for people over the age of 16 years with an established diagnosis of asthma.

Despite the emphasis on proactive care undertaken in most UK practices by asthma nurses[18] as part of the Chronic Disease Management programme[19] only about one-third of patients achieve an annual review.[20-1] Many reasons have been suggested to account for the reluctance of patients to attend for an asthma review but a common theme is a perception that their asthma is not serious enough to warrant the time involved in attending an asthma clinic.[20-1] Innovative ways of undertaking reviews will need to be considered if practices are to achieve the 70% target set by the quality indicators in the GMS contract.[1] A trial of telephone consultations has shown that this mode of consultation can increase the proportion of patients reviewed with no loss of asthma-related quality of life or patient satisfaction.[22] The shorter duration of telephone consultations suggests this may be an efficient way of delivering care. Other innovations, such as e-mail consultations, have yet to be evaluated, but may contribute to improving access to regular asthma reviews.

Monitoring of people with COPD

COPD is a condition in which deterioration is inevitable, particularly if the patient continues to smoke, so advice that patients should be reviewed regularly seems reasonable.[3,8] There is, however, no evidence to inform decisions about the most appropriate models of care. Issues that still need to be addressed include the frequency of recall appropriate for different severities of COPD, the important components of quality care and who should deliver that care.[23]

Reviews may include the following key components:

▶ **Reassessment of spirometry.** Monitoring the rate of decline of lung function detects those patients with accelerated deterioration (> 500 ml over five years) in whom specialist opinion may be considered,[3] and provides a reminder to review care in response to reducing lung function. In the absence of evidence, the GMS contract has pragmatically defined a quality indicator based on spirometry repeated bi-annually.[1]

▶ **On-going health promotion.** Smoking cessation advice is crucial, but encouragement to maintain an active lifestyle is also important.[24]

▶ **On-going assessment and optimisation of therapy.** The Medical Research Council (MRC) dyspnoea scale[25] (see Figure 10.2) is recommended for grading breathlessness, and alerting the clinician to increasing disability and the corresponding need for increased provision of bronchodilators.[3] The GMS contract[1] emphasises the importance of checking inhaler technique, at least bi-annually, in patients with COPD as their poor respiratory function can compromise the effective delivery of inhaled medication.

It is recommended that this dyspnoea scale should be recorded at every routine review for people with COPD.

▶ **Recognition and management of complications.** Depression is recognised as a significant complication of COPD and may need treatment. Severe COPD, the onset of cor pulmonale, or an oxygen saturation of < 92% suggests chronic hypoxia and should prompt referral for consideration of long-term oxygen therapy.[26]

▶ **Assessment of disability.** Additional social support may be needed as symptoms impact on activities of daily living.

Figure 10.2 **MRC Dyspnoea scale**[25]

Grade	Degree of breathlessness related to activities
1	Not troubled by breathlessness except on strenuous exercise
2	Short of breath when hurrying or walking up a slight hill
3	Walks slower than contemporaries on level ground because of breathlessness, or has to stop for breath when walking at own pace
4	Stops for breath after walking about 100 m or after a few minutes on level ground
5	Too breathless to leave the house, or breathless when dressing or undressing

Recent advances in the management of asthma and COPD

Recent advances

- Inhaled steroids are the recommended preventer drug for adults and children with asthma, but a trial of other treatments should be conducted before increasing the maintenance dose above 800 mg a day for adults or 400 mg a day for children.

- Inhaled steroids do not significantly affect the rate of decline in lung function in patients with COPD, but they can reduce the exacerbation rate in those with severe disease, for example, in people with an FEV_1 less than 50% predicted and who experience more than two exacerbations a year.

- Pulmonary rehabilitation improves exercise tolerance and quality of life in patients with moderate/severe COPD.

- COPD patients have palliative care needs that need to be addressed.

- The GMS contract sets targets for the provision of smoking cessation advice for patients with asthma and COPD.

Note: **All doses of inhaled steroids refer to beclomethasone given via a metered dose inhaler. (BDP≡)**
      Adjustment may be necessary for fluticasone, mometasone or other devices.

Asthma management

The BTS-SIGN asthma guideline reinforces the advice that inhaled steroids are the recommended preventer drug for adults and children,[2] although, it is now clear that, for many patients, the optimal maintenance dose may be 400 μg daily for adults or 200 μg for children (BDP≡). Recent advances have extended our understanding of the most appropriate options when low doses of inhaled steroids fail to adequately control symptoms. Much research has been devoted to identifying effective therapeutic regimes, but it is important not to overlook the need for a broad assessment when asthma control deteriorates. Patients may stop taking inhaled steroids, or decide to abandon the spacer device that ensured effective delivery of the drug. Environmental factors may be significant, either at home or work. Importantly, the deterioration may be due to the development of other medical conditions.

The link with rhinitis

The importance of the link between asthma and rhinitis has been highlighted by the *Allergic Rhinitis and its Impact on Asthma guidelines*.[27] A third of people with rhinitis will develop symptoms of asthma and over half of asthma suffers will also have rhinitis. This concept of 'one airway, one disease' has a number of implications for the primary care clinician. Enquiry about asthma symptoms should be part of the routine assessment of patients with rhinitis. Conversely, assessment and treatment of rhinitis should be part of routine asthma reviews. Some studies have suggested that treating the rhinitis with nasal steroids may improve asthma control.[28]

Although interventions designed to reduce house dust mite exposure in patients with perennial rhinitis may be of some benefit in improving nasal symptoms,[29] reducing allergen levels has not been shown to be an effective measure in adults with asthma.[30-1]

'Add-on' therapy for asthma

Recognition that, for many patients, increasing the dose of inhaled steroids confers little additional benefit whilst increasing the side effects has led to interest in alternative strategies for improving asthma control. Early suggestions that long-acting beta-agonists might be useful add-on therapy have been corroborated by a significant body of evidence.[32-4] The addition of a long-acting beta-agonist to a modest dose of inhaled steroids can reduce symptoms and the need for rescue medication, improve quality of life and reduce exacerbations.[33] This supports the recommendation in the BTS-SIGN guideline that adults should not increase their maintenance dose of inhaled steroid above 800 µg daily (BDP≡) without a trial of other therapy. The equivalent dose in children is 400 µg daily. The first choice 'add-on' therapy for adults and older children is a long-acting beta-agonist.[2]

This statement, however, belies the complexity of tailoring medication to individual circumstances.

> ▶ Adding formoterol to a low dose of budesonide was as effective as quadrupling the dose of budesonide for treating the symptoms due to 'mild'

loss of control. The number of 'severe' exacerbations, however, were controlled better by the high dose of inhaled steroids.[33]

▸ Leukotriene antagonists can reduce the symptoms of rhinitis,[35] raising the possibility that patients whose asthma has slipped out of control during the hay fever season may benefit from a treatment that can help both manifestations of their allergy.

▸ Both long-acting beta-agonists and leukotriene antagonists effectively reduce exercise-induced asthma[2] and a patient's preference for a tablet or an inhaler may be an important factor in selecting treatment. *BTS guideline 2003*

▸ In pre-school children long-acting beta-agonists appear to be less effective and leukotriene antagonists may be the better option.[36] *Paediatric 2001*

The clear message is the importance of assessing each patient individually, and monitoring the effect and side effects of any change in treatment.

Many questions, however, remain to be answered. Pragmatic studies are needed in primary care populations to allow for the influence of patient's preferences, compliance and inhaler technique on outcomes. Combination inhalers containing an inhaled steroid with a long-acting beta-agonist, with their potential for convenient dosage schedules but reduced ability to adjust individual drug doses, add yet another dimension to influence the clinician's decision.

Leukotriene receptor antagonists

Leukotriene antagonists are orally active drugs which block the action of the chemical mediators, cysteinyl leukotrienes. Recent trials suggest that they can improve asthma control in combination with inhaled steroids, and are currently recommended as first-line add-on therapy for children under five years old.[2,37] They reduce eosinophilic inflammation but are considerably less potent than inhaled steroids which remain the preventer treatment of choice in patients of all ages[2] though emerging evidence is exploring the role of leukotriene antagonists as preventer treatment for pre-school children with episodic, viral-induced wheeze.

Smoking cessation

Smoking is by far the most important cause of COPD and cessation is the only intervention that reduces the rate of decline in lung function.[10,38] Smokers have an increased severity of asthma symptoms and the children of smokers have an increase in respiratory disease.[39] A focus on smoking cessation is therefore amply justified.[1]

Brief advice from a general practitioner helps about 2% of smokers to quit.[40] By expecting primary care clinicians to record smoking status annually the quality indicators in the GMS contract aim to facilitate opportunistic smoking cessation advice.[1] The recommendations are summarised as:

▶ **Ask** about smoking and **Advise** cessation at every opportunity. General practitioners are committed to health promotion, but cite many barriers to incorporating smoking cessation activity into routine general practice, such as lack of time, inadequate training and a belief that advice may be ineffective.[41] There is a concern that the advice to 'ask about smoking at every opportunity' risks jeopardising the doctor–patient relationship and may be counter-productive.[42] More recent guidelines have modified this to 'ask at least once a year'.[43]

▶ **Assist:** The availability of pharmacological aids to smoking cessation has provided the general practitioner with a range of cost-effective products to provide practical support to a determined quitter.[44] Once a 'quit day' has been set prescribing nicotine replacement therapy or bupropion offers a natural opportunity to support the patient's attempt to stop by arranging follow-up for subsequent prescriptions. Both therapies approximately double the quit rate (see Box 10.3).

▶ **Arrange:** Local arrangements for providing support for people wishing to quit smoking will vary but are likely to include access to individual counselling or smoking cessation groups. Booklets can support advice given in a consultation and telephone helplines or websites may provide useful information.

Box 10.3 Therapeutic aids to smoking cessation

Nicotine replacement is available in a range of delivery systems for purchase over-the-counter or on prescription. All facilitate a controlled withdrawal by providing a background level of nicotine to reduce craving, either achieving a steady state (as with patches) or providing increased levels as required (as with gum). Patients who are pregnant or breast feeding, under 18 years of age, or with certain chronic conditions (such as cardiovascular disease, diabetes, hyperthyroidism, renal and hepatic disease) are advised to seek medical advice. Discussion should cover the risks and benefits of using nicotine replacement therapy which will deliver less nicotine, and none of the other harmful chemicals, that would be obtained from cigarettes. The most common side effects are topical irritation. Some patients experience sleep disturbance especially when using the 24-hour patches.

Bupropion is an antidepressant that reduces withdrawal symptoms. It is only available on prescription. It is contra-indicated in patients with a history of seizures, eating or bipolar disorders, pregnancy or breast feeding. A number of cautions and drug interactions need to be considered. It should be commenced one to two weeks before the quit date, using a reduced dose for the first six days. The drug is associated with a range of side effects: seizures occur in about 1 in 1,000.

COPD Management

The mainstay of the pharmacological treatment of COPD remains beta-agonists and anticholinergics.[3,8] These probably work, at least in patients with severe disease, by reducing hyperinflation rather than by bronchodilation and their efficacy is not predicted by improvements in lung function. Trials of treatment should therefore be based on symptomatic response rather than peak flow or spirometric reversibility. Use of higher doses of bronchodilators, ideally delivered from a metered dose inhaler via a spacer, may be limited in some patients by side effects. Long-acting beta$_2$-agonists provide sustained relief from symptoms and improve exercise tolerance. Recent evidence confirms their role in patients continuing to experience symptoms with short-acting bronchodilators.[45]

Tiotropium

Tiotropium is an anticholinergic drug with a very long duration of action which improves clinical outcomes, including reducing shortness of breath and the number of exacerbations.[46] It is administered regularly on a daily basis. The half-life of several days means that it may be a week before maximum benefit is achieved.

Inhaled steroids in COPD

Four major studies, using different inhaled steroids in patients with a range of disease severity have demonstrated that inhaled steroids do not reduce the accelerated decline in lung function in COPD.[9,47-9] Current guidelines, therefore, do not recommend the routine use of inhaled steroids in patients with COPD.[3,8] Response to a short course of oral steroids does not reliably predict benefit to long-term inhaled steroids.[9]

A large UK trial, which studied moderate/severe group of patients, showed a reduction in the exacerbation rate from 1.33 to 0.99 episodes per year, reflected in an improved quality of life.[9] This suggests that patients with moderate to severe disease (FEV$_1$ less than 50% of predicted) who have frequent exacerbations (e.g. more than two exacerbations per year) would benefit from using inhaled steroids. However, practical questions remain. Which inhaled steroid should be used and at what dose and via which delivery system? Side effects, particularly easy bruising and local oral symptoms,[9,48] may be a concern at the relatively high doses of inhaled steroids (BDP $\equiv$ 800 μg to 2000 μg daily) used in these studies.

Pulmonary rehabilitation

Patients with moderate to severe COPD will benefit from the multidisciplinary, holistic approach of pulmonary rehabilitation. Most programmes are
hospital based, though some are carried out in the community and a few
are based in primary care.[50] Details of each programme vary, but important
components include, an assessment of need, optimisation of therapy, exercise
training, an education programme and psychosocial support.[51] Pulmonary
rehabilitation can increase exercise tolerance, relieve breathlessness, reduce
hospital admissions and improve quality of life.[52] It should be offered to all
symptomatic patients (MRC dyspnoea grade 3 or more) with disability.

Palliative care

The prognosis in severe COPD is poor, only half the patients discharged from
hospital after an exacerbation survive for two years.[53] Regrettably the palliative care needs of this severely disabled group of patients are rarely met.[54] A
lack of opportunity to discuss end-of-life decisions denies patients the right
to prioritise palliative treatment (such as morphine to reduce dyspnoea)[55] and
potentially life-sustaining interventions (such as mechanical ventilation). The
'common sense' approach suggested by Abrahm may be a useful basis for
planning care.[56] This recognises the unpredictability of the terminal phase of
COPD and suggests that, rather than delay until death is imminent, discussion about palliative care should be offered as soon as it is recognised that
death could occur at any time due to ordinary intercurrent illness.

Oxygen therapy

Oxygen therapy is important both acutely, to treat asthma attacks or other
respiratory emergencies, but also to relieve the hypoxia that complicates severe
chronic obstructive pulmonary disease. Pulse oximeters are readily available
and relatively cheap; oximetry has been shown to be both feasible and useful
in primary care.[57] The need for long-term oxygen therapy should be considered in patients with severe COPD ($FEV_1 < 30\%$ predicted) and those with
peripheral oedema or polycythaemia. Screening in primary care would ensure
that all potentially eligible patients (those with an oxygen saturation of $< 92\%$)
are referred for formal assessment for long-term oxygen therapy.

Drugs on the horizon

Monoclonal anti-immunoglobulin E antibodies

Omalizumab is an anti-immunoglobulin E antibody that lowers free immu-
noglobin E (IgE) levels, reducing responsiveness to antigen challenge. In
patients with severe allergic asthma this can reduce symptoms and exacerba-

tion rates. Omalizumab is administered by sub-cutaneous injection at from two- to-four-weekly intervals. Despite the inconvenience this imposes, patients report an improved quality of life.[58]

Phosphodiesterase 4 inhibitors

Phosphodiesterase 4 (PDE 4) inhibitors are highly selective derivatives of theophylline. Early studies suggest they may have an anti-inflammatory effect in COPD and may improve lung function, possibly reducing exacerbation rates without the side-effect profile that limits the usefulness of theophyllines.

Self-management in asthma and COPD

Recent advances

- Patients with asthma should be offered self-management education that should focus on individual needs, and be reinforced by a written action plan.

- Every asthma consultation is an opportunity to review, reinforce and extend both knowledge and skills.

Asthma action plans

— cochrane 200?

The evidence that self-management education, including the provision of written asthma action plans, improves morbidity and reduce acute episodes is not new.[15] It is given the highest grade of recommendation by the BTS–SIGN guideline and was one of the key messages promoted after the launch of the guideline. Despite this only a minority of people with asthma have a written personal asthma action plan[20] possibly because self-management is seen as complex and time consuming to implement.[59] Some of the common questions about implementation raised by primary care clinicians are discussed below.

▶ **Should plans be based on symptoms or peak flows?** Most trials have _Thoren 2004_ included both symptoms and peak flows in their action plans. Trials which have compared these approaches have found them to be equivalent.[60] Clinicians may be guided by individual patient preference.

▶ **Should we advise patients to double their inhaled steroids at the onset of deterioration?** The studies that have contributed to the evidence base supporting self-management have included a step at which inhaled steroids should be increased. Evidence of limited effect of doubling inhaled steroids from studies of compliant patients poorly controlled on _MJAMSA BMJ 2006_ moderate doses has raised doubts about this strategy.[32–4, 61] However, in a trial of patients with mild-to-moderate asthma, Foresi et al showed that

200 µg of budesonide daily with a five-fold increase for one week at the onset of an attack, reduced exacerbations as effectively as taking 800 µg of budesonide throughout, and significantly better than the group maintained on 200 µg of budesonide.[62] Patients with mild asthma, often poorly compliant and on a low maintenance dose, should be encouraged to substantially increase (or recommence) inhaled steroids as soon as control slips.[61] *Thorax 2004*

▶ **Should patients have an emergency supply of oral steroids?** Delay is the commonest preventable factor in asthma deaths and prompt use of oral steroids is critical. Patients at risk of acute attacks may wish to accept responsibility for commencing a course of steroids when symptoms increase and bronchodilators become increasingly ineffective. A fall in peak flow to less than 60% of their best will confirm the need for action.

▶ **Doesn't this take time?** There is evidence that written action plans should be provided in the context of self-management education.[63] However, education should be seen as an on-going process that can be incorporated into normal care. An initial appointment with the practice asthma nurse should be supported by all health care professionals using every opportunity to review, refine and reinforce the advice.[2]

▶ **Will patients follow their action plans?** Patients vary in the autonomy they wish to accept and plans need to be adapted accordingly. Qualitative data suggests that patients adapt their action plans in the light of experience, reinforcing the concept of self-management education as an on-going process.[64] *BMJ 2002*

An example of a suitable personal asthma action plan, available from Asthma UK is shown in Figure 10.3.

Self management in COPD

Self-management for patients with COPD has been less well studied. In a trial of secondary care patients, implementing self-management plans as part of an intensive education programme reduced acute admissions by 39%,[65] though other trials have not confirmed this benefit.[66] A smaller study in primary care patients showed changes in self-management behaviour.[67] Further research is needed to identify the most appropriate type of action plan for patients with COPD.

Figure 10.3 **Personal asthma action plan**

ACTION PLAN

Be in control

Symptoms are:	Peak Flow is:	Action is:
No symptoms		Normal – continue your treatment or talk to your doctor/nurse about taking less treatment
Getting a cold, symptoms during daytime and/ or nightime		Take .... of ....(times a day) and blue inhaler for relief of symptoms
Out of breath Blue inhaler does not help		Continue as a above and start steroid tablets .... mgs x .... and contact ....
Too breathless to speak		This needs emergency action straight away. See back page

This Asthma Action Plan is part of a range of 'Be in Control' resources available from the Asthma UK (www.asthma.org.uk)

Delivery of care for people with respiratory disease

Recent advances

- Current provision for respiratory health care and allergy services does not meet reasonable patient expectations.
- GPwSIs in respiratory disease may facilitate the development of services within PCOs to bridge this gap.

In January 2003 an alliance of UK medical charities, organisations and professional bodies with an interest in the provision of respiratory medicine published a report, *Bridging the Gap.*[68] This document defined 'reasonable patient expectations' and provided checklists for primary and secondary care professionals working with PCOs to deliver high quality, integrated respiratory health care. Current services will need to be developed and new initiatives encouraged if these aims are to be met.

General Practitioners with a Special Interest

Publication of the NHS Plan[69] signalled the creation of GPwSIs as a means of cost-effectively reducing waiting lists for specialist opinions and for specific procedures such as endoscopy. The key concepts underpinning the role of GPwSIs, as defined by the Royal College of Physicians and Royal College of General Practitioners, emphasised the importance of maintaining a primary care perspective while encouraging the development of defined specialist competencies to meet local health care needs.[70]

The General Practice Airways Group published a discussion paper defining and broadening the potential roles for a respiratory GPwSI to include: leading the strategic planning within a PCO from a primary care perspective; setting quality standards for respiratory care; and providing clinical expertise for conditions most common in general practice (e.g. asthma, COPD, 'chest infections', allergies).[71] These concepts have now been embodied in a guideline for a respiratory GPwSI.[72] Many of the services discussed below could come within the remit of a respiratory GPwSI.

Spirometry services

Recognition of the importance of spirometry and the availability of relatively cheap, electronic spirometers has stimulated considerable interest in undertaking spirometry within general practices. In 2001, two-thirds of practices in the UK owned a spirometer.[73] There are concerns, however, about the quality of spirometry undertaken in primary care[74] particularly as a recent survey observed that in a quarter of general practices spirometers were used by staff with no formal training.[73] Strategic planning of spirometry services, either at practice or PCO level will need to address issues of quality as well as capacity in order to meet the demands of the GMS contract[1] for objective diagnosis and monitoring of COPD.

Hospital at home

Respiratory disease is responsible for one in eight emergency hospital admissions,[75] and is a major contributory factor in the winter bed crisis.[76] There is considerable interest in the concept of 'Hospital at Home', and recent trials have suggested that about one-third of admissions can be prevented,[77] and lengths of stay halved[78] with supported discharge and nurse-led home care. Patient satisfaction with these schemes is high.[79]

Allergy services

The increasing incidence of allergic disease, including asthma and rhinitis, has exposed the inadequate provision of allergy services in the UK. In their report *Containing the Allergy Epidemic*, the Royal College of Physicians recommend that allergy services should be co-ordinated in a regional allergy centre, but recognises the frontline role of primary care and advocates improved training of GPs and practices to meet the increased demand.[80]

References

1. NHS Confederation, British Medical Association. *New GMS Contract 2003: investing in general practice.* London: BMA, March 2003

2. The British Thoracic Society/Scottish Intercollegiate Guideline Network. British Guideline on the management of asthma. *Thorax* 2003; **58 (S1)**: i1–i94

3. National Institute for Clinical Excellence. CG12 chronic obstructive pulmonary disease – management of chronic obstructive pulmonary disease in adults in primary and secondary care. London: NICE, March 2004

4. Martinez F D. Development of wheezing disorders and asthma in pre-school children. *Paediatrics* 2002; **109**: 362–7

5. Stephenson P. Management of wheeze and cough in infants and pre-school children in primary care. *Prim Care Respir J* 2002; **11(2)**: 42–4

6. Cochran D. Diagnosing and treating chesty infants. *BMJ* 1998; **316**: 1546–7

7. Stewart A L, Greenfield S, Hays R D, *et al.* Functional status and well-being of patients with chronic conditions: results from the medical outcomes study. *JAMA* 1989; **262**: 907–13

8. Global Strategy for the diagnosis, management, and prevention of chronic obstructive pulmonary disease. NHLBI/WHO Global Iniative for Chronic Obstructive Lung Disease (GOLD) Workshop summary. *Am J Respir Crit Care Med* 2001; **163**: 1256–76

9. Burge P S, Calverley P M A, Jones P W, *et al.* on behalf of ISOLDE. Randomised, double blind, placebo controlled study of fluticasone propionate in patients with moderate to severe chronic obstructive pulmonary disease: the ISOLDE study. *BMJ* 2000; **320**: 1297–303

10. Anthonisen N R. The Lung Health Study: Effects of smoking intervention and the use of an inhaled anticholinergic bronchodilator on the rate of decline of FEV1. *JAMA* 1994; **272**: 1497–505

11. Badgett R G, Tanaka D J. Is screening for chronic obstructive pulmonary disease justified? *Preventive Med* 1997; **26**: 466–72

12. Calverley P M A. COPD: early detection and intervention. *Chest* 2000; **117 (S2)**: 365S–71S

13. van Schayck C P, Loozen J M C, Wagena E, *et al.* Detecting patients at high risk of developing chronic obstructive pulmonary disease in general practice: cross sectional case finding study. *BMJ* 2002; **32**: 1370–3

14. Stratelis G, Jakobsson J, Molstad S, Zetterstrom O. Early detection of COPD in primary care: screeing by invitation of smokers aged 40 to 55 years. *Br J Gen Pract* 2004; **54**: 201–6

15. Gibson P G, Powell H, Coughlan J, *et al.* Self-management education and regular practitioner review for adults with asthma (Cochrane Review). In: *The Cochrane Library*, Issue 3, 2003. Oxford: Update Software

16. Pearson M G, Bucknall C E, eds. *Measuring clinical outcome in asthma: a patient focussed approach.* London: Royal College of Physicians, 1999

17. Jones K, Clearly R, Hyland M. Predictive value of a simple asthma morbidity index in a general practice. *Br J Gen Pract* 1999; **49**: 23–6

18. National Health Service, England and Wales. *The National Health Service (General Medical Services) Regulations* 1992. London: HMSO, 1992

19. Jones R C M, Freegard S, Reeves M, *et al*. The role of the practice nurse in the management of asthma. *Prim Care Respir J* 2001; **10**: 109–11

20. Price D, Wolfe S. Delivery of asthma care: patient›s use of and views on healthcare services, as determined from a nationwide interview survey. *Asthma J* 2000; **5**: 141–4

21. Gruffydd-Jones K, Nicholson I, Best L, *et al*. Why don't patients attend the asthma clinic? *Asthma Gen Pract* 1999; **7**: 36–8

22. Pinnock H, Bawden R, Proctor S, *et al*. Accessibility, acceptability and effectiveness of telephone reviews for asthma in primary care: randomised controlled trial. *BMJ* 2003; **326**: 477–9

23. Price D, van der Molen T. The Aberdeen primary care COPD research needs statement. March 2001. *Prim Care Respir J* 2001; **10**: 47–9

24. Chavannes N, Vollenberg J J H, van Schayck C P, *et al*. Effects of physical activity in mild to moderate COPD: a review. *Br J Gen Pract* 2002; **52**: 574–8

25. Fletcher C M, Elmes P C, Fairbairn M B, *et al*. The significance of respiratory symptoms and the diagnosis of chronic bronchitis in a working population. *BMJ* 1959; **2**: 257–66

26. Roberts C M, Bulger J R, Melchor R, *et al*. Value of pulse oximetry in screening for long-term oxygen therapy requirement *Eur Respir J* 1993; **6**: 559–62

27. Bousquet J van Cauwenberge P, Khaltaev N for the ARIA group. Allergic rhinitis and its impact on asthma. *J Allergy Clin Immunol* 2001; **108s**: S147–S333

28. British Society for Allergy and Clinical Immunology. *Rhinitis Management Guidelines 3rd Edition*. London: Dunitz, 2000

29. Sheikh A, Hurwitz B. House dust mite avoidance measures for perennial allergic rhinitis (Cochrane Review). In *The Cochrane Library*, Issue 2, 2004. Chichester, UK: John Wiley & Sons, Ltd

30. Gotzsche P C, Johansen H K, Burr M L, *et al*. House dust mite control measures for asthma (Cochrane Review). In *The Cochrane Library*, Issue 2, 2004. Chichester, UK: John Wiley & Sons, Ltd

31. Woodcock A, Forster L, Matthews E, *et al*. Control of exposure to mite allergen and allergen-impermeable bed covers for adults with asthma. *N Eng J Med* 2003; **349**: 225–36

32. Walters E H, Walters J A E, Gibson, M D P. Inhaled long acting beta agonists for stable chronic asthma (Cochrane Review). In: *The Cochrane Library*, Issue 2, 2004. Chichester, UK: John Wiley & Sons, Ltd

33. Pauwels R A, Lofdahl C G, Postma D S, *et al*. (FACET) Effect of inhaled formoterol and budesonide on exacerbations of asthma. *N Engl J Med* 1997; **337**: 1405–11

34. Shrewsbury S, Pyke S, Britton M. Meta-analysis of increased dose of inhaled steroid or addition of salmeterol in symptomatic asthma (MIASMA). *BMJ* 2000; **320**: 1368–73

35. Meltzer E O, Malmstrom K, Lu S, *et al*. Concomitant montelukast and loratidine as treatment for seasonal allergic rhinitis: a randomised, placebo controlled clinical trial. *J Allergy Clin Immunol* 2000; **105**: 917–22

36. Knorr B, Franchi L M, Bisgaard H, *et al*. Montelukast a leukotriene recepter antagonist, for the treatment of persistent asthma in children aged 2 to 5 years. *Pediatrics* 2001; **108**: E48

37. Ducharme F M. Anti-leukotrienes as add-on therapy to inhaled glucocorticosteroids in patients with asthma: systematic review of current literature. *BMJ* 2002; **324**: 1545–8

38. Fletcher C, Peto R. The natural history of chronic airflow obstruction *BMJ* 1977; **1**: 1645–8

39. Cook D G, Strachan D P. Health effects of passive smoking. 10: Summary of effects of parental smoking on the respiratory health of children and implications for research. *Thorax* 1999; **54**: 357–66

40. Raw M, McNeill A, West R. Smoking Cessation Guidelines for Health Professionals – A guide to effective smoking cessation interventions for the health care system. *Thorax* 1998; **53**: S1–S18

41. McAvoy B R, Kaner E F, Lock C A, *et al*. Our Healthier Nation: are general practitioners willing and able to deliver? A survey of attitudes to and involvement in health promotion and lifestyle counselling. *Br J Gen Pract* 1999; **49**: 187–90

42. Coleman T, Murphy E, Cheater F. Factors influencing discussion of smoking between general practitioners and patients who smoke: a qualitative study. *Br J Gen Pract* 2000; **50**: 207–10

43. West R, McNeill A, Raw M. Smoking cessation guidelines for health professionals: an update. *Thorax* 2000; **55**: 987–99

44. National Institute for Clinical Excellence. Guidance on the use of nicotine replacement therapy (NRT) and bupropion for smoking cessation. *Technology Appraisal Guidance No. 39*. London: NICE, March 2002

45. Drug and Therapeutics Bulletin. Managing stable chronic obstructive pulmonary disease. *Drug Ther Bull* 2001; **39**(11): 81–4

46. Drug and Therapeutics Bulletin. Tiotropium for chronic obstructive pulmonary disease. *Drug Ther Bull* 2003; **41**(2): 15–16

47. Vestbo J, Sorensen T, Lange P, *et al*. Long-term effect of inhaled budesonide in mild and moderate chronic obstructive pulmonary disease: a randomised controlled trial. *Lancet* 1999; **353**: 1819–23

48. Pauwels R A, Lofdahl C G, Laitenen L A, *et al*. for EUROSCOP. Long-term treatment with inhaled budesonide in persons with mild chronic obstructive pulmonary disease who continue smoking. *N Engl J Med* 1999; **340**: 1948–53

49. The Lung Health Study Research Group. Effect on inhaled triamcinolone on the decline in pulmonary function in chronic obstructive pulmonary disease. *N Eng J Med* 2000; **343**: 1819–23

50. Jones R C M, Copper S, Riley O, *et al*. A pilot study of pulmonary rehabilitation in primary care. *Br J Gen Pract* 2002; **52**: 567–8

51. Lacasse Y, Wong E, Guyatt GH, *et al*. Meta-analysis of respiratory rehabilitation in chronic obstructive pulmonary disease *Lancet* 1996; **348**: 1115–19

52. Cambach W, Wagenaar RC, Koelman T W, *et al*. The long-term effects of pulmonary rehabilitation in patients with asthma and chronic obstructive pulmonary disease: a research synthesis. *Arch Physical Med Rehabilitation* 1999; **80**: 103–11

53. Connors A F, Dawson N V, Thomas C, *et al*. Outcomes following acute exacerbation of chronic obstructive lung disease. The SUPPORT investigators. *Am J Respir Crit Care Med* 1996; **154**: 959–67

54. Gore J M, Brophy C J, Greenstone M A. How well do we care for patients with end stage chronic obstructive pulmonary disease? A comparison of palliative care and quality of life in COPD and lung cancer. *Thorax* 2000; **55**: 1000–6

55. Jennings A-L, Davies A N, Higgins J P T, *et al*. A systematic review of the use of opioids in the management of dyspnoea. *Thorax* 2002; **57**: 939–44

56. Abrahm J L, Hansen-Flaschen J. Hospice care for patients with advanced lung disease. *Chest* 2002; **121**: 220–9

57. Jones K, Cassidy P, Killen J, *et al*. The feasibility and usefulness of oximetry measurements in primary care. *Prim Care Respir J* 2003; **12**: 4–6

58. Buhl R. Omalizumab (Xolair) improves quality of life in adult patients with allergic asthma: a review. *Respir Med* 2003; **97**: 123–129

59. Thoonen B P A, Jones K P, van Rooij H A, *et al*. Self-treatment of asthma: possibilities and perspectives from the practitioner's point of view. *Family Practice* 1999; **16**: 117–22

60. Gibson P G, Powell H. Written action plans for asthma: an evidence-based review of the key componenets. *Thorax* 2004; **59**: 94–99

61. FitzGerald J M, Becker A, Sears M R, *et al*. Doubling the dose of budesonide versus maintenance treatment in asthma exacerbations. *Thorax* 2004; **59**: 550-556

62. Foresi A, Morelli M C, Catena E for the Italian Study Group. Low-dose budesonide with the addition of an increased dose during exacerbations is effective in long-term asthma control. *Chest* 2000; **117**: 440–6

63. Toelle B G, Ram F S F. Written individualised management plans for asthma in children and adults (Cochrane Review). *Cochrane Library*, Issue 3, 2003. Oxford: Update Software

64. Douglas J, Aroni R, Goeman D, *et al*. A qualitative study of action plans for asthma. *BMJ* 2002; **324**: 1003–5

65. Bourbeau J, Julien M, Maltais F, *et al*. Reduction of hospital utilisation in patients with chronic obstructive pulmonary disease. *Arch Intern Med* 2003; **163**: 585–91

66. Monninkhof E, van der Valk P, van der Palen J, *et al*. Effects of a comprehensive self-management programme in patients with chronic obstructive pulmonary disease. *Eur Respir J* 2003; **22**: 815–20

67. Watson P B, Town G I, Holbrook N, *et al*. Evaluation of a self-management plan for chronic obstructive pulmonary disease. *Eur Respir J* 1997; **10**: 1267–71

68. The Respiratory Alliance. *Bridging the Gap 2003*. www.gpiag.org/news/bridging.php (last accessed July 2004)

69. Department of Health. *The NHS Plan: a plan for investment, a plan for reform*. London: HMSO, 2000

70. Royal College of General Practitioners and Royal College of Physicians. *General Practitioners with special interest*. London: RCGP and RCP, March 2001

71. Wiliams S, Ryan D, Price D, *et al*. General Practitioners with a special clinical interest: a model for improving respiratory disease management. *Br J Gen Pract* 2002; **52**: 838–43

72. Department of Health. *Guidelines for the appointment of General Practitioners with a Special Interests in the delivery on clinical services: Respiratory Medicine*. London: HMSO, April 2003. www.dh.gov.uk/PolicyAndGuidance/OrganisationPolicy/PrimaryCare/GPsWithSpecial Interests (accessed July 2004)

73. Jones R C M, Freegard S, Reeves M, *et al*. The role of the practice nurse in the management of chronic obstructive pulmonary disease. *Prim Care Respir J* 2001; **10**: 106–8

74. Eaton T, Withey S, Garrett J, *et al*. Spirometry in Primary Care practice. The importance of quality assurance and the impact of spirometry workshops. *Chest* 1999; **116**: 416–23

75. British Thoracic Society. *The Burden of Lung Disease*. November 2001. http://www.brit-thoracic.org.uk/docs/BurdenofLungDisease.pdf (accessed July 2004)

76. Damiani M, Dixon J. *Managing the Pressure. Emergency Hospital admissions in London 1997–2001*. London: The Kings Fund, 2002

77. Davies L, Wilkinson M, Bonner S, *et al*. Hospital at home versus hospital care in patients with exacerbations of chronic obstructive pulmonary disease: prospective randomised controlled trial. *BMJ* 2000; **321**: 1254–8

78. Cotton M M, Bucknall C E, Dagg K D, *et al*. Early discharge for patients with exacerbations of chronic obstructive pulmonary disease: a randomised controlled trial. *Thorax* 2000; **55**: 902–6

79. Ojoo J C, Moon T, McGlone S, *et al*. Patients' and carers' preferences in two models of care for acute exacerbations of COPD: results of a randomised controlled trial. *Thorax* 2002; **57**: 167–9

80. Royal College of Physicians. *Containing the Allergy Epidemic*. London: Royal College of Physicians, 2003

Resources

Guidelines for the management of respiratory disease

Asthma
▷ The British Thoracic Society / Scottish Intercollegiate Guideline Network. British Guideline on the management of asthma. *Thorax* 2003; **58 (S1)**: i1–i94.
The BTS / SIGN 2004 Update of British Guideline on the Management of Asthma may be downloaded from: www.brit-thoracic.org.uk and www.sign.ac.uk

▷ GINA Workshop Report. Global Strategy for Asthma Management and Prevention. (Updated November 2003). Available at: www.ginasthma.com

Asthma and Rhinitis
▷ Bousquet J van Cauwenberge P, Khaltaev N for the ARIA group. Allergic Rhinitis and its Impact on Asthma. *J Allergy Clin Immunol* 2001; **108 S**: S147–S333

Rhinitis
▷ British Society for Allergy and Clinical Immunology. *Rhinitis Management Guidelines* 3rd Edition. London: Dunitz, 2000

Chronic Obstructive Pulmonary Disease
▷ National Institute for Clinical Excellence (NICE). National clinical guideline on the management of chronic obstructive pulmonary disease in adults in primary and secondary care. National Collaborating Centre for Chronic Conditions. *Thorax* 2004; **59 (S1)**: 1–232 available from: www.nice.org.uk

▷ Global Strategy for the diagnosis, management and prevention of chronic obstructive pulmonary disease. *GOLD Workshop summary: updated 2003*. Available from: www.goldcopd.com

Smoking cessation

▷ British Thoracic Society. Smoking Cessation guidelines. *Thorax* 1998; **53**: S1–S19

▷ British Thoracic Society. Smocking cessation guidelines for health professional: an update. *Thorax* 2000; **55**: 987–99

▷ National Institute for Clinical Excellence. *Guidance on the use of nicotine replacement therapy (NRT) and bupropion for smoking cessation.* 2002. Technology Appraisal Guidance No 39 March 2002

Respiratory organisations and useful websites

▷ **British Thoracic Society** • www.brit-thoracic.org.uk
A range of guidelines for the management of respiratory disease is available from the BTS website. The latest update of the asthma guideline may be downloaded. Case studies, slides and posters to facilitate the implementation of the guideline are also available.

▷ **Scottish Intercollegiate Guideline Network** • www.sign.ac.uk
SIGN have a wide range of guidelines and Quick Reference Guides available on their website including the latest update of the asthma guideline (No. 63). Resources to support implementation of this guideline may also be downloaded.

▷ **General Practice Airways Group** • www.gpiag.org
The GPIAG is a professional organisation that promotes primary care respiratory medicine. Their website includes a practical supplement to complement the BTS SIGN asthma guideline and ready-made audit tools to facilitate implementation. Other resources include opinion sheets on key aspects of asthma and COPD care and diagnosis 'stickers'.

▷ **International Primary Care Respiratory Group** • www.theipcrg.org
The IPCRG is developing international primary care guidelines and their website provides access to a range of resources including opinion sheets on spirometry and validated questionnaires for monitoring COPD.

▷ **Respiratory GPwSI** • www.dh.gov.uk/policyandguidance/organisationpolicy/ primarycare/gpswithspecialinterests
Guidelines for the appointment of GPwSIs in the delivery of clinical services: Respiratory Medicine, 2003.

▷ **Asthma UK** • www.asthma.org.uk
Asthma UK produces the *Be in Control* range of resources that can be used to provide written action plans.

▷ **British Lung Foundation** • www.britishlungfoundation.org
The BLF website includes useful resources to support clinicians caring for patients with a range of respiratory diseases.

▷ **National Respiratory Training Centre** • www.nrtc.org.uk
The NRTC is an independent education and research institution, which provides accredited education and training in respiratory and allergic disease for health professionals.

▷ **Respiratory Education and Training Centre** • www.respiratoryetc.com
The RETC is an independent training organisation offering a broad spectrum of nationally recognised respiratory courses for primary and secondary health care professionals.

CHAPTER 11

Gastrointestinal Diseases

R Chaudhary, S Ghosh

RECENT ADVANCES ▼

- Incidence of oesophageal adenocarcinoma continues to increase. This is likely to be related to gastro-oesophageal reflux but endoscopic surveillance of Barrett's oesophagus remains controversial.

- Dyspepsia management guidelines should reduce endoscopic workload but advocate *H. pylori* test and treat for dyspeptic patients in the absence of alarm symptoms.

- Novel diagnostic methods such as wireless capsule endoscopy permit visualisation of the entire small intestine.

- Colonoscopy for screening and surveillance of colorectal cancer is often overused and should follow clearly defined guidelines.

- New therapies in inflammatory bowel disease such as infliximab in Crohn's disease offer hope to patients refractory to conventional therapy, and may reduce hospitalisation and surgery.

Gastrointestinal diseases are common and significant advances in evidence-based management have been made. Gastro-oesophageal reflux disease (GORD) and irritable bowel syndrome (IBS) are the most frequent gastro-intestinal afflictions. This chapter reviews the major increments in knowledge guiding current clinical practice and the areas of uncertainties. Changes in diagnostic modalities with introduction of virtual colonoscopy and capsule endoscopy, new therapies such as 5-hydroxytryptamine (5-HT) modulators in

IBS, infliximab in Crohn's disease and increasing incidence of cancers such as oesophageal adenocarcinoma are rapidly altering gastroenterology practice and referral patterns. The advances in costly diagnostic procedures and therapeutic agents lead to significant challenges in delivering a high standard of service, and rigorous health economic data is essential to guide evidence-based practice.

Oesophageal cancer and Barrett's oesophagus

Key messages

- Oesophageal adenocarcinoma has been increasing in incidence in the UK.

- This is likely to be related to chronic gastro-oesophageal reflux disease and development of Barrett's oesophagus.

- Barrett's surveillance remains controversial with no proven survival outcome studies.

- Improvements in the detection of dysplasia/early cancers and development of local therapy techniques are likely to offer advances in the future.

- Chemoprevention with aspirin / NSAIDs / COX-2 inhibitors may give the best hope of providing an impact on a population-wide basis.

Oesophageal cancer is the sixth most common cancer worldwide. It accounts for 6700 deaths per year in the UK, two-thirds of which are diagnosed in the over 65-year-old patients.[1] The clinical outcome is poor with a five-year survival rate of around 5%. The two main categories are squamous cell carcinoma and adenocarcinoma. The incidence of adenocarcinoma of the oesophagus is rising (doubling in ten years in the Western world). This climb has been linked to the increasing incidence of Barrett's oesophagus. There is a strong association between symptoms of gastro-oesophageal reflux and oesophageal adenocarcinoma. Among persons with recurrent reflux symptoms, the odds ratio (OR) for oesophageal adenocarcinoma is 7.7 (95% confidence interval (CI) = 5.3 to 11.4) and among those with long-standing, severe reflux symptoms, the OR is an astonishing 43.5 (95% CI = 18.3 to 103.5).[2]

Barrett's oesophagus (columnar-lined oesophagus with intestinal metaplasia) is a consequence of GORD and results from a change from the normal squamous epithelium to intestinal metaplastic columnar epithelium within the oesophagus.[3] Approximately 5% of people with reflux symptoms are found to have Barrett's oesophagus. The diagnosis is made endoscopically with histological confirmation made by appropriate biopsies. Dysplasia is the first step in the neoplastic process and is the best current indicator of the risk of cancer.

The progression from low- to high-grade dysplasia, followed by adenocarcinoma, is documented but not inevitable. The risk of developing a cancer in a segment of Barrett's is approximately 0.5% per year (Figure 11.1). Routine surveillance of Barrett's (Box 11.1) has been advocated because it represents a pre-malignant lesion.

Figure 11.1 Barrett's oesophagus with development of oesophageal adenocarcinoma

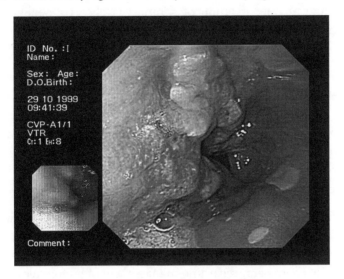

Box 11.1 **The rationale for the surveillance of Barrett's oesophagus**

	Reflux			Intervention	
	⇩			⇩	
Squamous	⇔ Intestinal	⇔ Low-grade	⇔	High-grade	⇔ Adenocarcinoma
Epithelium	Metaplasia	Dysplasia		Dysplasia	

Surveillance controversy

The practice of routine surveillance of Barrett's oesophagus remains controversial[4-5] for the following reasons:

▶ The number of people identified as to having Barrett's oesophagus represent a small fraction of those that develop adenocarcinoma. Barrett's surveillance has not convincingly demonstrated an impact on survival outcome.

▶ Endoscopic appearances may be normal despite high-grade dysplasia or adenocarcinoma in situ. Current recommendations are for quadrantic biopsies at 2 cm intervals depending on the length of the Barrett's. Random biopsy may lead to sampling error with areas of focal dysplasia or cancer missed.

▶ Traditionally a Barrett's segment has been defined as 3 cm or more in length and there has been little consensus on whether short segments Barrett's oesophagus (< 3 cm) requires surveillance.

▶ Pathological interpretation of samples is observer-dependent with current recommendations suggesting two specialist gastrointestinal pathologists to corroborate significant histology findings.

▶ On finding high-grade dysplasia up to 30% may have a synchronous undetected cancer due to sampling error. Oesophagectomy has therefore been the recommendation in cases of high-grade dysplasia but carries a definite mortality (> 3%) and significant morbidity, especially in an elderly target population. On the other hand, a policy of careful frequent biopsies and/or endoscopic ablation has also some supportive literature especially in those at high risk for surgical resection.

▶ Despite the natural history, progression to carcinoma is not inevitable and dysplasia may regress. We are currently unable to predict who will progress to adenocarcinoma and who will not. As a result there is a degree of controversy regarding management of high-grade dysplasia.

Nevertheless, evidence suggests that cancers identified through Barrett's surveillance are detected earlier allowing the opportunity of early intervention. In one survey, three-quarters of responding UK gastroenterologists advocate Barrett's surveillance, though practice varies widely.[6]

Clearly surveillance should be performed on appropriate patients, i.e. those who would undertake regular surveillance endoscopy and are suitable candidates for oesophageal resection. Intervention has to be tailored to the individual patient with local ablative therapies considered (ideally as part of a trial) as an alternative to oesophagectomy depending on local expertise. Currently, no universally accepted national guidelines for screening Barrett's oesophagus are available in the UK, and gastroenterologists vary from a completely nihilistic approach to screening, to enthusiastic adoption of US guidelines[7] (Table 11.1).

Table 11.1 **Current surveillance recommendations**
(American College of Gastroenterology) [7]

- Three-yearly surveillance in Barrett's cases following two surveillance endoscopies demonstrating no dysplasia.
- Yearly endoscopy in low-grade dysplasia after two initial six-monthly surveillance examinations.
- In high-grade dysplasia confirmation by two expert GI pathologists is required. Repeat endoscopy to look for mucosal irregularities (amenable to endoscopic mucosal resection) and for repeat intensive biopsies is recommended. Multi-focal dysplasia would require intervention. Patients with focal dysplasia may have three-monthly endoscopic surveillance.
- Maintenance with proton pump inhibitor for symptom control and mucosal healing.

Despite the problems with surveillance future developments in the early detection and treatment of oesophageal cancer seem promising.

Advances in detection of Barrett's oesophagus

A number of new techniques now promise earlier detection of neoplastic changes permitting targeted biopsies, and this clearly is the way forward with further refinement of the technology.[8–9] Dye spraying or staining techniques (chromoendoscopy) may enable the endoscopist to correctly identify areas of Barrett's oesophagus for biopsy. Examples include methylene blue staining, which stains goblet cells of the intestinal mucosa, and Lugol's stain, which stains squamous epithelium and is not taken up by intestinal metaplasia, dysplasia or tumour growth. Improvements in endoscopic technology, such as magnification endoscopy, increasingly allows the appreciation of minor superficial irregularities and thereby the detection of subtle, discrete mucosal lesions. Spectroscopy, narrow-band imaging and fluorescence detection are other techniques currently in development. It is hoped that they will improve the chances of identifying areas of concern. A combination of chromoendoscopy and magnification endoscopy may improve targeted biopsy, increasing dyplastic and early neoplastic pick-up. Endoscopic ultrasonography is now well established as the most accurate method of staging tumour extent and nodal involvement in oesophageal carcinoma (Figure 11.2).

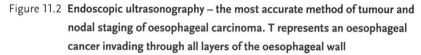

Figure 11.2 **Endoscopic ultrasonography – the most accurate method of tumour and nodal staging of oesophageal carcinoma. T represents an oesophageal cancer invading through all layers of the oesophageal wall**

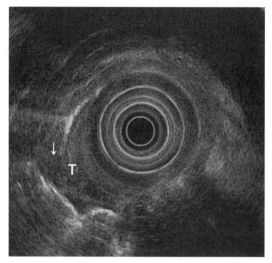

Investigation of the molecular changes that predispose to the development of a cancer may provide a means of identifying the 'at-risk' individuals in whom surveillance is most warranted. One possibility involves screening for one or even a panel of genetic abnormalities (such as mutation of the tumour suppresser gene p. 53). Flow cytometry of cytology samples may be useful to identify cells with abnormal chromosomal numbers and identify predisposition to cancer progression. Currently, no molecular technique is considered to be superior to standard endoscopic biopsies.

Treatment

Both endoscopic and medical therapies have been reported in Barrett's oesophagus with or without dysplastic changes, but no therapy is well established as standard.[10–11] Various ablative therapies of dysplastic areas or cancer have been reported but definitive randomised trial evidence and acceptance is awaited. Examples include photodynamic therapy, electrocoagulation therapy (e.g. argon plasma coagulation) and laser therapy. There are concerns regarding these techniques including recurrence, complications such as stricturing and the possibility of sub-mucosal buried Barrett's (possibly dysplastic) tissue. Further studies are on-going but the potential for a proven local ablation technique that could be used in cases of high grade dysplasia or even early cancers is real.

Endoscopic mucosal resection enables piecemeal resection of a segment of Barrett's or an early cancer whilst allowing a large tissue sample for pathological assessment. It may also be combined with other ablative therapies such as argon plasma coagulation or photodynamic therapy. More studies are needed to further evaluate its use in the treatment of dysplasia and early adenocarcinoma in Barrett's. This technique offers the prospect of a cure by local therapy and may provide an important alternative, in selected cases, to oesophagectomy, especially in frail, elderly patients.

Drugs

The role of proton pump inhibitors (PPIs) in the management of Barrett's remains uncertain. The possibility that PPIs could normalise the pH within the oesophagus and reduce the insult on the epithelium that stimulates proliferation is interesting. There is some data to suggest that PPIs may reduce the rate of dysplasia in Barrett's epithelium or even cause regression of Barrett's. More work is necessary to clarify these possibilities. The use of anti-reflux surgery to achieve similar goals has been disappointing. Currently PPIs are used for symptom control, rather than treatment of Barrett's oesophagus.

Both aspirin and non-steroidal anti-inflammatory drugs (NSAIDs) have been shown to reduce the incidence of carcinoma of the oesophagus. One case-control study demonstrated a reduction in odds-ratio in oesophageal cancer of more than one-third. Large studies are underway to investigate this further. These protective effects may be due to the suppression of cyclo-oxygenase 2 (COX-2) levels in Barrett's epithelium. COX-2 is now known to be widely expressed in cancers and acts in tumour angiogenesis and inhibits apoptosis. It is possible that chemoprevention of adenocarcinoma of the oesophagus may offer the simplest measure with greatest impact, given the frequent occurrence of Barrett's oesophagus in the general population, but considerable further research is required.

Cost-effectiveness of Barrett's oesophagus surveillance and screening has been determined by several groups and recent computer modelling (Markov) determined incremental cost-effectiveness of bi-annual endoscopy to be £9,275 per life-year saved.[12]

Dyspepsia

Dyspepsia refers to the symptom of chronic or recurrent pain or discomfort centred in the upper abdomen. It generally encompasses numerous diagnoses such as GORD (15–25%), gastric and duodenal ulcer disease (15–25%) and also functional dyspepsia (previously known as non-ulcer dyspepsia – 60%). Dyspepsia may be accompanied by symptoms such as nausea, retching, belching, bloating and abdominal fullness. Forty percent of people suffer from dyspepsia in any year, half of whom self-medicate. Dyspepsia accounts for up to 5% of all primary care physician visits. Over the counter remedies in the UK cost £88.5 million in 1999 and the NHS cost of all dyspepsia drugs in England and Wales in 1998 was £520 million (60% on PPIs).[13]

Management guidelines on this common and costly problem were recently issued from the Scottish Intercollegiate Guidelines Network (SIGN).[14] They emphasise that it is important to exclude pathology from surrounding organs in addition to the upper gastrointestinal tract. If symptoms are consistent with reflux then management is as for GORD. It is concluded that alarm features are almost always present in upper gastrointestinal cancer and are therefore useful to determine referral for specialist opinion. In line with the British Society of Gastroenterology (BSG)[15] the SIGN guidelines have increased the age threshold (used to detect cancers) from 45 to 55 years.

The SIGN guidelines, in agreement with the BSG, now advocate a 'test and treat' *Helicobacter pylori* strategy. *H. pylori* is known to be associated with 95% of duodenal ulcers and 70% of gastric ulcers. Eradication of *H. pylori* reduces ulcer disease, the risk of gastric cancer and benefits approximately 10% of functional dyspeptics. This improvement in dyspepsia, through the eradication of *H. pylori*, was demonstrated in the MRC trial that randomised two weeks of omeprazole against two weeks of *H. pylori* treatment (omeprazole, metronidazole and amoxicillin). Dyspepsia resolved in one year at 7% (PPI) against 21% (*H. pylori* eradication).[16] This result is consistent with the largest meta-analysis that examined nine trials and suggested a 9% reduction in the number of dyspeptic patients following eradication.

The other major change is a reduction in the emphasis on endoscopy in dyspepsia. In the over-55 age group (in whom upper gastrointestinal cancer is more common) first-line endoscopy for simple new onset dyspepsia (i.e. in the absence of alarm symptoms) is now not recommended. A treat and test policy is advocated instead. However, if the test is negative or symptoms persist or recur after eradication then referral is considered. In the under-55 age bracket a working diagnosis of functional dyspepsia can be assumed without referral for endoscopy as repeated invasive investigations are felt to be counterproductive.

Test and treat is a non-invasive approach, which compared with prompt endoscopy leads to similar clinical outcomes whilst reducing endoscopy workload.[17] Only 23% (95% CI = 12 to 44%) of patients allocated to *H. pylori* test-and-treat required endoscopy over a one-year follow-up. The UK still has relatively high *H. pylori* prevalence making test-and-treat the most cost effective policy. However, test-and-treat leads to symptom resolution in fewer than

50% of infected un-investigated dyspepsia patients.[18] A combined analysis of two randomised, double-blind studies (ORCHID and OCAY, n=718) investigating the effect of *H. pylori* eradication on symptoms of functional dyspepsia found no difference in response between *H. pylori* negative and positive patients.[19]

Empiric acid-suppression therapy is often used in the initial management of dyspepsia in primary care, and superior symptom relief is obtained by the use of a PPI compared to a H_2 receptor antagonist.[20] Such therapy may also be tried in functional dyspepsia, where a trial of *H. pylori* eradication therapy may also be considered. A summary algorithm of the management of dyspepsia is presented in Figure 11.3.

Figure 11.3 **Management of dyspepsia algorithm based on SIGN guidelines**[14]

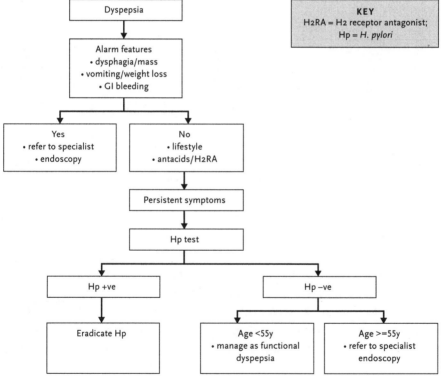

The new NICE guideline, CG17 *Dyspepsia: Managing dyspepsia in adults in primary care*, published August 2004, recommends that routine endoscopy in patients of any age presenting with dyspepsia and without alarm features is not necessary.

Obscure gastrointestinal bleeding

Key messages

- Obscure gastrointestinal bleeding is a difficult clinical problem and may require recurrent admission / investigation / transfusion.

- The diagnostic tests utilised and the extent of investigation of obscure bleeding must be tailored to the individual depending on the patient's duration and severity of bleeding, co-morbidity and previous investigation.

- After normal endoscopy and colonoscopy a small bowel source is likely.

- Enteroscopy has been the main investigative tool with a reasonable diagnostic yield and capability of therapeutic intervention.

- In cases of ongoing bleeding selective angiography may localise the source and enable treatment by embolisation.

- Capsule endoscopy is a novel form of imaging technology that provides a safe and useful diagnostic tool.

The advent of wireless capsule endoscopy has generated considerable excitement and also queries from patients regarding whether this may replace the more invasive conventional endoscopy. Currently however the main application of this technique is in the diagnosis of a small intestinal bleeding source.

Gastrointestinal bleeding is a common clinical problem. In the acute setting a source can often be identified and treatment instituted as necessary following adequate resuscitation. In approximately 5% of cases no cause is identified and bleeding continues overtly intermittently or an occult basis (often presenting as an iron deficiency).[21] Obscure bleeding may be defined as bleeding of unknown origin (after normal upper and lower endoscopy) that persists or recurs. These patients often present a diagnostic challenge.

Further investigation may include repeat upper endoscopy (and small bowel biopsy to rule out coeliac disease) and colonoscopy (with terminal ileoscopy) in the first instance. If normal the source is often in the small bowel. Radiographic imaging has traditionally been the first line of small intestine investigation with either small-bowel follow-through or an enteroclysis (or small bowel enema). The latter is more sensitive but may cause more patient discomfort and entails more radiation. Diagnostic yields are poor – of the order of 5–10%. They may demonstrate small bowel tumours / polyps, diverticular disease and inflammatory small bowel conditions.

Table 11.2 **Causes of obscure gastrointestinal bleeding according to site**

Upper tract	Small bowel	Colon
Erosions in H. hernias	Angiodysplasia	Angiodysplasia
Angiodysplasia	Small bowel tumours	Diverticular bleeding
Oesophageal varices	Small bowel ulcers/erosions	Portal colopathy
Gastric vascular ectasia	Crohn's disease/coeliacs	
	Small bowel diverticulosis	
	Dieulafuoy's	
	Meckels diverticulum	
	Radiation enteritis	
	Haemobilia	

Common causes of small bowel bleeding vary according to age with Meckel's diverticulum in the young, small bowel tumours in the middle-aged and angiodysplasia in the elderly. In view of the fact that the majority of small bowel bleeding is from angiodysplastic lesions (70%), enteroscopy has been advocated as the investigation of choice in obscure bleeding.[22-3] Push enteroscopy allows detection of these mucosal lesions and endotherapy as well as re-examination of the upper tract but is limited in the distal extent reached. Intra-operative enteroscopy remains an alternative in persistent difficult cases. Yield at push enteroscopy is from 30 to 70%.

With intermittent overt blood loss 99 mTc scans or angiography could be used to localise the site during an episode. Selective angiography is more technically difficult but provides superior localisation as well as therapeutic options with embolisation. Selective angiography requires a bleeding rate of 0.5ml/min to identify a source. In the absence of active bleeding angiography may still be useful in identifying small bowel tumours or angiodysplasia by their angiographic characteristics. A computed tomography (CT) scan may be helpful, for example, in diagnosing small bowel tumours, portal hypertension or aorto-enteric fistulae.

Visualisation of the small bowel has been recently advanced by the advent of wireless capsule endoscopy. Each single-use capsule is about the size of a large tablet (11 mm × 26 mm) and can be swallowed with water. It contains a camera, lens, battery, light source and transmitter. Two images per second are transmitted by the capsule to the portable data recorder attached to a waist-belt. The patient has an array of sensors placed on the abdomen that track the location of the capsule as it is propagated through the gut by peristalsis. The capsule is passed in the stools unless there is a stricture causing hold-up. The data is downloaded from the data-recorder at the end of the study to a workstation for interpretation. Capsule endoscopy appears well tolerated by patients. Contraindications include pregnancy and bowel obstruction/strictures.

Initial data for the use of capsule endoscopy in cases of obscure bleeding is promising. It was found to be superior to small bowel radiography[24]– the barium study was diagnostic in 20% of cases compared to 45% definite diagnoses with the capsule and suspected diagnoses in a further 40% (but not definite). Other studies confirm a diagnostic yield of about 60%.[25-6] Initial indications are that long-term outcomes such as transfusions, procedures and hospitalisation are significantly improved. Clearly wireless endoscopy offers no therapeutic option and endoscopic or surgical intervention is often required. Capsule endoscopy has rapidly gained acceptance as a valid tool in obscure bleeding. The capsule gives poor oesophageal, gastric and colonic views. Technological modifications to improve upper gastrointestinal and colonic images are under investigation. New areas of application are being investigated including the assessment of small bowel Crohn's disease. Capsule endoscopy has been used to investigate NSAID induced small bowel strictures and ulcers. It appears we have been underestimating the frequency of common small bowel injury secondary to NSAIDs.

Figure 11.4 **Capsule endoscopy showing small intestinal ulceration due to NSAID**

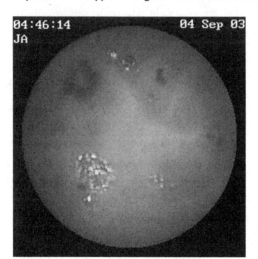

Osteoporosis in gastrointestinal diseases

Considerable research over the past decade has firmly established the association of several gastrointestinal diseases with osteopaenia. Osteopaenia is currently considered to be a significant problem in inflammatory bowel disease (IBD), coeliac disease, post-gastrectomy state and chronic liver disease, especially primary biliary cirrhosis. IBD is now well recognised to be associated with osteopaenia, though generally the effect is relatively modest. Overall, the prevalence of osteoporosis (T score < -2.5) in IBD is approximately 15%. Both corticosteroid use and inflammatory disease activity are associated with osteopaenia, but vitamin D deficiency is uncommon. In a survey of British General Practice using the General Practice Research Database, 231,778 fracture cases and 231,778 age- and sex-matched controls were studied. Patients with IBD had an increased risk of vertebral fracture (OR 1.72, 95% CI = 1.13 to 2.61) and hip fracture (OR 1.59, 95% CI = 1.14 to 2.23). The risk of hip fracture was greater in patients with Crohn's disease compared with patients with ulcerative colitis.[27] Only 13% of patients with IBD who sustained a fracture were on any form of bone-protective therapy. Osteoporosis is also more common in untreated coeliac disease than in the general population, with a prevalence of approximately 28% at the spine and 15% at the hip (AGA). Osteoporosis and osteomalacia may both occur post-gastrectomy and the prevalence of osteoporosis may be particularly high (32–42%).

Dual energy X-ray absorptiometry (DEXA) scans are used to diagnose and risk stratify osteopaenia in gastrointestinal diseases. Quantitative ultrasonography of the calcaneum has recently emerged as a valuable inexpensive, portable, radiation-free tool for assessing bone density. IBD patients considered to be at risk, coeliac patients a year after initiation of gluten free diet and post-gastrectomy patients ten years after surgery, should undergo DEXA scans to assess bone mineral density. Corticosteroid therapy should be kept to a minimum in IBD patients and steroid sparing drugs such as azathioprine considered early. In ileal Crohn's disease, budesonide with low systemic side-effects may be preferable to prednisolone. Correction of nutritional deficiencies is necessary in all gastrointestinal diseases including vitamin D, vitamin K and calcium supplementation. Vitamin D and calcium supplementation should be given to those at high risk of osteoporosis or those with established osteoporosis. Bisphosphonates are approved for use in patients who cannot withdraw from corticosteroids after three months of use, and in patients with known osteoporosis or atraumatic fractures.[28] Oestrogen therapy must be balanced against significant risks, which have been well publicised recently. A selective oestrogen receptor modulator may be used for prevention or treatment of osteoporosis in postmenopausal women, but this decision should be taken in a specialised osteoporosis clinic.

The general indications for DEXA scan and principles of management of osteoporosis in gastrointestinal diseases are summarised in Tables 11.3 and 11.4.

Table 11.3 **General indications for DEXA scan in gastrointestinal diseases**

IBD	Coeliac disease	Post-gastrectomy state
Prolonged steroid use (>3 month consecutive or recurrent courses)	All adults one year after gluten-free diet	Low trauma fracture
Low trauma fractures		Post-menopausal female or male aged >50
Post-menopausal female or male aged >50		Hypogonadism 10 years after surgery
Hypogonadism		

Table 11.4 **General management approach to osteopaenia in gastrointestinal diseases**

T-score >-1
Calcium/vitamin D
Weight-bearing exercise
Stop smoking
Avoid alcohol excess
Minimise steroids
Correct hypogonadism
T score -2.5 to -1
As above *plus*
If prolonged steroids, consider bisphosphonates
Repeat DEXA in 1–2 years
T score <-2.5 (or vertebral compression fractures)
Bisphosphonates
Exclude other causes of low bone mineral density, e.g. osteomalacia
Consider bone clinic referral

Colorectal cancer

Colorectal cancer is common, affecting approximately 30,000 people each year in UK, with an average five-year survival rate of 40%.[29] Early diagnosis improves prognosis and there is consensus about the requirement to screen people at increased risk of colorectal cancer. Within the resources currently available in the UK, people with a lifetime risk of less than one in ten do not generally qualify for screening. The standard method of screening is colonoscopy, and patients should be aware of the balance between reasonable risk reduction and detrimental effects of screening both specific to colonoscopy (perforation, haemorrhage, death) and general (i.e. anxiety, false alarm, false reassurance and over-diagnosis).

Follow-up after colorectal resection for carcinoma is common, but the benefits are uncertain. It is considered reasonable to perform a colonoscopy five years after surgery and thereafter at five-yearly intervals up to the age of 70 years.[30] During the first two years after surgery, liver imaging (CT scan, ultrasonography) may be offered to asymptomatic patients under the age of 70 years. The role of carcinoembryonic antigen (CEA) monitoring is uncertain. In Scotland, a randomised controlled trial showed that discharge to GP-based follow-up after colorectal resection was no worse than hospital surgical outpatient follow-up. Furthermore, the increased GP workload was only two extra surgery attendances per doctor per year and the majority of GPs were willing to undertake this work.[31]

Given that colorectal adenomas are very common and one-third of the population may develop a colorectal adenoma by the age of 60, colonoscopic surveillance after polypectomy should be advised, judiciously taking into account patient preferences, co-morbidity and age and the level of risk. In patients with only one or two small (< 10 mm) adenomas, five-yearly surveillance until one negative examination should suffice and indeed it may be acceptable to have no follow-up at all. Those with larger, < 10 mm adenomas or three or four small adenomas may require more frequent follow-up colonoscopies every three years until two consecutive colonoscopies are negative.[32] Only occasionally in the presence of five or more adenomas, or three or more adenomas with at least one being ≥ 10 mm is more frequent colonoscopy warranted. Many departments in the UK frequently perform colonoscopies unnecessarily, thus increasing patient waiting time. The cut-off age for stopping surveillance depends primarily on patient wishes and co-morbidity but is usually around the age of 75 years.

It is recommended that referrals from the community based solely on family history of colorectal cancer should be centralised to permit proper audit and the Regional Genetics Service might be well placed to provide a point of referral. Many referrals are however generated on minimal symptoms and a family history and serve as population screening by proxy. Patients with one first degree relative aged < 45 years affected by colorectal cancer or those with two affected first degree relatives may be considered for surveillance and referral to Clinical Genetics Service.[33] Such surveillance would generally involve a colonoscopy at initial consultation or between the ages of 35–40 years whichever is the later, and further colonoscopy at the age of 55 years.

A summary of the current key British Society of Gastroenterology guidelines are provided in Tables 11.5 and 11.6. The wider US recommendations are mentioned in Table 11.7.

Table 11.5 **British Society of Gastroenterology (BSG) recommendations for colonoscopic follow up after detection of adenomas**

Low risk 1–2 adenomas, <1 cm	None or five years *till 1 neg.*
Intermediate risk 3–4 adenomas or at least one >1 cm	Every three years *till 2 consq. neg*
High risk >5 adenomas or >3 adenomas (one >1 cm)	Annual followed by every three years

Table 11.6 **BSG Recommendations for family groups**

Relatives affected	Recommendation
Two first degree relatives or one first degree relative <45 years with colorectal cancer	Colonoscopy at first consultation or at age 35–40 years, whichever is later. If clear, repeat colonoscopy at age 55 years.
More than two first degree relatives affected or at risk of HNPCC*	Colonoscopy aged 25 years, or five years before earliest colorectal cancer. Gastroscopy at age 50 years, or five years before earliest gastric cancer in family. Two-yearly colonoscopy and gastroscopy. Refer to clinical genetics.

* HNPCC = Hereditary non-polyposis colon cancer

Table 11.7 **US recommendations for colorectal cancer screening in average risk population**

General population	FOBT & sigmoidoscopy every 3–5 years or colonoscopy every 10 years, beginning at age 50 years.
Subjects with 1st degree relatives with CRC	FOBT annually & sigmoidoscopy every 3–5 years or colonoscopy every 10 years, begining at age 40 years.

Significant advances in CT scans, providing 'virtual' imaging of the colon, now offers a realistic hope of non-invasive screening for colonic polyps and cancers. Virtual colonoscopy or CT colonography is a rapidly advancing technique in which imaging data from CT is computer-processed to generate two and three dimensional views of the colon and rectum (Figure 11.5).

Figure 11.5 **Virtual colonosopy images of the colon showing a polyp**

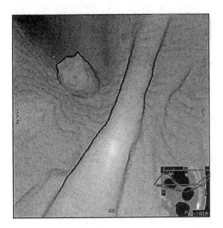
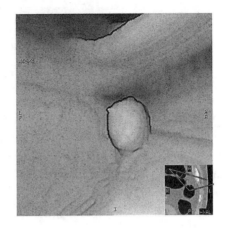

The sensitivity of primary three-dimensional virtual colonoscopy has been found to be 93.8% for polyps at least 10 mm in diameter, 93.9% for polyps at least 8 mm in diameter and 88.7% for polyps at least 6 mm in diameter.[34] Patient acceptance of virtual colonoscopy is high. Ideally, detection of polyps at virtual colonoscopy should lead to colonoscopy on the same or next day enabling preparation for colon cleansing only once prior to virtual colonoscopy. Further advances in this technology is expected, and this promises to be a valuable additional tool for colorectal cancer screening.

Chemoprevention of colorectal carcinoma is an area of intense research. Cohort and case control studies have consistently showed a risk reduction of 40–50% associated with aspirin use. A large randomised controlled trial in US on 1121 patients with a recent history of colorectal adenomas assigned to placebo (n=372), 81 mg of aspirin (n=377) or 325 mg of aspirin (n=372) demonstrated moderate chemopreventive effect of low-dose aspirin. Unadjusted relative risks of any adenomas were 0.81 (95% CI=0.69 to 0.96) in the low-dose aspirin and 0.96 (95% CI=0.81 to 1.13) in the 325 mg aspirin groups compared with placebo.[35] A smaller European study on 272 patients[36] with history of colorectal adenomas showed that daily soluble aspirin (160 or 300 mg/day) to be associated with reduction of risk for recurrent adenomas found at colonoscopy one year after starting treatment, with a relative risk of 0.73 (95% CI=0.52 to 1.04). The chemopreventive effect of 325 mg of aspirin in 635 patients with previous colorectal carcinomas recruited in a randomised placebo-controlled trial was more impressive, with an adjusted relative risk of 0.65 (95% CI=0.46 to 0.91) compared with placebo for recurrence of adenomas.[37] Longer follow-up data is required, and the optimum dose of aspirin is unclear.

Irritable bowel syndrome

Irritable bowel syndrome (IBS) is a common functional disorder characterised by abdominal pain or discomfort accompanied by symptoms of disturbed defaecation. From 35 to 41% of symptomatic gastrointestinal outpatients are diagnosed to have functional gastrointestinal disorders, of which IBS is the most common diagnosis.[38-9] In south-west England, the prevalence of IBS in females (aged 25–69 years) was 13% and in males (aged 40–69 years) was 5%.[40] IBS is characterised by three inter-related physiological abnormalities, though none is specific and unique enough to IBS to be useful as diagnostic tool (Figure 11.6).

Figure 11.6 **Three inter-related physiological abnormalities in irritable bowel syndrome**

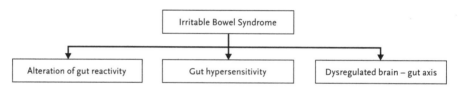

Patients with IBS seen at referral centres usually have greater psychological disturbances than those seen in primary care or non-patients in the community. In many patients a positive diagnosis of IBS may be made safely rather than achieving a diagnosis of exclusion. Alarm symptoms that must be excluded are shown in Box 11.2. The Rome II diagnostic criteria is useful not only for recruiting patients into trials, but also as a guide towards a positive diagnosis (Box 11.3).[41]

Box 11.2 **Alarm symptoms/signs which must be excluded prior to reaching a diagnosis of irritable bowel syndrome**

- Fever
- Weight loss
- Blood in stool (rather than just on wiping)
- Nocturnal diarrhoea disturbing sleep
- Family history of inflammatory bowel disease/colon carcinoma
- Abnormal physical findings, such as abdominal mass

- Abnormal rectal examination/sigmoidoscopy

- Anaemia

- Elevated C-reactive protein/Erythrocyte Sedimentation rate (ESR)

Box 11.3 **Rome II criteria for diagnosis of irritable bowel syndrome**

Abdominal pain/discomfort that has at least two out of the following three features for at least 12 weeks out of the preceding one year:

1. Relieved on defaecation.

2. Onset of pain associated with a change in frequency of stool.

3. Onset of pain associated with a change in stool form.

The following symptoms cumulatively support the diagnosis of irritable bowel syndrome

1. Abnormal stool frequency.

2. Abnormal stool form.

3. Straining, urgency or a feeling of incomplete evacuation.

4. Passage of mucus.

5. Bloating or a feeling of abdominal distension.

Though altered gastrointestinal motility may be frequently demonstrated in IBS, this is not diagnostic. Currently there is considerable research attention to visceral hypersensitivity, which is considered by many, but not all, researchers as a hallmark of IBS. Understanding of the neurohumoral modulation of gut sensitivity is opening the avenue for research into a number of therapeutic targets. Neural control of the gut is represented at multiple levels (Figure 11.7) permitting a whole range of physical, emotional, psychological and immunological triggers to alter gut sensitivity and motility. More recently, evidence of subtle inflammation and alteration of gut immune function have been described in IBS and especially post-infectious IBS patients. These have included increased number of mast cells,[42] lymphocytic infiltrates of myenteric plexus and lamina propria with increased interleukin 1b messenger RNA,[43] and an increase in enterochromaffin cells.[43] This raises the possibility that in a subset of IBS patients, such as post-infectious IBS which develops in 7–30% of patients recovering from bacterial gastroenteritis,[44] subtle inflammation and resultant alteration of afferent receptors may underlie the pathogenesis.

Figure 11.7 **Levels of neural regulation of the gut relevant in irritable bowel syndrome**

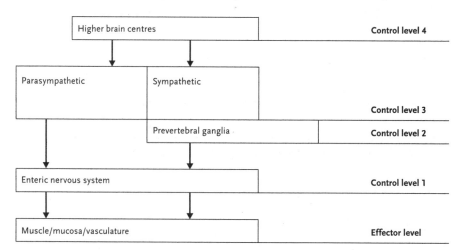

There is abundant evidence that IBS patients have significantly poorer quality of life than the general population. Reassurance, education and over-the-counter medications generally suffice for patients with mild symptoms, often managed in the community. Patients with moderate symptoms often require pharmacological and or psychological treatments (hypnotherapy, relaxation techniques). Pharmacological therapies include antidepressants which may alter visceral sensitivity and pain threshold. Tricyclic antidepressants, are often used in doses lower than antidepressant doses, but selective serotonin re-uptake inhibitors (SSRIs) may be better tolerated. Newly available agents acting on the 5-HT receptor may help abdominal pain, and choice depends on whether stool habits are primarily diarrhoeal (alosetron) or constipation (tegaserod). Alosetron hydrochloride, a selective 5-HT₃ antagonist, has shown moderate efficacy in relieving abdominal pain and normalising bowel frequency and urgency in female patients with diarrhoea-predominant IBS.[45] A significant adverse event, ischaemic colitis, occurring in 0.1–1% of patients, led to withdrawal of the drug from the market in November 2000, followed by re-approval in spring 2002 by the FDA under restrictive guidelines. A further 5-HT₃ antagonist, cilansetron, has shown similar efficacy to alosetron, but has also worked in male patients and awaits phase III trials. The 5-HT₄ agonists in contrast are effective in constipation predominant IBS, the prototype drug being the partial agonist tegaserod. The 5-HT modulators are not currently licensed in UK. The very small proportion of patients with severe and refractory symptoms may require expert psychological support and involvement of a multidisciplinary pain team.[46]

Inflammatory bowel disease

Key messages

- Biological therapies such as infliximab will play an increasing role in the management of Crohn's disease.

- Reduction in hospitalisation and surgery may offset some of the expense of infliximab therapy.

- There is an increasing trend to use immunomodulatory drugs such as azathioprine in IBD as steroid sparing agents.

Most of the advances have occurred in Crohn's disease (CD). CD is a chronic, relapsing inflammatory disorder of the gastrointestinal tract of unknown aetiology. Both genetic factors and environmental triggers are involved in disease initiation, while gut commensal bacterial flora are required for disease perpetuation. Identification of *NOD2/CARD 15* gene mutations and its association with ileal CD confirm both the genetic basis and the heterogeneity of genotype–phenotype associations.[47-8] CD is medically incurable and unlike ulcerative colitis, CD is not surgically curable. The prevalence of CD in the Western world is approximately 50–100 / 100,000 population and in UK the prevalence is 62.5217 / 100,000. The annual incidence is about 6–8 / 100,000 population. The pathogenesis of the chronic inflammation is related to significant intestinal mucosal immune dysregulation.

Table 11.8 **Course of Crohn's disease after therapy**

Country	Cohort	Reference	Indicator	Outcome
Sweden	N = 196 (1979–1987)	Munkholm *et al*[49]	Immediate outcome after 30 days; Prolonged outcome 30 days after therapy stopped	Complete remission 48%, partial remission 32%, no response 20% Prolonged steroid response 44%, steroid dependent 36%, steroid resistant 20%
Norway	N = 232 (1990–93)	Moum *et al*[50]	One year relapse rate	47% relapsed, 10% of whom had chronic relapsing course
Olmstead county, Minnesota USA	N = 173 (1970–93) Population-based	Faubion *et al*[51]	Immediate (30 days) after 1st course of therapy; 1 year outcome	Complete remission 58%, partial remission 26%, no response 16% Prolonged response 32%, steroid dependent 28%, surgery 38% (only 43% ever received steroids)

Conventional therapy with corticosteroids is disappointing in the long-term (Table 11.8)[49–51] and associated with considerable adverse effects. In the last decade the management of CD has altered rapidly with a more widespread and aggressive use of immunosuppressive medications such as 6-mercaptopurine/ azathioprine and methotrexate. Furthermore, less reliance is placed on corticosteroids, especially in paediatric practice where defined formula diets are widely used in Europe. It is important to consider the different components of analysis of this complex disease to decide on the optimal course of management (Box 11.4).

Box 11.4 Components of clinical analysis for a patient with Crohn's disease

- disease inflammatory activity
- extent and distribution of chronic destructive inflammation
- mechanical obstruction
- abscess or fistulation
- nutritional status/osteopaenia
- iatrogenic problems
- extraintestinal disease
- psychosocial factors

The term biological agents is often used to refer to engineered synthetic antibodies, cytokines and growth factor peptides with potent effects on the immune system and repair processes. Nucleic-acid-based therapies such as antisense oligonucleotides and gene therapies may also be included under the umbrella term of biological agents. Infliximab, the chimeric monoclonal antibody to Tumour Necrosis Factor (TNF) is the prototype of such agents and has been licensed for use in CD disease for over four years. Most new agents will now be judged against the therapeutic efficacy standards set by infliximab.

Infliximab

Infliximab is a chimeric IgG1 monoclonal antibody that is approximately 75% human and 25% murine. Infliximab has been shown to be effective in the treatment of moderate to severe active and fistulizing CD. The principal use of infliximab is in treating patients not responding to conventional therapies or developing unacceptable side effects. This is a significant advance in the management of CD, and despite its high cost, may reduce hospitalisation, surgery and morbidity of CD not responding to conventional drugs.

Serious and opportunistic infections may occur after anti-TNF therapy. Infliximab therapy has been associated with tuberculosis, histoplasmosis, listeriosis and aspergillosis and similar problems have been reported with the use of etanercept in rheumatoid arthritis.

The NICE guidelines (Box 11.5) currently govern the use of infliximab in CD in UK,[52] but increasing use of maintenance therapy is likely.

Box 11.5 **NICE recommendations for infliximab use in Crohn's disease (Issue April 2002; review May 2005)**

- severe active CD (CDAI ≥ 300)
- refractory to AZA, 6-MP, MTX
- surgery inappropriate. Fistulizing disease needs to have all the other criteria
- repeated episodic therapy provided other criteria met

References

1. Allum W H, Griffin S M, A Watson, *et al.* Guidelines for the management of oesophageal and gastric cancer. *Gut* 2002; **50 (S5)**: v1–v23

2. Lagergren J, Bergstrom R, Lindgren A, *et al.* Symptomatic gastroesophageal reflux as a risk factor for esophageal cancer. *N Engl J Med* 1999; **340**: 825–31

3. Guindi M, Riddell R H. The pathology of epithelial pre-malignancy of the gastrointestinal tract. *Best Pract Res Clin Gastroenterol* 2001; **15**: 191–210

4. Corley A, Levin T R, Habel LA, Weiss N S, *et al.* Surveillance and survival in Barrett's adenocarcinomas: A population based study. *Gastroenterology* 2002; **12**: 633–40

5. Craanen M E, Kulpers E J. Advantages and disadvantages of population screening and surveillance of at-risk groups. *Best Pract Res Clin Gastroenterol* 2001; **15**: 211–26

6. Mandall A, Playford R J, Wicks A C. Current Practice in surveillance strategy for patients with Barrett's oesophagus in the UK. *Aliment Pharmacol Ther* 2002; **17**: 1319–24

7. Sampliner R E and the Practice Parameters Committee. Practice guidelines on the diagnosis, surveillance, and the therapy of Barretts surveillance. *Am J Gastroenterol* 2002; **97**: 1888–95

8. Rollins A M, Sivak M V. Potential new endoscopic techniques for the earlier diagnosis of pre-malignancy. *Best Pract Res Clin Gastroenterol* 2001; **15**: 227–47

9. Slehria S, Sharma P. Barrett Esophagus. *Curr Opin Gastroenterol* 2003; **19(4)**: 387–93

10. Shami V M, Waxman I. Endoscopic Treatment of Early Gastroesophageal Malignancy. *Curr Opin Gastroenterol* 2002; **18**: 587–94

11. Pech O, Gossner L, May A, Ell C. Management of Barrett's oesophagus, dysplasia and early adenocarcinoma. *Best Pract Res Clin Gastroenterol* 2001; **15**: 267–84

12. Sonnenberg A, Soni A, Sampliner R E. Medical decision analysis of endoscopic surveillance of Barrett's oesophagus to prevent oesophageal adenocarcinoma. *Aliment Pharmacol Ther* 2002; **16**: 41–50

13. National Institute for Clinical Excellence. Technology Appraisal Guidance No. 7: Proton pump inhibitors in the treatment of dyspepsia. London: NICE, 2000

14. Scottish Intercollegiate Guidelines Network. *Dyspepsia: A national clinical guideline.* Edinburgh: SIGN, March 2003

15. British Society of Gastroenterology. *Dyspepsia Management Guidelines.* (Updated April 2002). London: BSG, 2002

16. McColl K, Murray L, El-Omar E, Dickson A, *et al.* Symptomatic Benefit from eradicating helicobacter pylori infection in patients with nonulcer dyspepsia. *N Engl J Med* 1998; **339**: 1869–74

17. Delaney B C, Innes M A, Deeks J, *et al.* Initial management strategies for dyspepsia (Cochrane Review). In: *The Cochrane Library.* Issue 4. Oxford: Update Software, 2002

18. Laine L, Schoenfeld P, Fennerty M B. Therapy for *Helicobacter pylori* in patients with nonulcer dyspepsia: a meta-analysis of randomised, controlled trials. *Ann Intern Med* 2001; **134**: 361–69

19. Veldhuyzen van Zanten S J, Talley N J, Blum A L, *et al.* Combined analysis of the ORCHID and OCAY studies: does eradication of *Helicobacter pylori* lead to sustained improvement in functional dyspepsia symptoms? *Gut* 2002; **50 (S4)**: iv26–iv30

20. Jones R H, Baxter G. Lansoprozole 30 mg daily versus ranitidine 150 mg b.d. in the treatment of acid-related dyspepsia in general practice. *Aliment Pharmacol Ther* 1997; **11**: 541–6

21. Zuckermann G R, Prakash C, Askin M P, Lewis B S. AGA technical review on the evaluation and management of occult and obscure gastrointestinal bleeding. *Gastroenterology* 2000; **118**: 201–21

22. Van Gossum A. Obscure digestive bleeding. *Best Pract Res Clin Gastroenterol* 2001; **15**: 155–74

23. Shields S J, Van Dam J. In pursuit of the hidden, the occult, and the obscure. *Gastroenterology* 1999; **117**: 273–5

24. Costamagna G, Shah S K, Riccioni M E, Foschia F, *et al.* A prospective trial comparing small bowel radiographs and video capsule endoscopy for suspected small bowel disease. *Gastroenterology* 2002; **123**: 999–1005

25. Leighton J, Sharma V, Malikowski M, Fleischer D. Long term clinical outcomes of capsule endoscopy in patients with obscure gastrointestinal bleeding. *Am J Gastroenterol* 2003; **98**: S300

26. Faigel D O, Fennerty M B. Cutting the cord for capsule endoscopy. *Gastroenterology* 2002; **123**: 1385–7

27. Van Staa T-P, Cooper C, Brusse L S, *et al.* Inflammatory bowel disease and the risk of fracture. *Gastroenterology* 2003; **125**: 1591–7

28. American Gastroenterological Association Medical Position Statement (unsigned). Guidelines on osteoporosis in gastrointestinal diseases. *Gastroenterology* 2003; **124**: 791–94

29. Cairns S, Scholefield J H. Guidelines for colorectal cancer screening in high risk groups. *Gut* 2002; **51 (SV)**: v1–v2

30. Scholefield J H, Steele R J. Guidelines for follow up after resection of colorectal cancer. *Gut* 2002; **51 (SV)**: v3–v5

31. Florey CV, Yule B, Fogg A, *et al*. A randomized trial of immediate discharge of surgical patients to general practice. *J Public Health Med* 1994; **16**: 455–64

32. Atkin W, Saunders B P. Surveillance guidelines after removal of colorectal adenomatous polyps. *Gut* 2002; **51 (SV)**: v6–v9

33. Dunlop M. Guidance on large bowel surveillance for people with two first degree relatives with colorectal cancer or one first degree relative diagnosed with colorectal cancer under 45 years. *Gut* 2002; **51 (suppl V)**: v17–v20

34. Pickhardt P J, Choi J R, Hwang I, *et al*. Computed tomographic virtual colonoscopy to screen for colorectal neoplasia in asymptomatic adults. *N Engl J Med* 2003; **349**: 2191–200

35. Baron J A, Cole B F, Sandler R S, *et al*. A randomised trial of aspirin to prevent colorectal adenomas. *N Engl J Med* 2003; **348**: 891–9

36. Benamouzig R, Deyra J, Martin A, *et al*. Daily soluble aspirin and prevention of colorectal adenoma recurrence: one-year results of the APACC trial. *Gastroenterology* 2003; **125**: 328–36

37. Sandler R S, Halabi S, Baron J A, *et al*. A randomised trial of aspirin to prevent colorectal adenomas in patients with previous colorectal cancer. *N Engl J Med* 2003; **348**: 883–90

38. Mitchell C M, Drossman D A. Survey of the AGA membership relating to patients with functional gastrointestinal disorders. *Gastroenterology* 1987; **92**: 1282–4

39. Russo M W, Gaynes B N, Drossman D A. A national survey of practice patterns of gastroenterologists with comparison to the past two decades. *J Clin Gastroenterol* 1999; **29**: 339–43

40. Heaton K W, O'Donnell L J D, Braddon F E M, *et al*. Symptoms of irritable bowel syndrome in a British urban community: consulters and nonconsulters. *Gastroenterology* 1992; **102**: 1962–7

41. Thompson W G, Longstreth G F, Drossman D A, *et al*. C. Functional bowel disorders and D. Functional abdominal pain. In: Drossman D A, Talley NJ, Thompson W G, Whitehead W E, Corazziari E, (eds). *Rome II: Functional gastrointestinal disorders: diagnosis, pathophysiology and treatment*. 2 ed. McLean, V A: Degnon Associates, 2000; 351–432

42. O'Sullivan M, Clayton N, Breslin N P, *et al*. Increased mast cells in the irritable bowel syndrome. *Neurogastroenterol Motil* 2000; **12**: 449–57

43. Spiller R C, Jenkins D, Thornley J P, *et al*. Increased rectal mucosal neuroendocrine cells, T lymphocytes, and increased gut permeability following acute Campylobacter enteritis and in post-dysenteric irritable bowel syndrome. *Gut* 2000; **47**: 804–11

44. Neal K R, Hebden J, Spiller R. Prevalence of gastrointestinal symptoms six months after bacterial gastroenteritis and risk factors for development of the irritable bowel syndrome: postal survey of patients. *BMJ* 1997; **7083**: 779–82

45. Camilleri M, Mayer E A, Drossman D A, *et al*. Improvement in pain and bowel function in female irritable bowel patients with alosteron, a 5-HT_3 receptor antagonist. *Aliment Pharmacol Ther* 1999; **13**: 1149–59

46. American Gastroenterological Association Medical Position Statement (unsigned). Irritable Bowel Syndrome. *Gastroenterology* 2002; **123**: 2105–07

47. Bonen D K, Cho J H. The genetics of inflammatory bowel disease. *Gastroenterology* 2003; **124 (2)**: 521–36

48. Ahmad T, Armuzzi A, Bunce M, *et al.* The molecular classification of the clinical manifestations of Crohn's disease. *Gastroenterology* 2002; **122 (4)**: 854–66

49. Munkholm P, Langholz E, Davidsen M, Binder V. Frequency of glucocorticoid resistance and dependency in Crohn's disease. *Gut* 1994; **35 (3)**: 360–2

50. Moum B, Ekbom A, Vatn M H, *et al.* Clinical course during the 1st year after diagnosis in ulcerative colitis and Crohn's disease. Results of a large, prospective population-based study in southeastern Norway, 1990–93. *Scand J Gastroenterol* 1997; **32 (10)**: 1005–12

51. Faubion W A, Loftus E V, Harmsen W S, Zinsmeister A R, Sandborn W J. The natural history of corticosteroid therapy for inflammatory bowel disease: a population based study. *Gastroenterology* 2001; **121 (2)**: 255–60

52. National Institute for Clinical Excellence. *Guidance on the use of infliximab for Crohn's disease. Technology Appraisal Guidance No. 40.* London: N ICE, April 2002

Further reading

AGA Technical Review on Irritable Bowel Syndrome (unsigned). *Gastroenterology* 2002; **123**: 2108–31

AGA Technical Review on Osteoporosis in Gastrointestinal Diseases (unsigned). *Gastroenterology* 2003; **124**: 795–841

CHAPTER 12

Neurology

Leone Ridsdale, Andrew Dowson, Greg Rogers

KEY MESSAGES	▶ **Neurological problems are common in primary care, particularly headache and epilepsy.**
▶ HEADACHE	• A diagnostic screen for headache can be conducted using a brief four-item questionnaire.
	• Migraine is the default diagnosis for patients with episodic, disabling headache.
	• Management strategies should be tailored to the patient's individual needs, by eliciting illness severity and the patient's preferences and co-morbidities.
	• Optimal management may be obtained with long-term follow up and a team approach to care.
▶ EPILEPSY	• With a list size of 2000 people an average GP will see a new patient with epilepsy every 1–2 years and should have 10–20 patients on his/her list with an established diagnosis of epilepsy.
	• An accurate history must be obtained from the patient and a witness, as the diagnosis of epilepsy is largely made on the basis of the history alone.
	• An attempt should always be made to classify the seizure type and epilepsy syndrome as this has implications for management and prognosis.

RECENT ADVANCES ▼

► HEADACHE

- National guidelines now exist for the management of migraine in primary care.

- Principles of headache practice have been agreed for international use.

- A framework for the implementation of a service for General Practitioners with a Special Interest (GPwSIs) in Headache has been produced by the DoH/RCGP.

► EPILEPSY

- Intermediate care, such as that provided by a GPwSI and/or an epilepsy specialist nurse, offers a new resource in the treatment of epilepsy.

Introduction

In the NHS the number of neurologists per head of population is low, with one neurologist for a population of 140,000.[1] Other European countries have one neurologist for a population of between 8000 and 38,000.[2] Neurologists in the UK divide their week working in district hospitals and neurological centres. This has made community team-building more challenging. The shortage of neurologists together with a focus on tertiary centres can be linked to less training in neurology for those doctors who train and work in district hospitals and primary care. In this context, doctors complain of a lack of confidence and competence in neurology, amounting to neurophobia.[3]

Nevertheless, disorders of the nervous system are common and GPs need to be open to potential learning gaps, particularly for conditions that they see frequently in primary care. What are the commonest neurological disease groups for which patients consult GPs? The RCGP morbidity statistics are shown in Table 12.1.[4]

Table 12.1 **Incidence and prevalence of neurological disorders over one year (1991–1992)**

Disease group	New or first ever episodes	Period prevalence
Migraine	94	115
Cerebrovascular disease	51	71
Neuropathy	33	36
Intervertebral disc disorders	26	39
Epilepsy	12	36
Dementia	8	18
Parkinson's disease	5	15
Multiple sclerosis	2	7

Source – **General Practice Morbidity Survey (1995)**[4]

Neurological disorders tend to be chronic, and represent the category of disease most likely to lead to disability. Table 12.1 shows that disorders such as epilepsy, dementia, Parkinson's disease and multiple sclerosis are particularly likely to require frequent attendance with a doctor.

Perceived lack of neurological expertise may lead to referral of patients, when some problems could be managed in general practice. For example, patients with migraine and other headache are the commonest group of new referrals seen by neurologists, accounting for about 25% of new appointment spaces.[5] Epilepsy is one of the commonest serious neurological disorders seen in general practice, in A&E and in hospital. Managing diabetes presents similar challenges to managing epilepsy, and specialists have created teams that educate and link-up care in the community. But patients with epilepsy have frequently not been advised and monitored by their GP or any other doctor.[6] Approximately 10% of people with epilepsy have attacks that are difficult to control, and poor management has been implicated in the fact that people with epilepsy are at three times the risk of suffering sudden unexpected death.[7] Good pro-active advice in the context of an integrated service provided by doctors and nurses may reduce A&E attendance, hospitalisation and mortality from epilepsy.

In view of the frequency and workload implications of migraine/headache disorders and the epilepsies, we have focused the rest of this chapter on recent advances in their diagnosis and management.

Epidemiology of migraine and other headaches

Headache is the commonest neurological condition, with about 70% of the general population reporting one or more headaches per month. Over 60% of the adult population have experienced tension type headaches (TTH),[8] while in population-based studies, the prevalence of migraine has been shown to be about 12% worldwide.[9] The other common major headache subtype is chronic daily headache (CDH), which affects about 4% of adults.[10] Other headache subtypes are relatively scarce, affecting 0.1% or less of adults.

Migraine starts during childhood and adolescence, peaks in prevalence during early middle age and declines in prevalence as sufferers move into old age.[9] Migraine is about three times more common in women than in men, affecting about 15% and 6%, respectively.[9] Migraine is also common in children. Overall, about 10% of children aged 5–15 years have migraine, rising from < 5% in those aged five years to 15% or more in those aged 12 years and older.[11] Migraine without aura is much more common than migraine with aura, accounting for about 90% of sufferers. Most sufferers who do have aura symptoms also suffer from attacks of migraine without aura.[9]

Overview of diagnosis
International Headache Society criteria
The International Headache Society (IHS) has published comprehensive diagnostic criteria for migraine, as shown below.[12]

▶ The occurrence of five or more lifetime headache attacks with similar features lasting from 4–72 hours each, patients being symptom-free between attacks.

▶ The presence of two or more of the following headache features:
  ▷ moderate to severe pain
  ▷ pain on one side of the head
  ▷ throbbing or pulsating headaches
  ▷ headaches exacerbated by routine activities (such as climbing stairs).

▶ The presence of one or more non-headache associated symptoms:
  ▷ aura symptoms, which must also satisfy additional strict criteria[12]
  ▷ nausea during the headache
  ▷ photophobia and/or phonophobia during the headache.

▶ The exclusion of secondary headaches, by a search for 'headache alarms', by history taking or physical examination.

These criteria are too strict and inflexible. For example, a patient with severe bilateral headache associated with photophobia and phonophobia can be diagnosed with migraine, even though they do not satisfy all the above criteria. Simpler and more user-friendly diagnostic criteria are needed for use by primary care physicians.

New diagnostic criteria for migraine

Recent initiatives by the UK Migraine in Primary Care Advisors (MIPCA) and the international Headache Care for Practising Clinicians (HCPC) organisations have led to the development of a new diagnostic screening questionnaire for migraine (Figure 12.1).[13–14] The four-item questionnaire is based on key features of the IHS diagnostic criteria,[12] but takes advantage of recent research, which shows that high-impact episodic headaches are almost always due to migraine.[15] In this scheme, TTH, migraine and chronic headaches can be distinguished and additional questioning used to confirm the diagnoses.

Figure 12.1 **New screening questionnaire for headache diagnosis** [13–14]

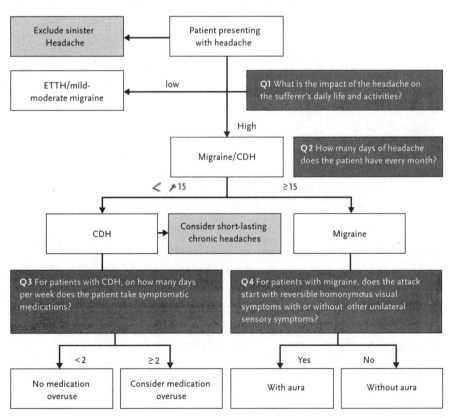

A crucial aspect of headache diagnosis is the exclusion of rare but potentially life-threatening secondary or sinister headaches. The HCPC organisation has developed new criteria for the exclusion of such headaches, which are simple to apply in primary care (Figure 12.2).[14]

Figure 12.2 **New algorithm for the exclusion of secondary (sinister) headaches**[14]

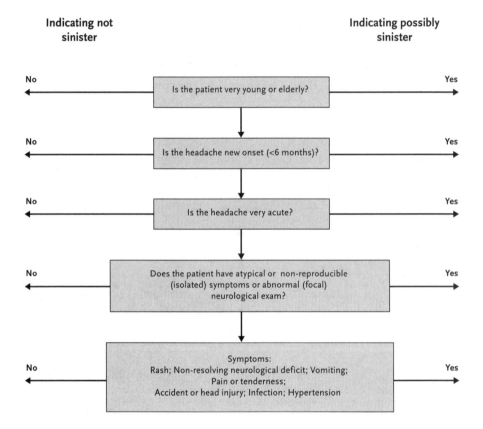

Overview of current management

Unfortunately, migraine and other headaches are under-diagnosed and under-treated in the UK.[16] Patients with significant medical needs frequently do not consult at all or lapse from care following their initial consultations, and many patients rely on ineffective over-the-counter medications.[17] The personal burden of headache to the sufferer and the economic burden on society are both high.[18] Much of the problem lies with currently-recommended care management strategies, which rely on the trial and error approach of step care.[19] This inevitably leads to delays in patients receiving effective care, and subsequent patient dropout.

The UK umbrella organisation Headache UK (comprising MIPCA, the British Association for the Study of Headache (BASH), the Migraine Trust, and the patient support organisations Migraine Action Association and Organisation for the Understanding of Cluster Headache) has recognised several deficiencies in headache management in the UK (see Box 12.1 below).[20]

Box 12.1 **Headache UK's assessment of the current status of headache services in the UK**[20]

- In today's primary care, the quality of headache services is unknown, and *ad hoc* services are generally performed on demand.

- Current headache services are unlikely to be adequate or cost-effective, with no national or local targets, little research or auditing undertaken, a lack of interest among GPs and neurologists, few professionals employed, and patients' access to healthcare restricted.

- Current NHS spending on the management of headache disorders is inadequate, unevenly distributed and not optimally managed.

- The lack of headache-interested specialist physicians results in patients suffering from long waiting lists, and often seeing a neurologist who has little training in headache management.

New initiatives for developing management guidelines

Recently, evidence-based guidelines for the management of migraine in primary care have been published in the UK,[13,21] USA,[22] and Canada,[23] and principles of care have been recommended for international use.[14] These principles are generic in scope, and can be summarised as follows:

▶ Set up a specific consultation for headache with the patient. Take a headache history, provide the patient with relevant information about their headaches and elicit their commitment to the care process.

▶ Conduct a differential diagnostic procedure.

▶ Provide management that is tailored to the patient's individual medical needs:
  ▷ Assess the severity of the patient's headache, in terms of its impact, frequency, duration, severity of the headache pain and any associated non-headache symptoms. Take account of the patient's preferences and co-morbidities in this process.
  ▷ Provide treatments that are appropriate to the patient's needs, using, wherever possible, therapies that have demonstrated objective evidence of favourable efficacy and safety. Rescue medications should be provided for treatment failure or breakthrough of symptoms.

▶ Provide proactive, long-term follow up for each patient, providing alternative treatments if the initial therapies have proved unsuccessful.

▶ Use physicians, nurses and other health care professionals in a team approach to the management of headache.

These principles can be used for all headache subtypes, with customisation of the medications prescribed. Figure 12.3 shows a management algorithm for migraine management.

Figure 12.3 **An algorithm for the management of migraine in primary care**[14]

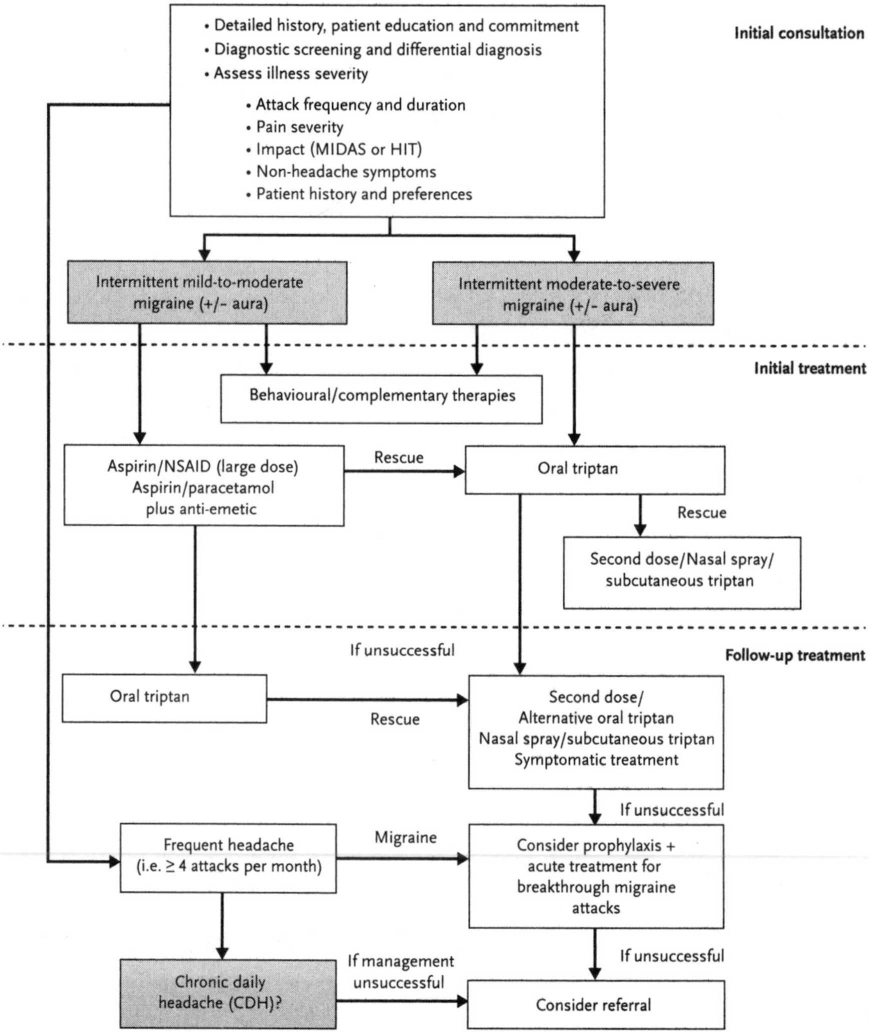

```
┌─────────────────────────────────────────────────┐
│ • Detailed history, patient education and commitment    Initial consultation
│ • Diagnostic screening and differential diagnosis
│ • Assess illness severity
│      • Attack frequency and duration
│      • Pain severity
│      • Impact (MIDAS or HIT)
│      • Non-headache symptoms
│      • Patient history and preferences
└─────────────────────────────────────────────────┘
```

Intermittent mild-to-moderate migraine (+/- aura)

Intermittent moderate-to-severe migraine (+/- aura)

Initial treatment

Behavioural/complementary therapies

Aspirin/NSAID (large dose) Aspirin/paracetamol plus anti-emetic — Rescue → Oral triptan

Rescue → Second dose/Nasal spray/ subcutaneous triptan

If unsuccessful

Follow-up treatment

Oral triptan — Rescue → Second dose/ Alternative oral triptan Nasal spray/subcutaneous triptan Symptomatic treatment

If unsuccessful

Frequent headache (i.e. ≥ 4 attacks per month) — Migraine → Consider prophylaxis + acute treatment for breakthrough migraine attacks

If unsuccessful

Chronic daily headache (CDH)? — If management unsuccessful → Consider referral

If unsuccessful

For migraine, acute and prophylactic medications may be required. Acute medications are needed for all patients; analgesic-based therapy can be given to patients with mild-to-moderate attacks and triptans to those with moderate-to-severe attacks and those who find analgesic-based therapy ineffective. Most patients find oral triptans effective, but nasal spray and subcutaneous formulations are available for those who require a more rapid onset of action or who cannot tolerate oral therapy due to nausea or vomiting. Patients should also be provided with rescue medication for when the original therapy fails. Prophylactic medications are needed for patients who suffer from frequent attacks (> 4 per month), and for those who do not achieve satisfactory treatment with, or who have concomitant co-morbidities that preclude the use of, appropriate acute medications. Suitable prophylactic medications include beta-blockers, pizotifen, the anticonvulsant sodium valproate and the anti-depressant amitriptyline (the latter two are not licensed for migraine in the UK but are listed in the BNF). Physicians should review the medications at follow up and switch them only if the existing medications are ineffective or are associated with significant side effects.[13-14]

Implications for practice

Implementation of these new guidelines for managing migraine should mean that the majority of sufferers can be managed in primary care, either by their own GPs, or by the new intermediate care service of GPwSI. A framework document for a GPwSI in headache service has been published[24] and we look forward to the full implementation of this service. Only complicated and refractory patients should need to be referred to a consultant neurologist, so saving the NHS significant costs and the patient significant waiting time.

Unresolved issues and future developments

Migraine management has been transformed over the past decade or so, thanks to the development of new therapies and the introduction of new guidelines. However, these initiatives have not yet been integrated into primary care, and migraine management is still suboptimal. The challenge is to educate GPs, nurses and other health care professionals on how to manage migraine and other headaches in the clinic. Initiatives are also needed to develop guidelines for chronic headaches, particularly CDH and cluster headache. The principles developed for migraine should prove invaluable for this purpose.

Epidemiology of epilepsy

Epilepsy is the most common serious neurological condition with a prevalence of between five and ten cases per 1000 persons in developed countries and the overall incidence around 50 cases per 100,000 persons.[25] There is a bimodal distribution for age of onset with peaks at both ends of life. Epilepsy is correctly termed a serious condition as it carries an increased mortality with up to a 1000 deaths a year being recorded in the UK.[26]

An overview of the diagnosis of epilepsy

An attempt should always be made to classify the seizure type and epilepsy syndrome as both may have implications for management and prognosis.[27] The current system of epilepsy classification, introduced in 1981 and revised in 1989, is summarised below.[28–9]

Box 12.2 **Epilepsy classification**

I. Partial seizures
A simple partial seizures (no loss of consciousness)

B complex partial seizures
  1. with impairment of consciousness at onset
  2. simple partial onset followed by impairment of consciousness

C partial seizures evolving to generalised tonic-clonic convulsions
II. Primary generalised seizures
Convulsive or non-convulsive with bilateral discharges involving sub-cortical structures
A absence B myoclonic C clonic D tonic E tonic-clonic F atonic
III. Unclassified epileptic seizures
Usually when an adequate description is not available

Diagnostic advances

The history and eyewitness account remain the mainstay of diagnosis of epilepsy. Focal seizures offer a history of a stereotypical aura and can often include automatisms with seizures tending to be asymmetrical. Primary generalised seizures, which often start in childhood or teenage years, have no aura, however, and the attacks are generally symmetrical. There is also a tendency for primary generalised seizures to be provoked by sleep deprivation, alcohol and in some cases by flashing lights.[27]

Most cases require neuro-imaging and the use of MRI has become widespread in the UK with several centres now offering functional MRI and single-photon emission computerised tomography (SPECT) scans. For an overview of these techniques and their clinical indication readers are directed to the professional pages of the National Society for Epilepsy website at www.e-epilepsy.org.uk.

Electroencephalography (EEG) is helpful but can only support a clinical diagnosis of epilepsy; a negative EEG does not exclude epilepsy. EEG has an important place in classifying the seizure type and is also one of several tools used in identifying the site of seizure onset, which has importance when epilepsy surgery is under consideration.

Pitfalls in diagnosis

The diagnosis of epilepsy has profound physical, psychological and economic implications for the patient. The Scottish Intercollegiate Guidelines Network (SIGN) advises that the diagnosis of epilepsy should be made by a neurologist or other epilepsy specialist: a specialist being defined as a consultant with expertise in epilepsy demonstrated by training and continuing education in epilepsy, as well as peer review of practice and regular audit of diagnosis. Epilepsy can be confused with several other causes of altered consciousness such as syncope, arrhythmia, panic attacks, or non-epileptic attack disorder (formerly referred to by the rather pejorative term pseudo-seizures). It is now recommended that a 12 lead ECG is performed in the assessment of all patients with a history of altered consciousness.

Advances in therapy

Amongst epileptologists there is a good deal of anecdotal evidence suggesting the superiority of the newer anti-epileptic drugs (AEDs) but there are few good quality clinical trials to support this belief. The discussion document on AEDs for adults released by NICE concludes that there is little good quality evidence from clinical trials to support the use of the newer monotherapy or adjunctive therapy AEDs over the older AEDs, or to support the use of one of the newer AEDs over another one. Whilst accepting that there is a need for more controlled trials, it is working practice to use broad spectrum AEDs for generalised epilepsy and narrow spectrum for focal epilepsy.[30]

Epilepsy service delivery

The National Clinical Audit of Epilepsy-related Death[7] identified the following areas in need of improvement:

▶ lack of management plans or structured review for people with epilepsy

▶ lack of re-referral to a specialist by the general practitioner for individuals needing reassessment

▶ lack of discussion with patients and families of the fatality risk of seizures

▶ deficiencies in the overall quality of epilepsy care in general practice and hospitals on a range of issues (54% of adults and 77% of children received inadequate care, and 42% of epilepsy deaths annually were potentially avoidable).

Further evidence that epilepsy care is in need of improvement is reflected by the epilepsy mortality rate, which has not improved over the past ten years (see below).

Table 12.2 **Mortality from epilepsy in the UK – figures taken from the annual reports of the Office of Population Censuses and Surveys**

	1991	1992	1993	1994	1995	1996	1997	1998
Male	502	515	414	411	433	513	487	502
Female	404	389	299	303	338	317	321	340

The mortality associated with epilepsy

Deaths seen in association with epilepsy fall into three groups:[31]

1. unrelated to epilepsy, such as neoplasms outside the central nervous system

2. underlying disease, such as cerebrovascular disease

3. epilepsy itself.

As well as dying as a result of physical trauma during a seizure, some people die without an obvious cause. This has been described as Sudden Unexpected Death from Epilepsy (SUDEP). The risk of SUDEP is closely related to seizure frequency, being considerably higher in patients who continue to have seizures than in those who are seizure free.[32]

Recent UK guidelines for epilepsy

The CSAG (Clinical Standards Advisory Group) report into Services for Patients with Epilepsy[33] found that only 52% of the community-based sample reported being seizure free. This compares to most epilepsy centres where seizure freedom of upwards of 70% is achieved.[34] From these figures it would seem reasonable to assume that at least 20% of patients in the community have the potential to become seizure free.

As seizure freedom correlates to improved quality of life and reduced mortality, a proactive model of care for epilepsy management is long overdue.[35] The SIGN Guidelines for Epilepsy were published in April 2003 and offer a very comprehensive and practical guide to best practice for epilepsy care.[36] NICE is expected to publish a review of newer AEDs and full guidance on the diagnosis, management and treatment of epilepsy in 2004.[37] Epilepsy is currently being evaluated within two separate National Service Frameworks – for long-term conditions and for children.

East Kent Health Authority included epilepsy alongside the other major disease categories in the Primary Care Clinical Effectiveness guidelines (Advanced PRICCE). They clearly illustrated the potential role of primary care in chronic disease management.[38]

The roles of primary and secondary care in the management of epilepsy

The past 50 years have seen the active treatment of epilepsy move from primary to secondary care. During this time there has been a move towards specialisation within secondary care with more physicians specialising in neurology. From this group some have specialised further to become epileptologists. The care provided by these specialists is excellent, however, it may reduce the number of clinicians who feel they have the competence and confidence to manage what is a common problem.[36] In parallel to this there has been a de-skilling of primary care.

The new GMS contract

The new GMS contract includes epilepsy in its Quality and Outcomes Framework and offers a resource to proactively manage epilepsy. It sets a target of 70% seizure freedom in the previous 12 months for people with epilepsy.

The potential role for GPwSIs in epilepsy

It is conceivable that as a result of the new GMS contract a large cohort of patients will be identified whose treatment needs improving. Referring the majority of these to current secondary care clinics could bring an already stretched service to a halt. One solution could be via GPwSIs in Epilepsy.[39]

With the remit to see patients already diagnosed as having epilepsy they could advise patients with epilepsy-related problems. This is being piloted in East Kent as a peripatetic service with a network of GPs currently being trained as GPwSIs in epilepsy.

The future for epilepsy care in the UK

Primary care is likely to play a pivotal role in the management of epilepsy, with patients who were formerly resigned to poor seizure control identified and sign-posted to further help. It is an illness that has been stigmatised by most communities, and it has caused suffering and unhappiness in the lives of many people for too long.

Conclusion

There has been some scepticism in the UK about the political fixation with waiting lists and national service frameworks. However, it may lead to a rethinking of the service provided for neurological patients. The NHS has traditionally managed with 10–20% of the number of neurologists available in other Western countries.[1-2] This means that neurology care has been fragmented. Doctors in primary care have attempted to find physicians in the district who can help them manage chronic, disabling conditions like stroke, dementia and Parkinson's disease. Neurologists now realise that they need to expand their numbers and link up more with district teams of doctors and nurses.[1-2] Can this turning outward by neurologists be linked-up to training for GPs and nurses with special interest? If this opportunity can be seized, people with neurological problems in the UK can look forward to better advice and care than they have had hitherto.

References

1. Association of British Neurologists, Service and Standards Subcommittee. *Job Planning and the New Consultant Contract*. London: ABN, 2003. www.theabn.org/downloads/jobplans-final-111103.pdf (accessed 17/09/2004)

2. Association of British Neurologists. *Acute neurological emergencies in adults*. London: ABN, 2002. www.theabn.org/downloads/AcuteNeurology.pdf (accessed 17/09/2004)

3. Schon F, Hart P, Fernandez C. Is clinical neurology really so difficult? *J Neurol Neurosurg Psych 2002*; **72**: 557–9

4. Royal College of General Practitioners, the Office of Population Censuses & Surveys, & the Department of Health. *Morbidity Statistics from General Practice. Fourth National Study 1991–1992*. London: HMSO, 1995

5. Wiles C M, Lindsay M. General practice referrals to a department of neurology. *J R Coll Physicians*. London 1996; **30**: 426–31

6. Ridsdale L, Robins D, Fitzgerald A, *et al.* Epilepsy monitoring and advice recorded: general practitioners' views, current practice and patients' preferences. *Br J Gen Pract* 1996; **46**: 11–14

7. Hanna N J, Black M, Sander J W, *et al. The national sentinel clinical audit of epilepsy related death: epilepsy – death in the shadows.* London: HSMO, 2002

8. Rasmussen B K, Jensen R, Schroll M, Olesen J. Epidemiology of headache in a general population: a prevalence study. *J Clin Epidemiol* 1991; **44**: 1147–57

9. Breslau N, Rasmussen B K. The impact of migraine: Epidemiology, risk factors, and co-morbidities. *Neurology* 2001; **56 (S1)**: 4–12

10. Silberstein S D, Lipton R B. Chronic daily headache. *Curr Opin Neurol* 2000; **13**: 277–83

11. Abu-Arefeh I, Russell G. Prevalence of headache and migraine in schoolchildren. *BMJ* 1994; **309**: 765–9

12. Headache Classification Subcommittee of the International Headache Society. The international classification of headache disorders. *Cephalalgia* 2004; **24 (S1)**: 1–160

13. Dowson A J, Lipscombe S, Sender J, *et al.* New guidelines for the management of migraine in primary care. *Curr Med Res Opin* 2002; **18**: 414–39

14. Dowson A J, Sender J, Lipscombe S, *et al.* Establishing principles for migraine management in primary care. *Int J Clin Pract* 2003; **57**: 493–507

15. Lipton R B, Cady R K, Stewart W F, *et al.* Diagnostic lessons from the Spectrum study. *Neurology* 2002; **58 (S6)**: 27–31

16. Lipton R B, Scher A, Steiner T J, *et al.* Patterns of healthcare utilization for migraine in England and the United States. *Neurology* 2003; **60**: 441–8

17. Lipton RB, Goadsby PJ, Sawyer JPC, *et al.* Migraine: diagnosis and assessment of disability. *Rev Contemp Pharmacother* 2000; **11**: 63–73

18. Clarke C E, MacMillan L, Sondhi S, *et al.* Economic and social impact of migraine. *Q J Med* 1996; **89**: 77–84

19. Steiner T J, MacGregor E A, Davies P T G. Guidelines for all doctors in the diagnosis and management of migraine and tension-type headache. London: British Association for the Study of Headache, 2000 www.bash.org.uk

20. Hope P. Organisation of headache services in the UK: Headache UK Executive Summary Document. Hansard; 22 January 2003

21. O'Flynn N, Ridsdale L. *Headache.* In: Marshall M, Campbell S, Hacker J, Roland M. *Quality Indicators of General Practice.* London: The Royal Society of Medicine Press, 2002

22. Bedell A W, Cady R K, Diamond M L, *et al.* Patient-centered strategies for effective management of migraine. Springfield, MI: Primary Care Network, 2000

23. Pryse-Phillips W E M, Dodick D W, Edmeads J G, *et al.* Guidelines for the diagnosis and management of migraine in clinical practice. *Can Med Assoc J* 1997; **156**: 1273–87

24. Department of Health. Guidelines for the appointment of general practitioners with special interests in the delivery of clinical services: *Headache.* London: Department of Health, April 2003
www.dh.gov.uk/assetRoot/04/07/97/63/04079763.pdf (accessed 17/09/2004)

25. Ridsdale L, Hart Y. *Towards better epilepsy care*. In: Jones R, Britten N, Culpepper L, *et al.* *Oxford Textbook of Primary Care*. Oxford: Oxford University Press, 2003

26. Kotsopoulos I A, van Merode T, Kessels F G, *et al.* Systematic review and meta-analysis of incidence studies of epilepsy and unprovoked seizures. *Epilepsia* 2002 Nov; **43 (11)**: 1402–9

27. Scottish Intercollegiate Guidelines Network (SIGN). Diagnosis and management of epilepsy in adults. A national clinical guideline. Edinburgh: SIGN, 2003. www.sign.ac.uk

28. The Proposal for revised clinical and electroencephalographic classification of epileptic seizures. From the Commission on Classification and Terminology of the International League Against Epilepsy. *Epilepsia* 1981; **22 (4)**: 489–501

29. Commission on Classification and Terminology of the International League Against Epilepsy. Proposal for a revised classification of the epilepsies and epileptic syndromes. *Epilepsia* 1989; **30**: 389–99

30. NICE discussion document on AEDs found at: www.nice.org.uk/pdf/HTA_Epilepsy_in_adults.pdf (accessed 17/09/2004)

31. Cockerell O C. The Mortality of Epilepsy. *Curr Opin Neurol* 1996; **9 (2)**: 93–6

32. Tomson T. Mortality in Epilepsy. *J Neurol* 2000; **247**: 15–21

33. Clinical Standards Advisory Group Services for people who have epilepsy. Report of a CSAG Committee chaired by Professor A Kitson at the request of UK Health Ministers and to the NHS. London: HMSO, 2000

34. Elwes R, Johnson A L, Shorvon S D, Reynolds E H, *et al.* The prognosis of seizure control in newly diagnosed epilepsy. *N Engl J Med* 1984; **311**: 944–7

35. Sperling M R, Feldman H, Kinman J, *et al.* Seizure control and mortality in epilepsy. *Ann Neurol* 1999 July; **46 (1)**: 45–50

36. Rogers G. The future of epilepsy care in general practice ... a role for the GPwSI? *Br J Gen Pract* 2002; **52**: 872–3

37. National Institute for Clinical Excellence. Epilepsy: the diagnosis and management of epilepsy in children and adults. NICE guideline. London: NICE, 2004 (in press) www.nice.org.uk/page.aspx?0=20119 (accessed 15/10/2004)

38. East Kent Health Authority – Primary Care Clinical Effectiveness (Advanced PRICCE). Standards for Treatment of Epilepsy. 2002 www.kentandmedway.nhs.uk/pdf/professional_pages/pricce/epilepsy.pdf (accessed 17/09/2004)

39. Department of Health. Guidelines for the appointment of General Practitioners with Special Interests in the Delivery of Clinical Services. *Epilepsy* London: HMSO, 2002 www.dh.gov.uk/assetRoot/04/08/28/68/04082868.pdf (accessed 17/09/2004)

CHAPTER 13

Musculoskeletal Disorders

Graham Davenport

▶ **KEY MESSAGES**
- Musculoskeletal (MSK) disease accounts for a large proportion of a general practitioner's (GP's) workload. Proper management can not only improve quality of care but also improve job satisfaction and reap rewards under the new contract.

- Osteoporosis creates a huge socio-economic burden of disease and disability. Identifying high-risk groups in primary care and using preventative treatment can result in a substantial reduction in morbidity and mortality from osteoporotic fractures.

- GPs need to present a unified lifestyle message that encompasses all the major diseases as well as osteoporosis.

- Prevention of falls in the elderly is a priority.

- Effective treatment of osteoporosis is available despite hormone replacement therapy no longer being recommended as first-line treatment.

- Calcium and vitamin D supplementation should be considered for all female nursing home residents.

- Osteoarthritis is eminently treatable in primary care with a number of management options for GPs, in addition to drug therapy.

- Non-steroidal anti-inflammatory drugs (NSAIDs) are widely used but selective cyclo-oxygenase inhibitors (coxibs) have a better safety profile and GPs should follow the National Institute for Clinical Excellence's guidance on their appropriate usage.

- Corticosteroid injections are cost-effective and have immediate benefits for patients. GPs will be rewarded under the new contract for provision of joint injections.

- Glucosamine and chondroitin have equivalent long-term efficacy to NSAIDs and are worth recommending to patients with mild knee osteoarthritis.

- Monitoring of disease-modifying drugs in rheumatoid arthritis patients in primary care is encouraged and rewarded under the new contract.

- Severe refractory rheumatoid arthritis patients may warrant referral for consideration of biologic therapy.

- Cardiovascular mortality is high in rheumatoid arthritis patients. Assessment of the cardiovascular risk and possible use of statins may reduce cardiovascular mortality in these patients.

- GPs should aim to help patients to achieve optimum quality of life by using a holistic approach and by allowing maximum choice and control over their disease.

Introduction

The Bone and Joint Decade (2000–2010) is an attempt to highlight the enormous socio-economic burden of musculoskeletal disease and to educate the public worldwide. As GPs we are only too aware of the distressing health consequences for the individual affected and the resultant suffering and disability.

GPs are very experienced in dealing with MSK conditions, which account for one in five of their consultations and are happy to manage them in general practice as long as they have sufficient support in terms of education, consultant back-up for difficult cases and adequate access to and availability of, ancillary services, such as physiotherapy.[1]

Although there is no National Services Framework (NSF) for musculoskeletal disease, the new contract for GPs encourages and rewards GPs to provide joint injections and monitoring of disease-modifying drugs for their patients. The NSF for Older People is an attempt to reduce the number of falls in the community and improve osteoporosis management, thereby preventing fractures.[2] NSF for older people 2001 (HMSO)

The aim of the Primary Care Rheumatology Society is to improve the quality of care to patients with MSK disease by supporting and providing educational activities for all GPs.[3] However, not all GPs have an interest or expertise in MSK medicine and the Government's plan to have 1000 GPs with special interests (GPwSIs) in place by 2004 will help to provide a seamless continuum between primary and secondary care to the ultimate benefit of patients.

This chapter focuses on areas of MSK disease and rheumatology where recent advances in understanding and treatment have changed the management of these conditions, namely: osteoporosis, osteoarthritis, and rheumatoid arthritis.

Osteoporosis

Osteoporosis is a global problem the prevalence of which is rapidly rising due to increased life expectancy and an ageing population. It is a progressive disease resulting in disabling fractures that cause substantial morbidity and mortality, impaired quality of life and a massive socio-economic burden (£1.7 billion costs in the United Kingdom).[4] The economic burden is equal to, if not greater than, that resulting from most of the other major diseases.[5]

Osteoporosis is most prevalent in postmenopausal women but, despite a one in three risk of developing osteoporosis during their lifetime, 80% of women do not feel it will affect them personally – as reported by the International Osteoporosis Foundation in their How Fragile is Her Future? survey.[6] This major European survey also found poor doctor–patient communication and a considerable variation in the availability of, and access to, diagnostic investigations as well as the medical treatment of osteoporosis. This presents major problems to health care education, in convincing these women of the benefits of identifying and treating asymptomatic osteoporosis.

The vertebral column is the most common site for osteoporotic fractures and these are associated with considerable morbidity and increased mortality over five years.[7–9] However, only a small proportion of vertebral fractures are presented clinically, and of the ones that are, only a proportion are detected by spinal imaging.[9] Studies have shown that 50% of women have had at least one vertebral fracture by the age of 80–4 years, but only 15% have had a vertebral fracture clinically diagnosed.[7,9–11]

Vertebral fractures are predictive of future fracture risk at the spine, hip and, to a lesser extent, at all other sites; 20% of women will have another fracture within a year of a vertebral fracture incident.[12–13] New vertebral fractures are associated with substantial increases in back pain and resulting functional disability in elderly women.[14] Prevention of new vertebral fractures should reduce the burden of back pain disability.

Key messages

- Osteoporosis is very common; affecting one in three women.

- Every GP will have approximately 100 osteoporotic patients.

- The most common osteoporotic fractures are vertebral and hip, both are associated with considerable morbidity and mortality.

- Twenty per cent of hip fracture patients will die within a year, and 50% remain permanently disabled.

The hip is the second most common fracture site. There is a one in six lifetime risk of hip fractures for postmenopausal women, with the majority occurring in women over the age of 80 years.[15–17] The morbidity and mortality of hip fractures is considerable, with one in five dying within one year of sustaining an osteoporotic fracture, and over 50% remain permanently disabled with an impaired quality of life.[18–19] Number needed to treat (NNT) analysis for women over 70 years with three risk factors was between 32 and 71 to prevent one hip fracture, assuming intervention reduced fracture rates by 30 or 50%.[20]

The annual cost of treating osteoporotic fractures in the UK is £1.7 billion and the average PCT of 100,000 patients will have costs of nearly £1.5 million. There are an estimated 3 million people with osteoporosis in the UK at present which means that each general practitioner has approximately 100 patients with the disease.[21–3]

Identification of high-risk groups in primary care

The lack of communication and co-ordination between primary and secondary care means that many patients with obvious risk factors are not being detected. For example, a recent retrospective study in Manchester assessed the proportion of patients with a low impact distal radial fracture who had had any investigation or treatment for osteoporosis prior to their subsequent hip fracture: 84% received no advice, investigation or treatment before they sustained their hip fracture.[24] An audit in primary care found that most patients who have an osteoporotic fracture are not started on treatment[25] despite the availability of guidelines in primary care.[26–7] Another study in primary care showed that, of patients who were identified as having osteoporosis, 66% were not diagnosed until they had sustained a fracture.[28]

Population screening is not cost effective but identification and scanning of high-risk groups can produce positive dual X-ray absorptiometry (DEXA) results in up to 50% of referrals.[29] The standard high-risk groups include those patients with low body weight, kyphosis, family history of maternal hip fracture, early menopause, hyperthyroidism, glucocorticoid therapy, smokers and those with a high alcohol intake.

Glucocorticoid therapy is an area that can be easily targeted in general practice. Bone loss with glucocorticoid therapy is greatest in the first six months of treatment with fractures often occurring in the first three months. One in six patients taking >7.5 mg glucocorticoids daily have a vertebral fracture within a year. This has led the Royal College of Physicians to issue guidelines on the management of glucocorticoid-induced osteoporosis (Box 13.1).[30]

Box 13.1 **RCP Guidelines for management of glucocorticoid-induced osteoporosis**

For patients aged over 65 years, or with a previous fragility fracture, the risk of osteoporosis is high; therefore, advise general measures and start treatment

- patients aged under 65 years without previous fragility fractures and who are starting oral glucocorticoids for more than three months should have their bone mineral density measured using dual X-ray absorptiometry:
  ▷ T score over 0: reassure and advise general measures
  ▷ T score 0–1.5: general measures and repeat BMD in 1–3 years
  ▷ T score less than 1.5: treat for osteoporosis

More recently, other high-risk groups have been identified. These include those with chronic mal-absorption problems such as Crohn's disease or coeliac disease, patients on anticonvulsant therapy and those with marked height loss.[31–4] Various tools for screening populations are being developed. These include the FRACTURE index, OSIRIS (Osteoporosis Index of Risk) and OST (Osteoporosis Self-assessment Tool) for determining the risk of osteoporosis and the PVFI (Prevalent Vertebral Fracture Index) for identifying the risk of undiagnosed vertebral fractures.[35–8] GPs need training in how to use such tools to identify those most at risk of fracture.

The use of different analytical techniques consistently identified women's age and body weight as key predictors for risk of osteoporosis.[39]

A structured audit programme initiated by the National Osteoporosis Society aims to identify those patients in primary care who are at highest risk of osteoporosis by using a risk assessment questionnaire and assessing high-risk patients using specialist nurses.[40] However, use of risk factor assessment has been shown in one study to result in identification of only 47% of the cases at high risk of osteoporosis.[29]

Ultrasonography provides a way of assessing bone strength without using ionising radiation, with other advantages of speed and low cost, which could prove useful in a primary care setting. Quantitative ultrasound measurement of the calcaneus was found to be as good as DEXA measurement of bone mineral density in predicting femoral neck fractures in a study of elderly women in residential care.[41] Another study showed ultrasound to be highly predictive of hip fractures in elderly women but it was also predictive of any fracture.[42] The position statement from the National Osteoporosis Society confirms the usefulness of quantitative ultrasound measurement as an independent risk factor for future osteoporotic fractures in post-menopausal women but recommends that confirmation of the diagnosis and monitoring of treatment is performed via axial (preferably hip) DEXA assessment of bone mineral density.[43] At present the method is being used as a means of screening populations prior to referral for DEXA and, compared with risk factor assessment, has a better specificity and predictive values.[44]

Peripheral X-ray absorptiometry of the distal forearm or calcaneus is also being used in primary care as a screening tool. The position statement from the National Osteoporosis Society states that, although forearm DEXA is especially predictive for Colles' fracture, it is less predictive than bone mineral density of the hip in predicting hip fracture risk in women over 65 years. It also recommends that monitoring of bone mineral density is best carried out by DEXA at the spine.[45]

Osteoporosis is defined in terms of bone mineral density, using WHO diagnostic cut-off values and, therefore, DEXA is the 'gold standard' for diagnosis.[46] The predictive value for fractures is greatest for DEXA at the hip but spinal DEXA is more useful for monitoring treatment. In the UK, recommendations are that DEXA is not used for population screening but for assessing high-risk groups.

The National Osteoporosis Society service framework for osteoporosis recommends that a PCT serving a population of 100,000 should have access to a bone densitometry service capable of providing 1000 DEXA scans per year.[23]

Many GPs do not have direct access to bone densitometry and have to refer patients via secondary care. In addition, the availability of DEXA scans is very limited in some areas which restricts the provision of an adequate osteoporosis service in primary care. The cost of developing an osteoporosis service in a PCT has been estimated at £174,000 allowing for 1000 scans on 100,000 populations.

Key messages

- Patients aged over 50 years with low fragility fractures should be offered treatment for osteoporosis.

- Patients aged over 65 years starting steroids should have concomitant osteoporosis treatment.

- Risk factor assessment identifies 50% of osteoporotic patients in primary care.

- Risk factors include age, low body weight, loss of height, family history of maternal hip fracture, early menopause, smoking, high alcohol intake, and mal-absorption problems.

- Primary care screening of women aged over 65 years with heel ultrasonography or peripheral dual X-ray absorptiometry (DEXA) can identify 90% of women with osteoporosis.

- Axial DEXA is still the 'gold standard' for diagnosis and is essential for monitoring treatment, but is not always available to primary care.

Prevention in primary care

Osteoporosis is a primary care disease and unless it is managed well in primary care, then fracture incidence and costs will continue to increase faster than the ageing population.[47] It is vital that, in the development of guidelines on the management of osteoporosis, it is stressed that prevention of osteoporosis is a crucial part of any programme. Primary care plays a pivotal role in the provision of lifestyle advice throughout life e.g. regarding diet and exercise, and also in the education of patients and doctors in the management of established disease and in the prevention of falls. Primary care offers lifestyle advice for many of the major diseases such as diabetes, coronary heart disease and malignancy.

There are many similar features such as smoking cessation advice, reduction of alcohol intake, aerobic exercise encouragement and healthy diet advice, which also apply to osteoporosis. It is vital to co-ordinate the approach to offering a lifestyle message that encompasses all the major diseases including osteoporosis. An important feature would be to ensure that dietary advice for diabetes and coronary heart disease does not compromise an adequate calcium intake essential for osteoporosis prevention.

Falls are common in the elderly with one person in two over 85 years living at home, falling at least once a year. Up to 10% of falls results in injury, usually a fracture with consequent high morbidity and mortality.[48] Therefore, preventing falls is important in reducing the fracture risk. This involves exercise programmes and home assessment to identify dangerous hazards such as loose carpets and iatrogenic causes such as multiple drug therapy. Hip protectors have been recommended as a way in which elderly persons can reduce their risk of suffering a fracture of the hip when they fall. Recent studies and reviews have cast doubt on their effectiveness[49–51] mainly as a result of their cosmetic appearance and discomfort that reduces compliance, especially in people living in the community.[52] High hip protector compliance is feasible but time intensive.[53] Exercise is important in the elderly: by increasing gait, balance, proprioception, reaction time, co-ordination, and muscle strength, the risk of falls can be reduced.[54–5] One study showed that the rate of falls was decreased by 30% in elderly women given a specific strength and balance training programme.[56] Other studies have shown that both past and present physical activity protects against hip fracture with up to 50% risk reduction.[57–9] Exercise prevents osteoporosis by increasing bone mass, density and strength.[60–1] It has its maximal effect if started at an early age.

Dietary advice in primary care is especially important to ensure that children and adolescents reach their maximum bone mass before adult life. Calcium and vitamin D intake is often inadequate in Western diets, which results in sub-maximal bone growth and adversely affects bone loss.[62] Low calcium intake in childhood is associated with increased osteoporosis risk in later life as well as an increase in fracture risk even in adolescents. Adequate calcium intake is important at all ages but especially in the elderly. In this age group, adequate protein intake and total nutrition is also important because malnutrition predisposes to falls.[48] Serum albumin levels are the single best predictor of survival or death after a hip fracture.[63]

Key messages

- Unified lifestyle message required from primary care.

- Prevention of falls in the elderly is a priority.

- Hip protectors are of doubtful benefit.

- Exercise not only increases bone mass and muscle strength but also improves gait, balance, and co-ordination.

- Dietary advice needs to be targeted at all age groups, including adolescents and the elderly.

Treatment in primary care

An adequate calcium intake (1000–1500 mg daily) is essential for postmenopausal women, by diet or supplements, which are available over the counter or on prescription. In addition, 800 IU of vitamin D is recommended for housebound elderly people because of the risk of sub-clinical vitamin D deficiency.

Although calcium and vitamin D alone are insufficient to treat established osteoporosis compared with the newer antiresorptive agents, there is still an important role for their use in the prevention of osteoporosis. Chapuy *et al* carried out a study in elderly mobile women living in French residential nursing homes. They have shown that the use of calcium and vitamin D reduced the risk of hip fractures although other studies have failed to produce a statistically significant conclusion.[54,64-5] Chapuy's recent study has supported his original findings that calcium and vitamin D3 reverse senile secondary hyperparathyroidism and reduce hip bone loss and the risk of hip fracture in elderly institutionalised women.[66]

A recent community study has shown that four monthly oral supplementation with 100,000 IU vitamin D, reduced osteoporotic fractures by 33%.[67] However, Meyer *et al* have also shown that the administration of 10 μg of vitamin D produced no reduction in hip fracture rates in nursing home residents.[68] Calcium and vitamin D supplementation has also been shown to improve body sway and therefore may prevent falls and subsequent non-vertebral fractures in elderly women.[54] This could also be the reason for the finding that an annual vitamin D injection can prevent fractures of the upper limbs and ribs but not other fractures.[69]

Meta-analysis of the efficacy of vitamin D in the prevention of osteoporosis in postmenopausal women shows that vitamin D with or without calcium decreases vertebral fractures and may decrease non-vertebral fractures.[70] Despite the possible differences between residents of French residential nursing homes and residents of English residential nursing homes, there appears to be sufficient evidence to recommend treatment of these residents with calcium and vitamin D.

The cost-effectiveness of treating women with osteoporosis is well documented.[71-4] The bisphosphonates are now considered first-line treatment for postmenopausal osteoporosis and are antiresorptive agents that reduce osteoclastic activity. Both alendronate and risedronate have excellent outcome data from large trials, which show that they significantly reduce the relative risk of vertebral and non-vertebral fractures by 40–50%.[75-8]

In view of the recent evidence regarding the cardiovascular and thromboembolic risks of long-term hormone replacement therapy(HRT),[79] guidelines have been issued by the Royal College of Physicians (Edinburgh).[80] It recommends that GPs should not prescribe HRT to asymptomatic women to prevent osteoporosis because the risks outweigh the benefits even in women at high risk of osteoporosis:

▶ HRT should not be used to prevent or treat cardiovascular disease

▶ women requiring HRT for menopausal symptoms should have their coronary heart disease risk assessed

▶ HRT is not recommended as first-line therapy for prevention and treatment of osteoporosis, except for women needing treatment for menopausal symptoms

▶ treatment should be assessed annually

▶ women with early menopause should take HRT up to the age of 50 years.

At present, 20% of current UK users are taking HRT to prevent osteoporosis but a large number of women are now coming off this treatment and guidance on the different treatments available to primary care for the management of women at risk of osteoporosis is a priority. A recent study has cast doubts on the effectiveness of hormone replacement therapy in osteoporosis prevention and shows that women who have continuously used hormone replacement therapy since the menopause are still at risk of osteoporosis and fractures.[81] In women with increased risk of breast cancer in whom HRT is contraindicated, the use of selective oestrogen receptor modulators (SERMs) has considerable benefit because of the dramatic reduction in risk of invasive breast cancer (76% during three years treatment).[82]

Compliance with drug taking is always a problem in elderly patients and the availability of once-weekly preparations of bisphosphonates is of considerable benefit.[83] Gastrointestinal intolerance can be a problem with the use of bisphosphonate preparations and once-weekly preparations are better tolerated than daily preparations.[84-5] Again, compliance can be a problem with the use of calcium and vitamin D preparations where the palatability of some formulations counterbalances any cost disadvantage.[86]

The main issues are: at what age to start treatment; which treatment to use for which age group; and duration of treatment. If a woman of 55 is found to have low bone mineral density then treatment for five years is going to have a marginal effect on her bone density at the age of 80 years when she is at greatest risk of sustaining a fracture.[87] There appears to be limited evidence for the long-term safety of these drugs over more than 12 years, and therefore, it is difficult to commit patients to life-long treatment at present.

Key messages

- Patients in residential nursing homes will benefit from calcium and vitamin D supplementation.

- Vitamin D has other benefits for neuromuscular co-ordination that may reduce the risk of falls.

- Bisphosphonates are the first-line treatment and once-weekly preparations improve tolerability and aid compliance.

- Hormone replacement therapy (HRT) is no longer an initial choice for osteoporosis treatment.

- Selective oestrogen receptor modulators (SERMs) may be a useful alternative in postmenopausal women where HRT is contraindicated. _ βαιοχι furd

- Treatment needs to be focused on the highest risk group – the elderly.

Advances in treatment

The development of teriparatide (recombinant human parathyroid hormone) is a major advance in osteoporosis treatment. It has a powerful effect on osteoblastic activity, which results in greater increases in bone mineral density compared with the bisphosphonates, and it reduces the relative fracture risk of vertebral and non-vertebral fractures by 50–65 %.[88] It requires daily injections and, in view of its costs, will probably be restricted to the management of severe osteoporotic cases in secondary care.

Another exciting area of research is in pro-osteoclastic cytokines, such as receptor-activating nuclear factor kappa B ligand (RANKL), which binds to its receptor (RANKL) on osteoclast precursors. Inhibition of RANKL results in prevention of bone loss and holds great promise in the future treatment of osteoporosis.[89]

Strontium ranelate has been found to have osteoblastic as well as anti-osteoclastic activity, and has been shown to be a well tolerated oral therapy with significant increases in bone mineral density compared with placebo in trials so far.[90]

Future strategy in primary care

Osteoporosis is not only a serious disease with considerable morbidity and mortality but also a major cause of disability and decreased quality of life, and a major cost to the NHS. It is largely a primary care disease, but requires co-operation between primary and secondary care as well as extensive education of both the general population and primary care teams.[91]

Early intervention is important and identifying high-risk patients is a priority but full-scale practice screening is not yet feasible. Methods of identification require awareness, opportunistic screening and computerised searches for high-risk groups. Immediate priority areas are the treatment of patients who have already sustained one or more osteoporotic fractures, urgent assessment of the need to co-prescribe antiresorptive agents to all patients on long-term glucocorticoid therapy and the prescribing of calcium and vitamin D to all housebound and institutionalised elderly patients.[23, 26-7] Prevention of the first fracture was the treatment goal for 97% physicians and provision of a unified lifestyle message by primary care is the first step in the battle against osteoporosis.[6]

Osteoarthritis

Osteoarthritis is the most common joint disorder in the world and the biggest single cause of disability.[92] In the UK, musculoskeletal problems account for around 25% of GPs' consultations, most of which are due to osteoarthritis.[93] Fifty-four per cent of people aged over 65 years and 10% of the population over the age of 50 have osteoarthritis of the knees.[94]

The main aims of a GP treating patients with osteoarthritis are to:

► reduce pain

► optimise function

► provide education and information

► advise about prevention of further damage

► allay patients' fears and reassure them.

What are the patient's fears and what do they want? Patients want to know that their pain is not due to cancer and that you can eliminate it for them. They want to know if their symptoms are going to get worse and whether they are going to become disabled. They want to know if you can help them carry out their usual activities, whether they can continue their work, and participate in sport.

In addition to education, GPs can help osteoarthritic patients in a number of ways including:

► provision of aids, appliances and orthoses

► referral to other health professionals e.g. physiotherapist, podiatrist, and occupational therapist

► use of drug treatment with topical preparations, analgesics, NSAIDs and coxibs, and with corticosteroid and hyaluronan injections.

Topical preparations

Application of creams can be useful if only one or two joints are involved. Capsaicin cream depletes the pain neuro-transmitter, substance P, and apart from occasional stinging and burning, is usually well-tolerated. Topical NSAID creams have been shown to be significantly more effective than placebo and have few adverse side effects.[95-6]

Drug therapy

Paracetamol remains first-line therapy in all age groups, not only for fever and pain, but in the management of osteoarthritis. In standard dosage, paracetamol has an excellent safety profile and rarely causes side effects.[97] Although some studies have raised the possibility of increased gastrointestinal complications with paracetamol, this has not been confirmed by other studies and paracetamol remains the initial choice of therapy in osteoarthritis.[98] However, studies have raised the possibility of a link between frequent paracetamol use and asthma in adults and children. One study has raised the possibility of a link between use of paracetamol in late pregnancy and the increased risk of wheezing in the offspring at 30–42 months.[99]

Although, NSAIDs have been shown to be superior to paracetamol in the treatment of hip and knee pain due to osteoarthritis, both drugs have similar benefits in terms of functional improvement.[100]

Non-steroidal anti-inflammatory drugs

Key messages

- Paracetamol remains the initial choice of therapy.

- All NSAIDs have gastrointestinal toxicity related to their COX-1 activity.

- Use the lowest dose of NSAID for the shortest time.

- For patients requiring long-term NSAIDs:
  - ▷ consider checking *Helicobacter pylori* status and possible treatment prior to starting NSAIDs
  - ▷ follow NICE guidelines for coxibs, which are equally efficacious and have a better safety profile
  - ▷ avoid NSAID and coxib treatment, if possible, for:
  - a) patients on low-dose aspirin, b) patients with hypertension, and c) elderly patients, at risk of heart failure.

NSAIDs are used extensively worldwide in the treatment of musculoskeletal problems, both inflammatory and non-inflammatory, and as analgesics for a multitude of conditions such as renal colic and dental pain.

Over 30 million people worldwide take NSAIDs regularly and 40% are over 60 years. In the UK, about 1.5 million people over 60 years take NSAIDs at any one time.[101] Twenty-four million prescriptions were issued for NSAIDs in

1993 (5% of all NHS prescriptions). The number of prescriptions is escalating due to the increasingly ageing population and the increase in osteoarthritis.

NSAIDs are responsible for 25% of the yellow card reports of suspected adverse drug reactions reported to the CSM. From 1964 to 1985, the CSM[102] received 3500 reports of upper gastrointestinal bleeding or perforation suspected of being caused by NSAIDs, of which 600 were fatal, the majority being in the elderly. The CSM concluded that serious gastrointestinal reactions with NSAIDs occur more commonly in the elderly, especially women, and are more likely to be fatal in this group. The CSM continues to remind GPs of the risks of gastrointestinal toxicity with NSAIDs.[103] In order to reduce these risks, patients should take the lowest dose of NSAID for the shortest duration, be aware that risks are highest in the elderly, make sure that the combination of aspirin and an NSAID is avoided if possible, and they should be aware that all NSAIDs, including ibuprofen and coxibs, have been associated with serious and fatal gastrointestinal reactions.

A nurse-based advice intervention reduced chronic NSAID use in primary care with 28% more patients in the intervention group either stopping NSAIDs or reducing the dosage by at least 50% compared with the control group.[104]

Approximately one-third of patients taking NSAIDs develop gastric or duodenal ulceration and the risks of ulcer complications such as gastrointestinal haemorrhage and perforation have increased three- to six-fold in recent years.[105] Two-thirds of patients on NSAIDs develop dyspeptic symptoms but there is little relationship between symptoms and endoscopically proven ulceration. Almost half of all patients with endoscopically proven ulcers are found to have no gastro-intestinal symptoms.[105] Every year, 12000 ulcer complications occur in the UK as a result of NSAID therapy.[106] The risk of a NSAID user developing a serious gastrointestinal complication is five to eight per 1000 patient years and the complication can occur at any time after starting the drug.[107]

NSAIDs users often are asymptomatic and often have no prior dyspepsia before developing a life threatening complication of a bleeding peptic ulcer.[108] For every 1200 patients taking NSAIDs for at least two months, one will die from gastroduodenal complications as a result of NSAID treatment.[109] On an individual practice level, a GP with a list size of 2500 would have three gastrointestinal emergency admissions per annum, of which one will be a NSAID user. One death will occur in a NSAID user every six years.[110]

Which NSAID should a GP use?

In low doses, different NSAIDs have different risks of serious gastrointestinal complications but this disappears at higher doses. For example, ibuprofen at 1200 mg/day is associated with less serious upper gastrointestinal complications than other NSAIDs but this is lost at higher doses of over 1800 mg / day.[111] The incidence of NSAID – induced bleeding ulcers could be reduced by two-thirds by substituting ibuprofen at 2.4 g/day, and to a negligible level by substituting ibuprofen at 1200 mg/day, for any other NSAID. High dosage of any NSAID increases the risk of dyspeptic symptoms by threefold.[112]

What about coxibs (selective cyclo-oxygenase 2 inhibitors)?

NSAIDs are associated with gastric mucosal injury that may result in peptic ulceration, upper gastrointestinal haemorrhage, and perforation.[113] Mucosal injury is thought to be mainly due to the inhibition of prostaglandins by NSAIDs. Prostaglandin synthesis is catalysed by two cyclo-oxygenase enzymes. Most NSAIDs are non-selective and inhibit the activity of the COX-1 enzyme in the stomach as much as the COX-2 enzyme, which is induced in the inflamed synovium. Prostaglandin synthesis stimulates the mucosal defence mechanisms and COX-1 inhibition results in the gastrointestinal complications of NSAIDs.[114] Coxibs have been developed that have selective COX-2 activity and provide the powerful anti-inflammatory action of standard NSAIDs with reduced gastrointestinal toxicity.

All coxibs have equivalent efficacy to NSAIDs in full dosage and may have a longer duration of action.[115] Four large studies have analysed the gastrointestinal safety of rofecoxib and celecoxib in over 39,000 patients with osteoarthritis or rheumatoid arthritis.[116–9] The results have shown that rofecoxib and celecoxib had significantly lower rates of gastrointestinal adverse events than those taking non-selective NSAIDs. Patients with multiple-risk factors or who were taking low-dose aspirin and corticosteroids as well as a coxib had a reduced risk of upper gastrointestinal events.

When should GPs use coxibs?

The improved gastrointestinal profile of coxibs has led NICE to issue recommendations on their usage: [120]

- ▶ patients aged over 65 years
- ▶ prior history of ulcers or gastrointestinal complications
- ▶ use of steroids or anticoagulants
- ▶ serious co-morbidity
- ▶ requirement for prolonged use of maximal doses.

Although coxibs have a better safety profile, 30–40% of patients will need their medication changed within six to 12 months for some reason.[121]

Cost-effectiveness of coxibs is related not just to a decrease of serious gastro-intestinal events treated in secondary care but also to the reduction in co-prescribing of gastro-protective agents with coxibs than NSAIDs.[122]

Unfortunately, rofecoxib was withdrawn at the end of September 2004 following new three-year data from the APPROVe (Adenomatous Polyp Prevention on Vioxx) trial, which showed an increased relative risk of confirmed cardio-vascular events, such as heart attacks and stroke, beginning after 18 months of treatment. As yet, there is no evidence that this a class effect of coxibs and retrospective analysis of extensive data has not revealed an increased cardiovascular risk with the use of celecoxib. Further studies are essential to investigate the long-term cardiovascular risks of all coxibs and GPs should review their patients on long-term NSAIDs and coxibs. Patients with a high cardiovascular risk should be prescribed low-dose aspirin and every attempt made to stop their NSAID or coxib and provide alternative treatment.

What should GPs do about Helicobacter pylori?

There is a strong association between *H. pylori* infection and upper gastro-intestinal disease. The strongest evidence for the role of *H. pylori* in peptic ulcer disease is the marked decrease in recurrence rates of ulcers following the eradication of infection, both for duodenal and gastric ulcers.[123] Consensus statements have recommended eradication of *H. pylori* as first-line therapy in *H. pylori*-associated gastric and duodenal ulceration.[124] With regard to NSAIDs, the evidence for treating *H. pylori* is equivocal. The interaction between NSAIDs and *H. pylori* infection on peptic ulcers is antagonistic, despite both being independent risk factors.[125] There is no evidence for *H. pylori* eradication in patients on NSAIDs but there may be benefit in eradicating *H. pylori* prior to starting long-term treatment with NSAIDs.[126-7]

What should GPs do about patients on low-dose aspirin?

Patients on low-dose aspirin for ischaemic heart disease (IHD) are still at risk of gastrointestinal complications. If possible, avoid treating these patients with NSAIDs and use simple analgesia instead. If it is essential to prescribe a NSAID then a coxib is preferable to minimise the gastrointestinal risks. Although the risks of gastrointestinal symptoms are greater with a coxib and aspirin than with a coxib alone, the risks are still better than a standard NSAID. Although some NSAIDs such as naproxen have an anti-platelet aggre-gation activity, it is not as profound as aspirin and it would be unwise to rely on naproxen to prevent vascular events in patients with IHD.

The cardioprotective effects of low-dose aspirin may be compromised by co-prescribing NSAIDs, but not by the intermittent use of NSAIDs. Therefore, this is another reason to avoid the combination of aspirin and NSAIDs, if possible.

Apart from gastrointestinal safety, are coxibs safer?

All NSAIDs can affect blood pressure significantly – both standard NSAIDs and coxibs.[128] NSAIDs, including coxibs can impair renal function and result in water and sodium retention in susceptible individuals, and they have been implicated in nearly 20% of hospital admissions with heart failure. The use of NSAIDs, including coxibs, should be avoided in patients with heart failure. If treatment is unavoidable, education of patients and careful monitoring is essential.[129-30]

Viscosupplementation

Three to five intra-articular injections of hyaluronic acid into an osteoarthritic knee at weekly intervals have been shown to provide pain relief and functional improvements for up to six months[131-3] although another study failed to show any benefit over physical therapy in knee osteoarthritis over three months.[134] However, there is no difference in efficacy between hyaluronic acid and corticosteroid injection into the joint at six months of follow-up.[135] There is some evidence that hyaluronic acid injections have a potential structure-modifying activity with arthroscopic findings showing less cartilage damage at six months than with corticosteroids.[136]

The disadvantages of hyaluronic acid injections are the need to give weekly injections, the cost, and the need for accuracy in giving the injection intra-articularly, as well as possible adverse side effects. There is still no clear understanding how it works as the hyaluronic acid is cleared from the joint within days but its clinical effects may be due to physiological changes as a result of its high molecular weight and the increased viscoelasticity within the joint.[137] It may have a place in the management of mild to moderate knee osteoarthritis in patients who cannot tolerate corticosteroids or who are awaiting total knee replacement. There is little evidence on the long-term benefits and safety of viscosupplementation.[138]

Corticosteroid injections have been used extensively for joint and soft-tissue problems in both primary and secondary care for many years. Their cost-effectiveness and immediate benefits to patients has been recognised by the government with their inclusion in the new contract, although long-term outcomes show little difference from other treatments, such as physiotherapy.

Although corticosteroids have been used for intra-articular injections for the last 30 years, most authorities recommend no more than three or four injections a year. There is no clear evidence that exceeding that number has a deleterious effect or results in a Charcot joint and a recent study has confirmed the safety of repeated corticosteroid injection for knee osteoarthritis.[139] In addition to the anti-inflammatory benefits of corticosteroids, joint aspiration is useful for diagnostic purposes to exclude sepsis and crystal arthropathies, as well as to relieve the pressure of a tense effusion.

Patellar taping of the knee in patients with patello–femoral osteoarthritis has been shown to reduce knee pain and self-reported disability significantly, and is a cheap and effective method of pain relief that can be taught to patients by the physiotherapist.[140] However, nearly all patients with symptomatic knee osteoarthritis benefit, including patients with isolated tibio–femoral osteoarthritis. It can be used in addition to drug treatment and exercise programmes, thereby increasing their benefits. Patients with knee osteoarthritis have reported pain reduction of up to 50% immediately after tape application. These benefits can be maintained in the short-term after treatment has been stopped.[141–2]

Glucosamine/chondroitin

Glucosamine, a naturally occurring aminoglycoside, is a precursor of glycosaminoglycans, an important constituent of articular cartilage. In vitro studies support its role in cartilage repair by stimulating synthesis of glycosaminoglycans.

A Cochrane review concluded that glucosamine had a clinical effect equivalent to NSAIDs and had a significantly better result than placebo, with an excellent side-effect profile.[143] Another review, a meta-analysis of placebo-controlled trials again found in favour of a beneficial effect of both glucosamine and chondroitin in pain relief, and functional improvement in patients with knee osteoarthritis.[144]

Possible disease-modifying effects of glucosamine have caused much interest as this is the first time any drug has been shown to have the possibility of slowing the disease progression of osteoarthritis. Two recent studies have shown significant joint space narrowing in knee osteoarthritis to be much less in patients on glucosamine compared with placebo.[145–6] More long-term studies are needed to confirm these findings. The consensus of the experts is that glucosamine and chondroitin are safe and cheap, with a possible equivalent efficacy to NSAIDs in the long-term (at least a month) and are therefore worth recommending to patients with mild-to-moderate knee osteoarthritis.[147]

As yet there is no standardisation of over-the-counter preparations, although the recommended dosage of glucosamine is 1500 mg daily. Although it has been suggested that glucosamine interferes with insulin resistance, a recent study has shown that it has no effect on the HbA1c concentration in Type 2 diabetics over three months.[148] There is some evidence that chondroitin could have a theoretical effect on the clotting time of some patients on anticoagulants.[149]

Exercise

There is extensive literature that supports the benefits of exercise in the osteoarthritic patient, especially for knee osteoarthritis,[150-1] but it is still an underused therapeutic intervention due to barriers such as patients' lack of knowledge about its benefit, attitudes about the appropriateness of exercise in the elderly and adverse environmental factors that limit exercise uptake.[152] It is important that GPs take these factors into account in order to tailor exercise regimes to the individual. Numerous successful schemes in the UK (exercise on prescription, for example) are active and not only provide mutual support, but allow the individual to start at the appropriate level of exercise.

Key messages

- The benefits of exercise in osteoarthritis cannot be stressed enough.

- Glucosamine/ chondroitin supplementation appears to be a safe and effective treatment, available over-the-counter, for knee osteoarthritis and may slow down disease progression.

- Patellar taping is a useful cost-effective method of pain relief for knee osteoarthritis.

- Corticosteroid and hyaluronic acid injections have a place in the short-term relief of pain and functional impairment of knee osteoarthritis.

Advances in the knowledge of osteoarthritis

Our knowledge of the pathogenesis of osteoarthritis has advanced through our understanding of the microanatomy and physiology of articular cartilage. Articular cartilage has always been thought of as an inert lubricating layer between joints but we now know that there is an active process of degradation and repair, and that chondrocyte metabolism is activated by physiological and pathological mechanical loads.

Articular cartilage is comprised of a collagen network, made up of chains of protein molecules, supported by a matrix of very large complex molecules called aggrecans whose three-dimensional shape enables them to retain water and gives shape, elasticity and strength to the cartilage. Aggrecans are comprised of proteoglycans, which themselves are made from many glycosaminoglycans molecules joined together by hyaluronic acid.

Matrix metalloproteinases (MMPs) are proteolytic enzymes that are involved in the constant breakdown and replacement of active matrix, which helps to maintain tissue integrity. If degradation exceeds renewal then the impaired collagen network leads to surface fibrillations – the initial stage in the progression to osteoarthritis. Further progression may depend on the mechanical load on the joint. Excessive expression of MMPs is known to occur in osteoarthritis and, therefore, there is much interest in the possible use of MMPs inhibitors that could prevent cartilage breakdown at an early stage before progression to osteoarthritis.[153-5]

The other main area of research is in the involvement of the cytokine pathways that are activated in osteoarthritis and lead to synovial inflammation. Some cytokines, notably interleukin-1 (IL-1) and tumour necrosis factor-alpha (TNF-alpha) are produced by the synovium and up-regulate MMPs. Inhibition of these cytokines may be of benefit in preventing progression in osteoarthritis.[156]

What does the future hold for NSAIDs and coxibs?
Nitric oxide-releasing NSAIDs (NO-NSAIDs)are derived from standard NSAIDs and are able to release nitric oxide over a long period of time. They have a good anti-inflammatory effect with minimal gastrointestinal and cardiovascular/renal toxicity.[157]

NSAIDs have been shown to have beneficial effects in the inhibition of colorectal carcinogenesis and possibly Alzheimer's disease and large-scale trials for both are currently underway.[158-9]

Rheumatoid arthritis

Rheumatoid arthritis is a chronic, progressive disease affecting one in 100 of the total UK population.[94] It causes joint pain and stiffness which can often lead to considerable loss of function with consequent disability. This means that each GP will have between 15 and 20 patients with rheumatoid arthritis and will see one new patient who has developed rheumatoid arthritis each year. There is still no national strategy to prioritise the care of patients with rheumatoid arthritis despite calls from the National Rheumatoid Arthritis Society, which has pointed out that rheumatoid arthritis is poorly resourced with too few specialists and that there are inequalities in the availability of new treatments, such as the anti-TNF alpha drugs.[160]

Changes in the new GP contract will encourage GPs to monitor patients on disease-modifying anti-rheumatic drugs and the increasing numbers of GPwSIs will hopefully shorten the prolonged wait between GP referral and secondary care rheumatology appointment. It has been shown that GPs are capable of taking over the management of rheumatoid arthritis follow-up and review following a recent DoH study that showed no detrimental effect on clinical outcome and had the benefits of cost-effectiveness as well as increased patient satisfaction.[161]

The initial priority with rheumatoid arthritis is to make the diagnosis and refer early in onset. Despite guidelines,[162] there is still considerable delay before many patients have a diagnosis and are started on disease-modifying drugs.[163]

Diagnosis can be very difficult in the early stages, with patients complaining of non-specific vague systemic symptoms, little active synovitis, and with no reliable diagnostic tests available. GPs also have to consider the differential diagnoses of viral arthralgia, osteoarthritis and other sero-negative arthropathies. Diagnosis of rheumatoid arthritis is easier when the classic symptoms and signs are present.[164]

At least four of these signs or symptoms should be present for six weeks:

▶ pain and swelling in at least three joint areas

▶ symmetrical presentation

▶ early morning joint stiffness for more than one hour

▶ involvement of metacarpophalangeal, proximal interphalangeal joints or wrists

▶ subcutaneous nodules

▶ positive rheumatoid factor

▶ radiological evidence of erosions.

In addition to starting disease-modifying drugs at an early stage, early intervention allows assessment by the multi-disciplinary team and education of patients to enable them to cope with their disease.

The main aims of treatment are to:

▶ control joint pain and swelling

▶ reduce permanent joint damage

▶ prevent loss of function and disability

▶ take a holistic approach to enable patients to gain control of their disease and improve the quality of their life.

Disease-modifying drugs not only improve the symptoms and reduce the inflammatory markers of rheumatoid arthritis, they also halt disease progression and minimise irreversible joint damage, resulting in improved outcome measures, quality of life and disability.[165] Although, most disease-modifying drugs are usually initiated in secondary care, the new GP contract provides for shared care monitoring of these drugs under enhanced services funding.

Initial treatment in rheumatoid arthritis is usually with sulphasalazine or methotrexate, which are equally efficacious in early rheumatoid arthritis. Patients who fail to respond adequately to initial therapy are changed to a different disease-modifying drug or given combination therapy but a proportion of patients have a sub-optimal response to all disease-modifying drugs. Unfortunately, disease-modifying drugs are also limited in efficacy by their toxicity, which results in many patients either failing to respond adequately or having to stop treatment because of side effects.

Biologic therapy

For patients who have failed to respond to disease-modifying drugs, the development of the new biologics, the anti-TNF alpha drugs, represent a major advance in the treatment of rheumatoid arthritis. These biologic drugs work by switching off the cytokine, TNF-alpha, which stimulates cells to produce the inflammatory response that results in the synovitis of painful swollen joints.

Three biological molecules have been developed: etanercept, infliximab (licensed for treatment in the UK) and adalimumab.

▶ Etanercept is a recombinant human TNF receptor fusion protein which binds to circulating or cell-bound TNF molecules and blocks the action of TNF-alpha. It has to be given subcutaneously twice weekly.

▶ Infliximab is a chimeric murine/human anti-TNF monoclonal antibody which binds to soluble as well as membrane-bound TNF and neutralises the effect of TNF-alpha. It has to be given by slow intravenous infusion at 0, 2 and 6 weeks and then 8-weekly intervals, and is used in combination with methotrexate.

▶ Adalimumab is a fully human anti-TNF monoclonal antibody and is given subcutaneously on alternate weeks.

They all have a very rapid onset of action compared with disease-modifying drugs and the majority of patients achieve a clinically significant response within the first two weeks of treatment.[166-8]

Patients' quality of life has been shown to be substantially improved, demonstrated by a significant reduction in health assessment questionnaire (HAQ) scores with all the anti-TNF drugs. These drugs have all been shown to prevent radiographic progression of the disease, as well as demonstrating sustained efficacy over four years associated with a lack of major toxicity.[169-70]

NICE guidelines recommend the use of etanercept and infliximab (the latter only in combination with methotrexate) as options for the treatment of adults who have continuing active rheumatoid arthritis that has not responded adequately to at least two disease-modifying drugs, including methotrexate (unless contraindicated).[171] Unfortunately, many rheumatologists are unable to follow these recommendations because of restricted funding or lack of specialist nurses and facilities.[172]

Toxicity of these drugs is very low and in general they are well-tolerated. Injection site reactions have occurred with etanercept and infusion-related side effects; for example, dyspnoea, fever, urticaria, have been reported with infliximab. There were no increases in the incidence of infections, serious or otherwise, during the clinical trials and long-term follow-up, but a number of cases of reactivation of tuberculosis have been reported with infliximab. There is a theoretical risk of malignancy and data suggests there may be an increased risk of lymphoma in rheumatoid arthritis patients treated with anti-TNF drugs but at present this is difficult to quantify because of confounding factors.[173]

Anti-TNF drugs have been shown to be highly effective in rheumatoid arthritis, with a rapid action, good risk–benefit ratio, and a sustainable response over four years, and deserve to be more widely available in the UK.[174] The high initial drug costs are offset by the long-term socio-economic savings produced by the prevention of disease progression.

Advances in treatment

Anakinra is the first interleukin antagonist available in the UK. Interleukin-1 (IL-1) is an important pro-inflammatory cytokine involved in the pathophysiology of rheumatoid arthritis. Anakinra is a recombinant IL-1 antagonist that produces a significant improvement in symptoms in rheumatoid arthritis, reduces radiological disease progression, and improves quality of life, as measured by the HAQ. It has a favourable risk–benefit profile.[175-7]

Anti-TNF alpha drugs are showing great promise in the treatment of other autoimmune diseases in addition to rheumatoid arthritis, particularly, in seronegative arthropathies such as ankylosing spondylitis and psoriasis.[178-9]

Rheumatoid arthritis and cardiovascular disease

Despite these advances in treatment, the mortality of rheumatoid arthritis does not appear to have altered over the last thirty years. Rheumatoid arthritis is associated with a significantly increased risk of cardiovascular disease resulting in increased co-morbidity and mortality.[180] The risk is similar to that associated with Type 2 diabetes and accounts for almost half of all deaths in patients with rheumatoid arthritis. In severe rheumatoid arthritis, the risk is equivalent to that from triple vessel coronary disease. This appears to be mainly due to ischaemic heart disease.[181] There is evidence that endothelial dysfunction secondary to rheumatoid vasculitis, results in accelerated athero-genesis.[182] Hypertension is common in rheumatoid arthritis and is significantly increased by NSAIDs and coxibs. GPs should be aware that using angiotensin-converting enzyme (ACE) inhibitors in patients taking NSAIDs may lead to nephrotoxicity.[183] Abnormal lipid profiles are common in patients with rheumatoid arthritis, and active rheumatoid arthritis is associated with reduction in high-density lipoprotein.

The use of statins has been shown to improve the lipid profile and reduce cardiovascular disease in general and their use in rheumatoid arthritis may not only reduce cardiovascular risks but may also have a beneficial immuno-modulatory and anti-inflammatory function on rheumatoid arthritis disease activity.[184]

Key messages

- Check rheumatoid arthritis patients for cardiovascular risk factors, especially blood pressure and lipids.
- Be aware of the effect of NSAIDs on blood pressure, and reduce dose if possible.
- Do not stop aspirin for cardiovascular protection, even if patients are on NSAIDs or coxibs, but try and use NSAIDs intermittently to avoid compromising the effectiveness of the aspirin.
- Avoid use of ACE inhibitors with NSAIDs, especially in the elderly.
- Consider the use of statins in rheumatoid arthritis.
- Encourage exercise.

Self-management

Encouraging patients to manage their own disease is a vital part of treatment. GPs have a critical role in helping, not only with all aspects of chronic disease management, but also with educational activities and directing patients to other sources of information and support.

The activities of the various arthritis charities have been instrumental in providing support to the individual. Arthritis Care set up a helpline service and introduced an arthritis self-management course, Challenging Arthritis.

This has led on to the Expert Patient Programme launched by the DoH. Expert patients and support groups are not just about managing the practical aspects of living with a chronic disabling condition. They enable patients to acknowledge, express and explore their fears and concerns and allow them to regain control over their disease.

In the absence of a National Services Framework, the Arthritis and Musculoskeletal Alliance (ARMA), composed of 27 member organisations, is developing over-arching standards of care for musculoskeletal services, which will help to guide policy makers as well as identify the quality of care that patients should be able to access.

Backwards into the future?

I see the future, not in terms of advances in new drug treatments, but one in which the individual patient retains full control of his / her disease, has instant access to all relevant information and to choice of treatment, which can be tailored to fit his / her special needs, has appropriate support from all the health care professionals and has the final decision in all aspects of his / her care. Our aim is to help the individual achieve the optimum quality of life. As GPs we have a pivotal and crucial role in ensuring patients receive the best possible care and providing this holistic approach, first advocated by Hippocrates, will enable primary care to face the challenges of musculoskeletal medicine in the 21st century.

References

1. Roberts C, Adebajo A O, Long S. Improving the quality of care of musculoskeletal conditions in primary care. *Rheumatology* 2002; **41 (5)**: 503–8

2. Department of Health, *National Services Framework for Older People*. London: HMSO, 2001

3. The Primary Care Rheumatology Society. See: www.pcrsociety.org.uk (accessed 17/09/2004)

4. Burgell R, Worley D, Johanssen A, *et al*. The cost of osteoporotic fractures in the UK: projection for 2000–2020 *J Med Econ* 2001; 4: 51–62

5. Reginster J Y. *The Osteoporosis Paradox: The Neglected Disease*. Belgium: International Osteoporosis Foundation Symposium, 7 December, 2000

6. International Osteoporosis Foundation. *How fragile is her future?* Switzerland: IOF, 2000

7. Ross P D. Clinical consequences of vertebral fractures. *Am J Med* 1997; **103 (S)**: 30S–43S

8. Nevitt M C, Thompson D E, Black D M, *et al*. Effect of alendronate on limited activity days and bed disability days caused by back pain in postmenopausal women with existing vertebral fractures. *Arch Intern Med* 2000; **160**: 77–85

9. Kado D M, Browner W S, Palermo L, *et al*. Vertebral fractures and mortality in older women: a prospective study. *Arch Intern Med* 1999; **159**: 1215–20

10. Cooper C, Atkinson E J, O'Fallon W M, Malton L J. Incidence of clinically diagnosed vertebral fractures: a population-based study in Rochester, Minnesota, 1985–1989. *J Bone Miner Res* 1992; **7**: 221–7

11. Melton L J III, Lane A W, Cooper C, *et al*. Prevalence and incidence of vertebral deformities. *Osteoporos Int* 1993; **3**: 113–19

12. Lindsay R, Silverman S L, Cooper C, *et al*. Risk of new vertebral fracture in the year following a fracture. *JAMA* 2001; **285 (3)**: 630–3

13. Melton L J, Atkinson E J, Cooper C, *et al*. Vertebral fractures predict subsequent fractures. *Ost Int* 1999; **10**: 214–21

14. Nevitt M C, Ettinger B, Black D M, *et al*. The association of radiographically detected vertebral fractures with back pain and function: a prospective study. *Am Int Med* 128; **10**: 793–800

15. Oden A, Dawson A, Dere W, *et al*. Lifetime risk of hip fractures is underestimated. *Ost Int* 1998; **8**: 599–603

16. Lauritzen J B, Schwarz P, Lund B, *et al*. Changing incidence and residual lifetime risk of common osteoporotic-related fractures. *Ost Int* 1993; **3**: 127–32

17. Cooper C. The crippling consequences of fractures and their impact on quality of life. *Am J Med* 1997; **103**: 12S–17S

18. Schurch M A, Rizzoli R, Mermillod B, *et al*. A prospective study on the socio-economic aspects of fracture of the proximal femur. *J Bone Miner Res* 1996; **11**: 1935–42

19. Koike Y, Imaizumi H, Takahashi E, *et al*. Determining factors of mortality in the elderly with hip fractures. *Tohoku J Exp Med* 1999; **188**: 139–42

20. Stewart A, Calder L D, Torgerson D J, *et al*. Prevalence of hip fracture risks in women age 70 years and over. *Q J Med* 2000; **93**: 677–80

21. Calculations based on prevalence of osteoporosis (from the NOS Primary Care Strategy) and the number of GP principals in post.

22. Dolan P, Torgerson D J. The cost of treating osteoporotic fractures in the United Kingdom female population. *Osteoporos Int* 1998; **8**: 611–17

23. National Osteoporosis Society. Accidents, Falls, Fractures, and Osteoporosis. A Strategy for Primary Care Groups and Local Health Groups. Bath: NOS, Jan 2000

24. Smith M G, Dunkow P, Lang D M. Treatment of Osteoporosis: missed opportunities in the hospital fracture clinic. *Osteoporos Int Symposium* Nov 2002; **13 (S3)**: S22

25. Torgerson D J, Dolan P. Prescribing by general practitioners after a osteoporotic fracture. *Ann Rheum Dis* 1998; **57**: 378–9

26. Primary Care Rheumatology Society. *Osteoporosis: minimum standards guidelines for PCR members*. Northallerton: PCRS, Feb 1999

27. Royal College of Physicians. *Osteoporosis: clinical guidelines for prevention and treatment*. London: Royal College of Physicians, 1999

28. Rowe R. The management of osteoporosis in general practice: results of a national survey. *Ost Review* 1999; **7 (2)**

29. Hughes R. *GP survey*. USA: American College of Rheumatology, 2000

30. Department of Health working group. Glucocorticoidinduced osteoporosis: guidelines for prevention and treatment. London: Royal College of Physicians, 2002

31. Klaus J, Ambrecht G, Steinkamp M, *et al.* High Prevalance of Osteoporotic Vertebral Fractures in patients with Crohn's Disease. *Gut* 2002. 51: 654–8

32. US study of Osteoporotic Fractures. *Am Soc Bone Miner Res* Sept 2002

33. University of Boston. Am Soc Bone Miner Res. Sept 2002

34. National Osteoporosis Society. *Osteoporosis in people with coeliac disease: recommendations.* Bath: NOS, Jan 2000

35. Black D M, Steinbuck M, Palermo L, *et al.* An assessment tool for predicting fracture risk in postmenopausal women. *Osteoporos Int* 2001; **12**: 519–28

36. Sedrine W B, Chevalier T, Zegels B, *et al.* Development and assessment of the osteoporosis index of risk (OSIRIS) to facilitate selection of women for bone densitometry. *Gynecol Endocrin* 2002; **16(3)**: 245–50

37. Sen S S, Geling O, Ross PD, *et al.* Validating the Osteoporosis self-assessment tool in New Zealand. *Osteoporos Int Symposium* 2002; **13(S3)**: S 38

38. Vogt T M, Ross P D, Palermo L, *et al.* Vertebral fracture prevalence among women screened for the fracture intervention trial and a simple clinical tool to screen for undiagnosed vertebral fractures. *Mayo Clin Proc* 2000; **75**: 888–96

39. Sen S S, Geling O, Messina O D, *et al.* Identification of Key Predictors for Osteoporosis through use of different analytical techniques. *Osteoporos Int Symposium* 2002; **13(S3)**: S 27

40. National Osteoporosis Society. *Nurse Initiative.* Bath: NOS, 2001

41. Hans D, Dargent-Moline P, Schott AM, *et al.* Ultrasonic heel measurements to predict hip fracture in elderly women: the EPIDOS Prospective Study. *Lancet* 1996; **348**: 511–14

42. Bauer D C, Gluer C C, Cauley J A, *et al.* Broadband ultrasonic attenuation predicts fractures strongly and independently of densitometry in older women. *Arch Int Med* 1997; **157**: 629–34

43. National Osteoporosis Society. *Position statement on the use of quantitative ultrasound in the management of osteoporosis.* Bath: NOS, Dec 2001

44. Hodson J, Marsh J. Quantitative ultrasound and risk factor enquiry as predictors of postmenopausal osteoporosis: comparative study in primary care. *BMJ* 2003; **326**: 1250–1

45. National Osteoporosis Society. *Position statement on the use of peripheral X-ray absorptiometry in the management of osteoporosis.* Bath: NOS, Nov 2001

46. National Osteoporosis Society. *Position statement on the reporting of dual energy x-ray absorptiometry (DEXA) bone mineral density scans.* Bath: NOS, Aug 2002

47. International Osteoporosis Foundation 2001. *Osteoporosis in the European Community. A call to Action*

48. Woolf A D, St John Dixon A. *Osteoporosis: A Clinical Guide.* 2nd ed. London: Dunitz, 1998

49. Parker M J, Gillespie L D, Gillespie W J. Hip protectors for preventing hip fractures in the elderly. Cochrane Database Syst Rev 2003; **(3)**: CD001255

50. Van Schoor N M, Smit J H, Twisk J W, *et al.* Prevention of hip fractures by external hip protectors: a randomized controlled trial. *JAMA* 2003; **289(15)**: 1957–62

51. Cameron I D, Cumming R G, Kurrle SE, *et al.* A randomised trial of hip protector use by frail old women living in their own homes. *Inj Prev* 2003; **9(2)**: 138–41

52. Birks Y F, Hildreth R, Campbell P, *et al.* Randomised controlled trial of hip protectors for the prevention of second hip fractures. *Age and Ageing* 2003; **32(4)**: 442–4

53. Burl J B, Centola J, Bonner A, Burque C. Hip protector compliance: a 13-month study on factors and cost in a long-term care facility. *J Am Med Dir Assoc* 2003; **4(5)**: 245–50

54. Pfeifer M, Begerow B, Minne H W, *et al.* Effects of a short-term vitamin D and calcium supplementation on body sway and secondary hyperparathyroidism in elderly women. *J Bone Miner Res.* 2000. **15 (6)**: 1113–18

55. Heinonen A, Kannis P, Sievanen H, *et al.* Randomised controlled trial of effect of high-impact exercise on selected risk factors for osteoporotic fractures. *Lancet* 1996; **348**: 1343–7

56. Campbell A J, Robertson M C, Gardner M M, *et al.* Randomised controlled trial of a general practice programme of home based exercise to prevent falls in elderly women. *BMJ* 1997; **315**: 1065–9

57. Joakimsen R M, Magmis J H, *et al.* Physical activity and predisposition for hip fractures: a review. *Osteoporos Int* 1997; **7**: 503–13

58. Slemendo C. Prevention of hip fractures: risk factor modification. *Am J Med* 1997; **103**: 655–73

59. Law M R, Wald N J, Meade T E. Strategies for prevention of osteoporosis and hip fracture. *BMJ* 1991; **303**: 453–9

60. Gutin B, Kasper M J. Can vigorous exercise play a role in osteoporosis prevention? *Osteoporos Int* 1992; **2**: 55–69

61. Kannus P, Haapasala H, Sankelo M, *et al.* Effect of starting age of physical activity on bone mass in the dominant arm of tennis and squash players. *Ann Intern Med* 1995; **123**: 27–31

62. Chapuy M C, Preziosi P, Maamer M, *et al.* Prevalence of vitamin D insufficiency in an adult normal population. *Ost Int* 1997; **7**: 439–43

63. Rico H, Revilla M, Villa L F, *et al.* Crush fracture syndrome in senile osteoporosis: a nutritional consequence. *J Bone Min Res* 1992; **7**: 317–19

64. Chapuy M C, Arlot M E, Duboeuf F, *et al.* Vitamin D and calcium to prevent hip fractures in elderly women. *N Engl J Med* 1992; **327**: 1637–42

65. Dawson-Hughes B, Harris S S, Krall E A, *et al.* Effect of calcium and vitamin D supplementation on bone density in men and women 65 years of age or older. *N Engl J Med* 1997; **337**: 670–6

66. Chapuy M C, Pamphile R, Paris, *et al.* Combined calcium and vitamin D3 supplementation in elderly women: confirmation of reversal of secondary hyperparathyroidism and hip fracture risk: the Decalyos II study. *Osteoporos Int* 2002; **13**: 257–64

67. Trivedi D P, Doll R, Khaw K T. Effect of four monthly oral vitamin D3 (cholecalciferol) supplementation on fractures and mortality in men and women living in the community: randomised double blind controlled trial. *BMJ* 2003; **326**: 469–72

68. Meyer H E, Smedshaug G B, *et al.* Can vitamin D supplementation reduce the risk of fracture in the elderly? A randomised controlled trial. *J Bone Miner Res* 2002; **17**: 709–15

69. Heikinheimo R J, Inkovaara J A, Harju E J, *et al.* Annual injection of vitamin D and fractures of aged bones. *Calcif Tissue Int* 1992; **51 (2)**: 105–10

70. Papadimitropoulos E, Wells G, Shea B, *et al.* Meta-analysis of the efficacy of vitamin D treatment in preventing osteoporosis in postmenopausal women. *End Review* 2002; **23 (4)**: 560–9

71. Ankjaer-Jensen J, Johnell O. Prevention of osteoporosis: cost-effectiveness of different pharmaceutical treatments. *Osteoporos Int* **6**: 265–73

72. Jonsson B. Targeting high-risk populations. *Osteoporos Int* 1996 **(S)**: S13–S16

73. Jonsson B, Kanis J, Dawson A, *et al.* Effect and offset of effect of treatment for hip fracture on health outcomes. *Osteoporos Int* 1999; **10**: 193–199

74. Tosteson A N A, Rosenthal D I, *et al.* Cost effectiveness of screening perimenopausal white women for osteoporosis: Bone densitometry and hormone replacement therapy. *Ann Intern Med* 113: 594–603

75. Bone H G, Hosking D, Devogelaer J P, *et al.* Ten years' experience with alendronate for osteoporosis in postmenopausal women. *N Engl J Med* 2004; **350(12)**: 1189–99

76. Black D M, Thompson D E, Bauer D C, *et al.* Fracture risk reduction with alendronate in women with osteoporosis: the Fracture intervention Trial. *J Clin Endocrin Metab* 2000; **85**: 4118–24

77. McClung M R, Geusens P, Miller P D, *et al.* Effect of risedronate on the risk of hip fracture in elderly women. *N Engl J Med* 2001; **344**: 333–40

78. Reginster J Y, Minne H W, Sorenson O H, *et al.* Randonised trial of the effects of risedronate on vertebral fractures in women with established postmenopausal osteoporosis. *Osteoporo Int* 2000; **11**: 83–9

79. Rossouw J E, Anderson G L, Prentice R L, *et al.* Risks and benefits of estrogen plus progestin in healthy postmenopausal women. Principal results from the Women's Health Initiative randomised controlled trial. *JAMA* 2002; **288**: 321–33

80. Royal College of Physicians of Edinburgh. *Consensus Conference on Hormone Replacement Therapy. Final Consensus Statement.* Edinburgh: Royal College of Physicians of Edinburgh, 2003. www.rcpe.ac.uk/esd/consensus/hrt_03.html

81. Nelson H D, *et al.* Osteoporosis and fractures in postmenopausal women using oestrogen. *Arch Intern Med* 2002; **162**: 2278–84

82. Cummings S R, Eckert S, Krueger K A, *et al.* MORE Randomised Trial. The effect of raloxifene on risk of breast cancer in postmenopausal women. *JAMA* 1999; **281**: 2189–97

83. Sackett D L, Snow J C. The magnitude of compliance and non-compliance. In: Haynes R B, Taylor W D, Sackett D L (eds), *Compliance in Health Care.* Baltimore: John Hopkins Univ Press, 1979: 11–22

84. De Groes P C, Lubbe D F, Hirsch L J, *et al.* Esophagitis associated with the use of alendronate. *N Eng J Med* 1996; **335**: 1016–21

85. Schnitzer T, Bone H G, Crepaldi G. Therapeutic equivalence of alendronate 70 mg once-weekly and alendronate 10mg daily in the treatment of osteoporosis. *Aging* (Milano) 2000; **12(1)**: 1–12

86. Rees T P, Howe I. A randomised, single blind crossover comparison of the acceptability of the calcium and vitamin D3 supplements Calcichew D3 Forte and AdCal D3 in elderly patients. *Curr Med Res* 2001; **16(4)**: 245–51

87. Fogelman I. Screening for osteoporosis. No point until we have resolved issues about long-term treatment. *BMJ* 1999; **319**: 1148–9

88. Neer R M, Arnaud C D, Zanchetta J R, *et al.* Effect of parathyroid hormone on vertebral bone mass and fracture incidence among postmenopausal women with osteoporosis. *N Engl J Med* 2001; **344**: 1434–41

89. Hofbauer L C, Heufelder A E. Role of receptor activator of nuclear factor-kappaB ligand and osteoprotegerin in bone cell biology. *J Mol Med* 2001; **79(5–6)**: 243–53

90. Meunier PJ, Roux C, Seeman E, *et al.* The effects of strontium ranelate on the risk of vertebral fracture in women with postmenopausal osteoporosis. *N Engl J Med* 2004; **350**: 459–68

91. European Commission. *Report on Osteoporosis in the European Community. Action for Prevention.* Luxembourg: Office for Official Publications of the European Communities, 1998

92. Department of Health NHS Executive. *Burdens of disease: a discussion document.* London: HMSO, 1996

93. Belsey J. Primary care workload in the management of chronic pain. A retrospective cohort study using a GP database to identify resource implications for UK primary care. *J Drug Assess* 2002; **5**: 153–64

94. Arthritis Research Campaign. Arthritis: the big picture. www.arc.org.uk/about_arth/bigpic.htm (accessed 17/09/2004)

95. Moore RA, Tramer M, Carroll D, *et al.* Quantitative systematic review of topically applied non-steroidal anti-inflammatory drugs. *BMJ* 1998; **316**: 333–8

96. Grace D, Rogers J, Skeith K, Anderson K. Topical diclofenac versus placebo: A double blind randomised clinical trial in patients with osteoarthritis of the knee. *J Rheumatol* 1999; **26**: 2659–63

97. Prescott LF. Paracetamol: past, present, and future. *Am J Ther* 2000; **7(2)**: 143–7

98. Singh G. Gastrointestinal complications of prescription and over-the-counter nonsteroidal anti-inflammatory drugs: a view from the Aramis database. *Am J Ther* 2000; **7(2)**: 115–21

99. Shaheen SO, Newson RB, Sheriff A, *et al.* Paracetamol use in pregnancy and wheezing in early childhood. *Thorax* 2002; **57(11)**: 958–63

100. Towheed TE, Judd MJ, Hochberg MC, Wells G. Acetaminophen for osteoarthritis. Cochrane Database Syst Rev 2003; **(2)**: CD004257

101. Langman MJS. Anti-inflammatory drugs and the gut-ulcerative damage and protection from damage. *Excerpta Medica* 1995; **72**: 1–8

102. CSM Update. Non-steroidal anti-inflammatory drugs and serious gastro-intestinal adverse reactions: 1. *BMJ* 1986; **292**: 614

103. CSM. Reminder: Gastrointestinal toxicity of NSAIDs. *Current Problems in Pharmacovigilance* 2003; **29**: 8

104. Jones AC, Coulson L, Muir K, *et al.* A nurse delivered advice intervention can reduce chronic non-steroidal anti-inflammatory drug use in general practice: a randomised controlled trial. *Rheumatology* (Oxford) 2002; **41(1)**: 14–21

105. Russell RI. Protection from NSAID-induced gastro-intestinal damage. *Inflammopharmacology* 1995; **3**: 327–33

106. Hawkey CJ. Non-steroidal anti-inflammatory drug gastropathy: causes and treatment. *Scand J Gastroenterol* 1996; **31(S220)**: 124–7

107. MacDonald TM, Morant SV, Robinson GC, *et al.* The risk of serious upper GI complications is constant with continuous NSAID therapy: results of a record linkage study in 52,382 exposed patients. *Gastroenterology* 1995; **108(4)**

108. Armstrong CP, Blower AL. Non-steroidal anti-inflammatory drugs and life-threatening complications of peptic ulceration. *Gut* 1987; **28**: 527–32

109. Tramer MR, *et al.* Quantitative estimation of rare adverse events which follow a biological progression: a new model applied to chronic NSAID use. *Pain* 2000; **85**: 169–82

110. Blower AL. Predicting GI Complications. Clinical Forum. *The Silent Risk.* 1996

111. Henry D, Mc Gettigan P. Epidemiology overview of gastrointestinal and renal toxicity of NSAIDs. *Int J Clin Pract Suppl* 2003; **(135)**: 43–9

112. Ofman JJ, Maclean CH, Straus WL, *et al.* Meta-analysis of dyspepsia and non-steroidal anti-inflammatory drugs. *Arthritis Rheum* 2003; **49(4)**: 508–18

113. Hawkey C J. Non-steroidal anti-inflammatory drugs and peptic ulcers. *BMJ* 1990; **300**: 278–84

114. Hawkey C J, Rampton D S. Prostaglandins and the gastro-intestinal mucosa: are they important in its function, disease or treatment. *Gastroenterology* 1985; **89**: 1162–88

115. Barden J, Edwards J E, McQuay H J, Moore R A. Single-dose rofecoxib for acute postoperative pain in adults: a quantitative systematic review. *BMC Anesthesiol* 2002; **2(1)**: 4

116. Bombardier C, Laine L, Reicin A, *et al*. Comparison of upper gastrointestinal toxicity of rofecoxib and naproxen in patients with rheumatoid arthritis. VIGOR Study Group

117. Lisse J R, Perlman M, Johansson G, *et al*. *Gastrointestinal tolerability and effectiveness of rofecoxib versus naproxen in the treatment of osteoarthritis: a randomized controlled trial. Ann Intern Med* 2003; **139**: 539–46

118. Silverstein FE, Faich G, Goldstein J L, *et al*. *Gastrointestinal toxicity with celecoxib vs nonsteroidal anti-inflammatory drugs for osteoarthritis and rheumatoid arthritis: the CLASS study: A randomised controlled trial*

119. Whelton A, Fort J G, Puma J A, *et al*. Cyclooxygenase-2-specific inhibitors and cardiorenal function: a randomised controlled trial of celecoxib and rofecoxib in older hypertensive osteoarthritis patients. *Am J Ther* 2001; **(2)**: 85–95

120. National Institute for Clinical Excellence. *Guidance on the use of cyclo-oxygenase (Cox) 2 selective inhibitors in the treatment of osteoarthritis and rheumatoid arthritis*. NICE Technology Apppraisal Guidance. London: NICE, 2001

121. Anonymous. Coxibs in arthritis: update July 2002. Bandolier. www.jr2.ox.ac.uk/bandolier/booth/Arthritis/coxib702.html (accessed 17/09/2004)

122. Moore A. Arthritis: should we be prescribing coxibs? *The New Generalist* 2003; **1(1)**

123. Rauss E A, Tytgat G N J. Eradication of Helicobacter pylori cures duodenal ulcer. *Lancet* 1990; **335**: 1233–5

124. Malfertheiner P. Current European concepts in the management of Helicobacter pylori infection: the Maastricht consensus report. *Gut* 1997; **41**: 8–13

125. Konturek P C, Konturek S J, Czesnikiewicz M, *et al*. Interaction of Helicobacter pylori and non-steroidal anti-inflammatory drugs on gastric mucosa and risk of ulcerations. *Med Sci Monit* 2002; **8(9)**: RA 197–209

126. Lee Y T, Chan F K L, Sung J Y, *et al*. Prevention of NSAID-induced ulcer by eradication of Helicobacter pylori. A prospective randomised study (abstract). *Gut* 1996; **39(S2)**: A26

127. Ng T M, Fock K M, *et al*. Helicobacter pylori and NSAIDs in bleeding gastric ulcer (abstract). *Gut* 1996; **39(S2)**: A2

128. Frishman W H. Effects of nonsteroidal anti-inflammatory drug therapy on blood pressure and peripheral oedema. *Am J Cardiol* 2002; **89(6A)**: 18D–25D

129. Bleumink G S, Feenstra J, Sturkenboom M C, Stricker B H. Nonsteroidal anti-inflammatory drugs and heart failure. *Drugs* 2003; **63(6)**: 525–34

130. Page J, Henry D. Consumption of NSAIDS and the development of congestive cardiac failure in elderly patients: an underrecognised public health problem. *Arch Intern Med* 2000; **160(6)**: 777–84

131. Miltner O, Schneider U, Siebert C H, *et al*. Efficacy of intraarticular hyaluronic acid in patients with osteoarthritis – a prospective clinical trial. *Osteo & Cart* 2002; **10(9)**: 680–6

132. Couceiro J M. Multicenter clinical trial on the efficacy of intra-articular hyaluronic acid in osteoarthritis of the knee. *Revista Espanola de Reumatologia Sabado* 2003; **30: (02)**: 57–65

133. Huskisson E C, Donnelly S. hyaluronic acid in the treatment of osteoarthritis of the knee. *Rheumatology* (Oxford) 1999; **38 (7)**: 602–7

134. Bayramoglu M, *et al*. Comparison of two different viscosupplements in knee osteoarthritis- a pilot study. *Clin Rheum* 2003; **22(2)**: 118–22

135. Redd B. AAOS: Hylan Injections show equal efficacy as Corticosteroids for Arthritis of the Knee. Annual Meeting of A AO S. (7/2/2003)

136. Frizziero L, Ronchhetti P. Intra-articular treatment of osteoarthritis of the knee: an arthroscopic and clinical comparison between sodium hyaluronate and methylprednisolone acetate. *J Orth Traum* 2002; (Abstract) **3 (2)**: 89–96

137. Moreland L W. Intra-articular hyaluronan and hylans for the treatment of osteoarthritis: mechanisms of action. *Arthritis Res Ther* 2003; **5 (2)**: 54–67

138. Espallargues M, Pons J M. Efficacy and safety of viscosupplementation with Hylanm G - F 20 for the treatment of knee osteoarthritis: a systematic review. *Int J Technol Assess Health Care* 2003; **19 (1)**: 41–56

139. Raynauld J, Buckland-Wright C, Ward R, *et al*. Safety and efficacy of long-term intra-articular steroid injections in osteoarthritis of the knee: A randomised, double-blind, placebo controlled trial. *Arth Rheum* 2003; **48 (2)**: 370–7

140. Cushnaghan, *et al*. Taping the patella medially: a new treatment for osteoarthritis of the knee joint? *BMJ* 1994; **308**: 753–5

141. Hinman R S, Crossley K M, McConnell J, Bennell K L. Efficacy of knee tape in the management of osteoarthritis of the knee: blinded randomised controlled trial. *BMJ* 2003; **327**: 135–8

142. Hinman R S, Bennell K L, Crossley K N, McConnell J. Immediate effects of adhesive tape on pain and disability in individuals with knee osteoarthritis. *Rheumatology* (Oxford) 2003; **42 (7)**: 865–9

143. Towheed T E, *et al*. Glucosamine therapy for treating osteoarthritis (Cochrane Review). In: The Cochrane Library, Issue 1, 2001. Oxford: Update Software

144. McAlindon, *et al*. Glucosamine and chondroitin for treatment of osteoarthritis. A systematic quality assessment and meta-analysis. *JAMA* 2000. **283**: 1469–73

145. Pavelka K, Gatterova J, Olejarova M, *et al*. Glucosamine sulphate use and delay of progression of knee osteoarthritis: a 3-year, randomised, placebo-controlled, double-blind study. *Arch Intern Med* 2002; **162**: 2113–23

146. Reginster J Y, Deroisy R, Rovati L C, *et al*. Long-term effects of glucosamine sulphate on osteoarthritis progression: a randomised, placebo-controlled clinical trial. *Lancet* 2001; **357**: 251–6

147. Anon. Is glucosamine worth taking for osteoarthritis? *Drug Ther Bull* 2002; **40 (11)**: 81–3

148. Scroggie D A, Albright A, Harris M D. The effect of glucosamine-chondroitin supplementation on glycosylated haemoglobin levels in patients with type 2 diabetes mellitus: a placebo, double-blinded, randomised controlled clinical trial. *Arch Intern Med* 2003; **163 (13)**: 1587–90

149. Brecher A S, Adamu M T. Coagulation protein function: enhancement of the anticoagulant effect of acetyaldehyde by sulphated glycosaminoglycans. *Dig Dis Sci* 2001; **46 (9)**: 2033–42

150. Fransen M, McConnell S, Bell M. Exercise for osteoarthritis of the knee or hip. Cochrane Database Rev 2003; **(3)**: C D 004286

151. Brosseau L, MacLeay L, Robinson V, *et al*. Intensity of exercise for the treatment of osteoarthritis. Cochrane Database Rev 2003; **(2)**: C D 004259

152. Heath J M, Stuart M R. Prescribing exercise for frail elders. *J Am Board Fam Pract* 2002; **15(3)**: 218–28

153. Martel-Pelletier J, Welsch D J, Pelletier J P. Metalloproteases and inhibitors in arthritis diseases. *Best Pract Res Clin Rheumatol* 2001; **15(5)**: 805–29

154. Masuhara K, Nakai T, Yamaguchi K, *et al.* Significant increases in serum and plasma concentrations of matrix metalloproteinases 3 and 9 in patients with rapidly destructive osteoarthritis of the hip. *Arthritis Rheum* 2002; **46(10)**: 2625–31

155. Marder G, Greenwald R A. Potential applications of matrix metalloproteinases in geriatric practice. *Isr Med Assoc J* 2003; **5(5)**: 361–4

156. Fernandez J C, Martel-Pelletier J P. The role of cytokines in osteoarthritis pathophysiology. *Biorheology* 2002; **39(1–2)**: 237–46

157. Bandarage U K, Janero D R. Nitric oxide-releasing nonsteroidal anti-inflammatory drugs: novel gastrointestinal-sparing drugs. *Mini Rev Med Chem* 2001; **1(1)**: 57–70

158. Garcia-Rodriguez L A, Huerta-Alvarez C. Reduced risk of colorectal cancer among long-term users of aspirin and nonaspirin nonsteroidal anti-inflammatory drugs. *Epidemiology* 2001; **12(1)**: 88–93

159. Etminan M, Gill S, Samii A. Effect of nonsteroidal anti-inflammatory drugs on the risk of Alzheimer's disease: systematic review and meta-analysis of observational studies. *BMJ* 2003; **327**: 128

160. *The Painful Truth: A consensus statement from the National Rheumatoid Arthritis Society.* National Rheumatoid Arthritis Society. Maidenhead: N RA S, July 2003

161. Kirwan J R. Outpatient workload. *Rheumatology* (Oxford) 2003; **42(10)**: 1269–70

162. Primary Care Rheumatology Society. Rheumatoid arthritis: a protocol for early referral and DMARD monitoring guidelines. 27/9/2001.

163. Emery P, Breedveld F C, Dougados M, *et al.* Early referral recommendation for newly diagnosed rheumatoid arthritis: evidence based development of a clinical guide. *Ann Rheum Disease* 2002; **61**: 290–7

164. Arnett F C, Edworthy S M, Bloch D A, *et al.* The American Rheumatism Association 1987 revised criteria for the classification of rheumatoid arthritis. *Arthritis Rheum* 1988; **31**: 315–24

165. Fries J F, Williams C A, Morfeld D, Singh G, *et al.* Reduction in long-term disability in patients with rheumatoid arthritis by diease-modifying antirheumatic drug-based treatment strategies. *Arthritis Rheum* 1996; **39**: 606–22

166. Weinblatt M E, Kremer J M, Bankhurst A D, *et al.* A trial of etanercept, a recombinant tumour necrosis factor receptor:Fc fusion protein, in patients with rheumatoid arthritis receiving methotrexate. *N Engl J Med* 1999; **340**: 253–9

167. Maini R, St Clair E W, Breedveld F, *et al.* Infliximab (chimeric anti-tumour necrosis factor alpha monoclonal antibody) versus placebo in rheumatoid arthritis patients receiving concomitant methotrexate: a randomised phase III trial. *Lancet* 1999; **354**: 1932–9

168. Lipsky P E, Van der Heijde D M, St. Clair E W, *et al.* Infliximab and methotrexate in the treatment of rheumatoid arthritis. Anti-tumour necrosis factor trial in rheumatoid arthritis with concomitant therapy study group. *N Engl J Med* 2000; **343**: 1594–602

169. Genovese M, Bathon J M, Martin R W, *et al.* Etanercept vs. methotrexate in early rheumatoid arthritis. Two-year radiographic and clinical outcomes. *Arthritis Rheum* 2002; **46**: 1443–50

170. Moreland L M, Cohen S B, Baumgartner S W, *et al.* Long-term safety and efficacy of etanercept in patients with rheumatoid arthritis. *J Rheumatol* 2001; **28**: 1238–44

171. National Institute for Clinical Excellence. *Guidance on the use of etanercept and infliximab for the treatment of rheumatoid arthritis.* Technology Appraisal Guidance No. 36. London: NICE, March 2002

172. Arthritis and Musculoskeletal Alliance. *ARMA Implementation of NICE Guidance on the use of Anti-TNF alpha Therapies for Adults with Rheumatoid Arthritis;* A report by ARMA, July 2003

173. Zatarain E, Chakravarty EF, Genovese MC. Rheumatoid Arthritis, TNF Inhibition, and the Risks of Lymphoma. *Int J Adv Rheum* 2003, 1(3): 91–6

174. Haraoui B, Keystone EC. Anti-TNF Therapy in Rheumatoid Arthritis: Were the Promises Fulfilled? *Int J Adv Rheum* 2003, 1(3): 82–90

175. Rubbert-Roth A, Perniok A. Treatment of patients with rheumatoid arthritis with the interleukin-1 receptor antagonist anakinra. *Z Rheumatol* 2003; 62(4): 367–77

176. Bresnihan B, Cobby M. Clinical and radiological effects of anakinra in patients with rheumatoid arthritis. *Rheumatology* (Oxford) 2003; 42(2)ii: 22–8

177. Cohen SB, Rubbert A. Bringing the clinical experience with anakinra to the patient. *Rheumatology* (Oxford) 2003; 42(2)ii: 36–40

178. Braun J, Pham T, Sieper J, *et al.* International ASAS consensus statement for the use of anti-tumour necrosis factor agents in patients with ankylosing spondylitis. *Ann Rheum Dis 2003;* 62(9): 817–24

179. Dubin DB, Tanner W, Ellis R. Biologics for psoriasis. *Nat Rev Drug Discov* 2003; 2(11): 855–6

180. Watson DJ, Rhodes T, Guess HA. All-cause mortality and vascular events among patients with rheumatoid arthritis, osteoarthritis, or no arthritis in the UK General Practice Research Database. *J Rheumatol* 2003; 30(6): 1196–202

181. Kitas GD, Erb N. Tackling ischaemic heart disease in rheumatoid arthritis. *Rheumatol* 2003; 42: 607–13

182. Bacon PA, Stevens RJ, Carruthers DM, Young SP, *et al.* Accelerate atherogenesis in autoimmune rheumatic diseases. *Autoimmun Rev* 2002; 1(6): 338–47

183. Adhiyaman V, Asghar M, Oke A, *et al.* Nephrotoxicity in the elderly due to co-prescription of angiotensin converting enzyme inhibitors and nonsteroidal anti-inflammatory drugs. *J R Soc Med* 2001; 94: 512–4

184. Kwak B, Mulhaupt F, Myit S, Mach F. Statins as a newly recognised type of immunomodulator. *Nat Med* 2000; 6: 1399–402

Further information

Primary Care Rheumatology Society • www.pcrsociety.org.uk

Arthritis Research Campaign (ARC) • www.arc.org.uk

Arthritis Care • www.arthritiscare.org.uk

Arthritis and Musculoskeletal Alliance • www.arma.uk.net

National Rheumatoid Arthritis Society • www.rheumatoid.org.uk

National Osteoporosis Society • www.nos.org.uk

British Society for Rheumatology • www.rheumatology.org.uk

CHAPTER 14

Mental Health

Alan Cohen

▶ KEY MESSAGES
- Common mental health problems are common – very common. They account for 30% of general practice consultations, and 90% of people with mental health problems are managed entirely in primary care.

- The management of depression and anxiety will be influenced significantly over the forthcoming 24 months by the publication and implementation of NICE guidelines.

- There is, however, little new money to provide for the successful management of these common and disabling conditions.

- These guidelines are more likely to be successfully implemented if the flexibilities of the new GMS contract are fully utilised.

- The new GMS contract makes clear that the physical health of people with a severe and enduring mental illness is the responsibility of primary care services – and that physical illness for people with schizophrenia and bi-polar affective disorder is a significant cause of morbidity and mortality in this group.

Mental health problems are common; 30% of all general practice consultations have a mental health component. Out of all those with mental health problems, 90% are managed entirely in primary care, and 30% of all people with a severe and enduring mental illness are managed entirely in primary care.[1]

Figure 14.1 **Costs associated with providing care for people with mental health problems**[2]

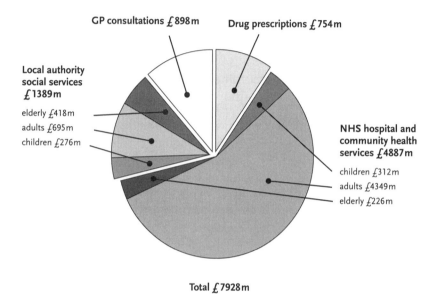

GP consultations £898m   Drug prescriptions £754m

Local authority social services £1389m

elderly £418m
adults £695m
children £276m

NHS hospital and community health services £4887m

children £312m
adults £4349m
elderly £226m

Total £7928m

The above diagram represents the costs to the public purse of providing mental health services in England for 2002–03. The disparity between the costs associated with specialist mental health services (who provide care for some 10% of people with mental health problems) compared with the estimated cost of general practice consultations is clear, and is an interesting example of the '80:20 rule'. What is more significant is that the majority of advances made in the field of mental health provision lies within the specialist care systems. It is in the nature of caring for people with mental health problems that there will be no new operation discovered to cure depression, no sudden blinding insight into the human genetic code that will prevent people becoming stressed at work. Advances in mental health tend to involve two broad areas, new medications, and the way that care is being delivered – the organisation of care, different teams, new workers etc.

More confusingly, the organisation of care, and the introduction of new ways of working seems to be geographically dependent. Devolution of central government to national assemblies has also meant that financial resources to fund organisational development is geographically dependent – so that resources for Northern Ireland services may be different to those available to English GPs. In England and Wales, the National Institute for Clinical Excellence (NICE) is the arbiter of new technologies and medications. A separate system exists for Scotland, with organisations such as the Scottish Intercollegiate Guideline Network (SIGN) providing advice about guidelines and their implementation, which can overlap in some areas with NICE. This survey of recent advances will therefore discuss recommendations that come from both centres, even though it is acknowledged that not all GPs may be able to access or implement such changes.

Even more inequitably, this review will also cover the policy changes that are being introduced as a consequence of the NHS Plan, in England. Whilst these changes are limited to England, their significance to the provision of primary care mental health services is profound, and need to be discussed.

Further to this, American research on the organisation of primary care will be included, since – unlikely as this may seem – it has an impact on the development of services in the UK.

This review will consider advances in the delivery of care in relation to both the management of common mental health problems, such as depression and anxiety, as well as the management of severe and enduring mental illness.

The new GMS contract has just been introduced, and for the first time there are specific incentives to improve the way that care is provided in primary care for people with severe mental illness and depression. This probably represents the most significant recent advance, and so when discussing the management of these conditions, the relevance to the new contract will be identified.

Common mental health disorders

These disorders include conditions such as depression, generalised anxiety, panic disorder, mixed anxiety with depression, adjustment disorder, and somatisation – all of which are the bread and butter of Monday morning surgery. Less common are post traumatic stress disorder, obsessive compulsive disorder, other phobias and eating disorders.

Table 14.1 **Prevalence of mental health disorders in primary care**

Diagnosis	Weekly prevalence per 1000 adults aged 16–64	No of patients on GP list of 1650 (assuming 63% of GP list is aged 16–64)	No of patients on GP list of 2000 (assuming 63% of GP list is aged 16–64)
Psychotic illness	4	4	5
Mixed anxiety and depression	92	96	116
Generalised anxiety	47	49	59
Depressive episode	28	29	35
All phobias	19	20	24
Obsessive compulsive disorder	12	12	15
Panic disorder	7	8	9
All neuroses	173	180	218
Drug dependence	42	44	53
Alcohol dependence	81	84	102

Data for ONS taken from the Psychiatric Morbidity Survey among adults living in private households, 2000[3]

The above table, drawn from the most recently available data, provides some evidence as to the extent of mental health morbidity in primary care. Over 10% of the patients on a GP's list will have a significant mental health problem. Up until 2000, there had never been a specific allocation of resources from within the mental health budget to provide support and care for these people. Counselling services, which are present in over 50% of PCTs, have always been funded from primary care sources, such as GP fund holding, or by moving resources from other services. It is therefore welcomed that the NHS Plan (2000)[4] in England, for the first time, identified a new resource for the provision of primary care mental health services, the new post of a graduate mental health worker, and promised the resources to develop these new roles.

In 1999 the National Service Framework for Mental Health[5] set standards for the role of primary care in the provision of mental health services. The standards required of primary are outlined in Box 14.1.

Box 14.1 **National Service Framework for Mental Health – standards two and three**

Standard two

Any service user who contacts their primary health care team with a common mental health problem should:

- have their mental health needs identified and assessed

- be offered effective treatments, including referral to specialist services for further assessment, treatment and care if they require it.

Standard three

Any individual with a common mental health problem should:

- be able to make contact round-the-clock with the local services necessary to meet their needs and receive adequate care

- be able to use *NHS Direct*, as it develops, for first-level advice and referral on to specialist helplines or to local services.

To support the implementation of these standards, the NHS Plan outlined a new post – that of graduate mental health worker – that was intended to support primary care to provide these services (Box 14.2).

Box 14.2 **Graduate mental health workers in primary care**

Most mental health problems are managed in primary care. One in four GP consultations are with people with mental health problems. So improving these services will have a major impact on the health and wellbeing of the population:

- one thousand new graduate primary care mental health workers, trained in brief therapy techniques of proven effectiveness, will be employed to help GPs manage and treat common mental health problems in all age groups, including children. In addition, 500 more community mental health staff will be employed to work with general practitioners and primary care teams, with NHS Direct, and in each accident and emergency department to respond to people who need immediate help. These staff will be able to call on crisis resolution teams if necessary

- by 2004, more than 300,000 people will receive extra help from the new primary care mental health workers and around 500,000 people will benefit from additional mental health staff working in frontline settings. These changes will ease pressure on GP services.

The process of implementing the introduction of these new workers is now well underway. Their role has been developed, the resources identified, and the training programmes commissioned. There are now twelve locations around England that are providing the training for these new workers.

The guidance published by the DoH in 2002,[6] described three main areas of work for these workers: client work, secondly practice work, and finally working with the wider community.

▶ **Client Work**: This means working with the individual patient, and includes a number of different types of talking therapy that are believed to have a significant evidence base. Thus these new workers will be able to provide a number of brief interventions such as interpersonal therapy. Brief interventions, of one sort or another, have been shown to be effective in a number of different conditions such as of health-risk behaviours including: smoking; problems with alcohol;[7] unexplained physical symptoms;[8] areas related to mental health such as sleep problems;[9] or regulation of long-term benzodiazepine or hypnotic drugs.[10] Cognitive behaviour therapy (CBT) has a strong evidence base for effectiveness in helping people with mild-to-moderate depression, and a slightly less strong evidence base for helping people with anxiety and panic disorder. Graduate workers will be expected to provide CBT to help manage these conditions. It is important here to emphasise the DoH's guidance, in that the intened role for these workers is to provide care to people who have been properly assessed by another professional. Graduate workers will not have the skills, or training, to be able to assess a person presenting to primary care with mental distress – that is predominantly the responsibility of the GP or the Community Mental Health Team (CMHT), but if subsequent treatment with CBT or some other form of brief talking therapy is required, then graduate workers may be appropriate to deliver that intervention.

It is interesting to note that the original NHS Plan description of the possible work of a graduate worker included not only what they might do, but whom they might work with – who their clients may be. In this context the NHS Plan and the subsequent guidance is clear that there is a role for these workers in caring for children with mental health problems. This should be considered very carefully following the advice from the Committee on Safety of Medicines that a number of antidepressants, specifically venlafaxine and paroxetine, should not be used in children and adolescents. Managing children and adolescents with depression requires a multi-disciplinary team response as the DoH guidance makes quite clear. There may be a role however for these workers in supporting children with some forms of behaviour disturbance.

▶ **Practice Work**: The intention here is to support practices in providing more effective care to people with mental health problems. This support may take many forms, from help and advice in completing practice audits, creating registers of people with particular conditions, to developing support groups of users to feedback information on the quality and quantity of services. There is also the opportunity for these workers to facilitate the development of closer working between both CMHT and Primary Health Care Team (PHCT), and between PHCTs to share services, knowledge and skills more effectively.

▶ **Working with the Wider Community**: There is a potential role for these workers to develop the strengths of the voluntary sector, by collecting information on available local services into a register which can be accessed by primary care teams. They may also take on a similar role with the statutory sector by developing maps of how to navigate mental health and social services care to ensure that the housing, educational, employment needs of individuals are being appropriately addressed by services, and that they can be accessed by primary care staff.

That the DoH has allocated a significant resource to primary care mental health services is to be applauded and supported. Inevitably, however, there have been questions as to the details of these new workers. This paper is not intended to be a critique of graduate mental health workers, and for those who are interested in further information, the CPC,[11] the Manchester Primary Care Research and Development Centre,[12] and the Counselling in Primary Care Trust[13] all have significant information and publications on this issue.

NICE guidelines

At the time of writing, the NICE guidelines on Depression[14] are available as a first draft consultation. By the time of publication the Depression and Anxiety Guidelines should both be available in their final forms (*due at the end of 2004*). It is therefore inappropriate to comment on their content at this point although even at this early stage there are two issues that should be highlighted. The first is the opportunity of linking the development of national guidelines to the national enhanced level of care in depression as described in the new GP contract, and secondly the concept of a stepped care approach to managing people with depression.

The recently approved GMS contract introduced many new concepts to the way that general practitioners are rewarded for providing a high quality service to their patients. A national enhanced level of service for people with depression is one of the innovations introduced.

Box 14.3 **Definition of enhanced services**

> **The contract document, at paragraph 2.13, states:**
>
> Enhanced services are:
>
> i. essential or additional services delivered to a higher specified standard, for example, extended minor surgery
>
> ii. services not provided through essential or additional services. These might include more specialised services undertaken by GPs or nurses with special interests and secondary care requirements, and innovative services that are being piloted and evaluated.

The guidance produced with the new contract set out the aims, definition, service outline and accreditation criteria. The clinical standards set are based on the Defeat Depression Campaign run jointly between the Royal College of General Practitioners and the Royal College of Psychiatrists. Since the current NICE guidelines for depression have not yet been finally approved and published, it is not yet possible to say how they may differ from the currently described best practice. One would hope that there will not be a great difference, but that the advisors to the contract conditions undertake to look at the guidelines when they are published and make any changes that may be appropriate. To link a nationally enhanced service to nationally agreed guidelines produced by NICE would be a very effective method of implementation, an issue that has bedevilled the use of guidelines for many years.

The guidelines have been developed by NICE for use in England and Wales; the contract negotiators will have to find a way to manage the fact that, as clinical evidence is updated, the recommendations from any guideline may vary between the four countries in the UK.

Stepped care

In 2001, Goldberg and von Korff[10] reviewed the structural changes needed to improve the care of people with depression. They describe twelve papers, randomised controlled studies since 1995, that tried to influence the behaviour of general practitioners, and analysed which elements of the interventions had been effective. The authors found that all twelve studies used treatment guidelines, screening and patient education, but that only seven studies had been successful in improving the outcome for the sufferer. The element of the interventions that consistently improved patient outcome was case management and access to a specialist mental health professional.

Case management in this context included active follow-up of the patient to ascertain if the treatment plan was being adhered to, and whether or not the depressive symptoms were improving, and then taking action – if adherence was poor or the patient was not improving – by appropriate referral to a mental health specialist. Such contacts with patients were often made by telephone follow-up, which provided a relatively low cost per case. The important message made by the authors was that to significantly influence the outcome of a common condition it is not sufficient just to provide treatment guidelines. Other structural changes are needed, such as case management, which sits between standard primary care services and standard secondary care/community mental health teams. The first draft of the NICE guidelines for depression introduce this concept as a stepped care programme in England and Wales.

Figure 14.2 **Depression: core interventions in the management of depression in primary and secondary care**

Inpatient team, crisis team, day hospital	Risk to life, severe self-neglect	Medication, combined treatments ECT
Mental health specialists	Treatment resistance and frequent references	Medication, complex psychological interventions
PCMHW, GP, GPwSI, Counsellor	Moderate or severe depression	Medication, brief psychological interventions, social support
GP, Practice Nurse, Practice Counsellor	Mild or moderate depression	Active review: self-help, computerised CBT, exercise
Primary Care Team	Recognition	Watchful waiting, assessment

National Institute for Clinical Excellence (2003) Draft NICE guideline, First consultation, September 2003. London: National Institute for Clinical Excellence.
Available from www.nice.org.uk/Docref.asp?d=86357

This model is important for it provides an organisational 'home' for the new workers described in the NHS Plan, both the new graduate workers (described in the above diagram as PCMHWs (Primary Care Mental Health Workers) and the GPwSI, the General Practitioner with a Special Interest. It leads to the natural development of a single team sitting between PHCTs and CMHTs made up of graduate workers, practitioners with a special interest (GPs or nurses), counsellors and GPs, who provided specialist care for patients who are not appropriate for secondary care services, but cannot be managed with confidence in primary care. The Sainsbury Centre for Mental Health is currently piloting this development in four PCTs in England.

Severe mental illness

Phelan,[15] in a recent *BMJ* editorial wrote, *'Over 60 years ago the BMJ reported an association between mental illness and poor physical health. Subsequent research, in many countries, has consistently confirmed that psychiatric patients have high rates of physical illness, much of which goes undetected.'*

Physical health of people with severe mental illness – the evidence base
Several articles have examined the increased mortality associated with mental illness, the most comprehensive of which is the meta-analysis undertaken by Harris and Barraclough[16] in 1998. They analysed 20 papers, covering a population of 36,000 from nine countries, that related specifically to schizophrenia. Using these data they calculated Standardised Mortality Rates (SMR) for this group as a whole and for specific causes of death. The SMR for males with schizophrenia for all causes of death was 156 (95% C I = 151 to 162) and for females with schizophrenia was 141 (95% C I = 136 to 146). The SMR for infectious diseases as a cause of death in people with schizophrenia was 455 for males and 490 for females. The SMR for respiratory diseases causing death was 214 for males and 249 for females. Whilst there was no specific mention of influenza as a direct cause of the increased mortality, significantly increased SMRs in both respiratory and infectious causes of death make such an infection significant (see Table 14.2).

Table 14.2 **SMR for people with schizophrenia**

SMR	All causes	Infectious diseases as the cause of death	Respiratory diseases as the cause of death
Males	156	455	214
Females	141	490	249

From Harris and Barraclough[16]

Harris and Barraclough also examined the conditions of 'Psychotic Disorder NOS' (DSM III R 298.90) and 'Bipolar Disorder' (DSM III R 296.4x– 296.70). The evidence in these groups is less detailed, and in some cases based on a single study. In the former group, the SMR for all causes was 199, and for the latter, 202. In the former group, the SMR for infectious diseases was 185, and for respiratory diseases, 191. In the latter group, the SMR for infectious diseases was 40, but the SMR for respiratory diseases was 1034. However, these results are based on a single study from Israel and Harris and Barraclough suggested that the certification of death criteria may be different from the other papers studied.

Table 14.3 **SMR for people with psychotic disorder NOS or bi-polar disorder**

SMR	All causes	Infectious diseases as the cause of death	Respiratory diseases as the cause of death
Psychotic Disorder NOS	199	185	191
Bipolar Disorder	202	40	1034

From Harris and Barraclough[16]

The conclusion that can be drawn from the meta-analysis undertaken by Harris and Barraclough is that people with severe and enduring mental illness (schizophrenia, psychosis, and bipolar disorder) have a significantly increased risk of death due to infections and/or respiratory disease.

Health promotion

There are few papers that describe the overall health of people with a severe and enduring mental illness, or provide an explanation for their increased mortality. Kendler[17] proposed an environmental model – based on a study of twins in the National Academy of Sciences, National Research Council Twin Registry – that the consequences of the illness on the lifestyle of people with schizophrenia, make them more likely to die from diseases, rather than trauma, or by suicide.

In the general population there is evidence that cigarette and heavy alcohol use,[16,18] poor diet,[19] and lack of exercise,[19] all contribute significantly to the increased mortality rates.

Kendrick[20] studied 101 people with a severe and enduring mental illness living in the community, and found that 26 were obese (BMA > 30), 53 were current smokers, and 11 were hypertensive. Twenty-one reported daily cough and sputum, 24 shortness of breath, 11 wheezing, and seven chest pain on exertion. These rates were significantly higher than population rates in a contemporary national survey. Nearly all the risk factors were recorded in the general practice records but few attempts to intervene were apparent. He concluded that primary care teams should make special efforts to tackle risk factors among this group.

Brown et al[19] reviewed the health of 179 local patients with schizophrenia over a 15-year period. They identified that 20 deaths were associated with cardiovascular or respiratory disease, and calculated the SMR at 225

(CI = 137 to 334). They also prospectively surveyed the lifestyles of 140 people with schizophrenia, and found that their diet was unhealthy (higher in fat and lower in fibre than the reference population), they took less exercise than the reference population, and also had significantly higher levels of cigarette smoking.

Burns and Cohen[21] looked at the quantity of health promotion data recorded in GP notes for people with a severe mental illness. They showed that although the consultation rate (consultations per year) was significantly higher than normal, 13–14 consultations per year, compared to an average consultation rate of three, the amount of data recorded for a variety of health promotion areas was significantly less than normal, even in those practices that were gaining extra remuneration for recording health promotion data for the general population.

HIV and hepatitis C

Data from the UK on the incidence and prevalence of either of these conditions in people with schizophrenia does not exist. However, there are a number of papers from the US that indicate that this is an area that will become significant. Published rates of HIV amongst psychiatric patients are from 3.1% to 23.9%, at least eight times higher than the general population.[22-3] These studies were both carried out on the East Coast of America, and there are no similar sero-prevalence studies for elsewhere in the US.

Rates of Hepatitis C (HCV) have been reported from Italy where it was found that 6.7% of 1180 patients were sero-positive.[24] Rosenberg[23] found that 19.6% of 751 psychiatric inpatients and outpatients were infected with HCV. On the West Coast of America, Meyer (in press) found that 20.3% of 508 inpatients were sero-positive. These rates should be compared to the rate found in the general population of 1.8%.

Since the studies are recent, and this is an emerging problem, explanations for the high rates are unclear. Theories proposed include the risk-taking behaviour associated with severe mental illness, as being the most likely explanation.

Diabetes and glucose intolerance

Reports as early as the 1920s[25] described the increased prevalence of diabetes in people with schizophrenia – hardly a recent advance! However, the advent of the phenothiazine group of medication to treat schizophrenia has increased the prevalence of diabetes, as it is believed to alter glucose–insulin homeostasis. Indeed chlorpromazine has been used to prevent hypoglycaemia in malignant insulinoma.

Diabetes seems more common in older people with schizophrenia. In 1996, Mukherjee[26] found an overall prevalence of 15% in 95 patients with schizophrenia but in patients under 50, there were no cases of diabetes. In those aged between 50 and 60, the rate was 12.9% and in those over 60 the rate rose to 18.9%. The prevalence rate in the general population is 2%.

The newer atypical antipsychotics and, in particular, olanzepine and clozapine, have been found to have an association with diabetes and impaired glucose metabolism.[27] The rates are clearly increased: around 12% of patients being treated with clozapine are likely to develop diabetes mellitus and a further 10% will have impaired glucose tolerance, based on the American Diabetic Association's interpretation of oral glucose tolerance tests – there are no studies from the UK with this type of data. Mechanisms are unclear, but insulin resistance, and/or an increase in central adiposity seem to be possible explanations. The significance, irrespective of the cause, is that patients with schizophrenia should have their urine checked annually for glucose, or have an annual fasting blood glucose assay, and that this is particularly true for older people.

There is some evidence from the US that people with schizophrenia and diabetes receive less good care than those with diabetes alone [personal communication – Drake]; once again there is no equivalent data from the UK to support or deny this early evidence.

New GMS contract

The relevance of the foregoing is that it provides the evidence base for supporting the quality and outcome framework in mental health, to reward general practitioners for attending to the physical health of the severely mentally ill.

To do so requires a register to be developed; this chapter is not the place to enter the ethical and practical debate that centres around creating registers in primary care – the interested reader is directed to the Sainsbury Centre for Mental Health Briefing Paper[28] on the GMS contract, which sets out some of the issues.

Having identified people with a severe and enduring mental illness, to earn the rewards the GP must attend to the physical health needs of these patients, by assessing their cardiovascular and respiratory systems, checking for impaired glucose metabolism, advising on drug and substance misuse, and advising on smoking and healthy living options. Interestingly, the issue of HIV or hepatitis C is not as yet mentioned in the guidance supplied by the BMA, but will no doubt begin to appear as patients start developing cirrhosis.

Summary

The GMS contract is probably the most significant recent advance in primary care mental health. It provides for the implementation of all the recent evidence and research around organisational care, and the physical health of the severely mentally ill, both of which are a major concern to primary care physicians and teams. It is to be hoped that this combination of evidence and implementation will really lead to improved care for two groups of people who in the past may not have always benefited as much as they could from health care services.

References

1. Sainsbury Centre for Mental Health Primary Solutions. London: Sainsbury Centre for Mental Health, 2002

2. Economic and social costs of mental illness. London: Sainsbury Centre for Mental Health, 2003

3. Singleton N, Bumpstead R, O'Brien M, *et al*. *Psychiatric Morbidity among Adults Living in Private Households, 2000: summary report*. London: Office of National Statistics, 2001

4. Department of Health. *The NHS Plan: A plan for investment, a plan for reform*. London: HMSO, 2000

5. Department of Health. *National Service Framework for Mental Health: Modern Standards and Service Models*. London: HMSO, 1999

6. Department of Health. *Fast-forwarding primary care mental health: graduate primary care mental health workers – best practice guidance*. London: HMSO, 2003

7. Montgomery P. & Dennis P. Cognitive behavioural interventions improve some sleep outcomes in older adults. Cochrane Database Systematic Review. 2003; CD003161

8. Morgan K, Dixon, S, Tomeny, M, Mathers N, and Thompson. *Psychological treatment for insomnia in the regulation of long-term hypnotic drug use*. London: HMSO, NHS R&D National Co-ordinating Centre for Health Technology Assessment (NCCHTA), 2002

9. Roth A & Fonagy P. *What works for whom? A critical review of psychotherapy research*. New York: The Guilford Press, 1996

10. Von Korff M. & Goldberg D. Improving outcomes in depression. *BMJ* 2001; **323**: 948–9

11. Counsellors and Psychotherapists in Primary Care. www.cpc-online.co.uk (accessed 18/11/2004)

12. Manchester Primary Care Research and Development Centre. www.npcrdc.man.ac.uk

13. The Counselling in Primary Care Trust. www.cpct.co.uk (accessed 18/11/2004)

14. National Institute for Clinical Excellence. www.nice.org.uk (accessed 18/11/2004)

15. Phelan M, Stradins L, Morrison. Physical Health of people with severe mental illness. *BMJ* 2001; **322**: 443–4

16. Harris E C, Barraclough B. Excess mortality of mental disorder. *Br J Psychiatry* 1998; **173**: 11–53

17. Kendler K S, Eaves L J. Models for the joint effect of genotype and environment on liability to psychiatric illness. *Am J Psychiatry* 1986; **143 (3)**: 279–89

18. Addington J, el-Guebaly N, Campbell W, Hodgins D C, Addington D. Smoking cessation treatment for patients with schizophrenia. *Am J Psychiatry* 1998; **155**: 974–6

19. Brown S, Birtwistle J, Roe L, Thompson C. The unhealthy lifestyle of people with schizophrenia. *Psychol Med* 1999; **29**: 697–701

20. Kendrick T, *et al.* Randomised controlled trial of teaching general practitioners to carry out structured assessments of their long-term mentally ill patients. *BMJ* 1995; **311**: 93–8

21. Burns and Cohen. Item of Service payments for general practitioner care of severely mentally ill patients: does the money matter? *Br J Gen Pract* 1998; **48**: 1415–6

22. Cournos F, and McKinnon K. HIV seroprevalence amongst people with severe mental illness in the United States: a critical review. *Clin Psychol Rev* 1997; **17**: 259–69

23. Rosenberg S D, Goodman L A, Osher F C, *et al.* Prevalence of HIV, hepatitis B, and hepatitis C in people with severe mental illness. *Am J Public Health* 2001; **91**: 31–7

24. Cividini A, Pistorio A Regazzetti A, *et al.* Hepatitis C virus iinfection amongst institutionalized psychiatric patients: a regression analysis of risk. *J Hepatol* 1997; **27**: 455–63

25. Braceland F J, Meduna L J, Vaichulis J A. Delayed action of insulin on schizophrenia. *Am J Psychiatry* 1945 **102**: 108–110

26. Mukherjee S, Decina P, Boola V, *et al.* Diabetes mellitus in schizophrenic patients. *Compr Psychiatry* 1996; **37**: 68–73

27. Henderson D C. Atypical anti-psychotic induced diabetes mellitus: how strong is the evidence? *CNS Drugs* 2001; **16**: 1–13

28. *Investing in General Practice – The new General Medical Services Contract for GPs. Policy Briefing 21.* London: The Sainsbury Centre for Mental Health, 2003

CHAPTER 15

Older People

Steve Iliffe, Danielle Harari, Cameron Swift

▶ **KEY MESSAGES**

- The available evidence does not support population screening for morbidity and disability in later life, especially amongst asymptomatic individuals.

- The previous contractual obligation, expressed as the '75 and over checks', represented bad policy based on thin science.

- The National Service Framework for Older People creates opportunities for enhancing the quality of primary care for older people.

- The question is how to focus clinical attention on the often complex problems of co-morbidity without lapsing into a check-list approach to health needs assessment.

RECENT ADVANCES ▼

- The enhancement of clinical skills coupled to case finding appears a rational approach to timely identification of tractable problems.

- We advocate a pragmatic 'best buy' approach to clinical interventions in a limited number of clinical domains.

- This will allow general practitioners and their teams to offer a systematic health promotion programme to their older patients, to organise their own approach to case finding, and to structure thinking about managing multiple pathologies and co-morbidities.

- The next logical step is to develop systematic case management, in which practice nurses may play the central role.

The new contract for general practice has quietly deleted the obligation to offer annual assessments of health to all people aged 75 and over, ending 13 years of bad policy based on thin science. The National Service Framework for Older People creates opportunities for enhancing the quality of primary care for older people, and general practitioners with a specialist interest in ageing and health may catalyse change at local level. The question is how to focus clinical attention on the often complex problems of co-morbidity, to maximum effect, without lapsing into a culture that delegates the tasks to insufficiently trained nurses who follow a check-list approach to health needs assessment. In this chapter we offer a clinical perspective on primary care for older people that emphasises the diagnostic role of the general practitioner in case-finding, and the case-management role of the practice nurse. The 17 clinical domains discussed here are common, important and tractable problems identified in the preparation of an evidence base for a European study of health-risk assessment in older people,[1] presented to fit UK circumstances. The domains and the evidence were investigated and debated by a multi-disciplinary and multinational group of clinicians, and presented to general practitioners in three European countries for their critical appraisal. Differences in medical cultures, in methods of health care financing and in the relationships between generalists and specialists generated different national interpretations of the evidence. In this chapter we present the UK perspective. Because the NHS already has age-related policies on immunisation against influenza and pneumococcal pneumonia, cervical cancer screening and mammography for breast cancer, we have excluded them from the discussion. For the same reason we have not included medication review (as required by the National Service Framework for Older People) as a separate theme.

Where the grading of any supporting evidence is clear this is indicated using the scale **A–D** based on established guidelines:[2] A-evidence from meta-analysis of randomised controlled trials (RCTs), or from at least one RCT; B-evidence from at least one controlled trial without randomisation or quasi-experimental study; C-evidence from descriptive studies; and D-evidence from expert committee reports or opinions.

For each of the 16 clinical domains we have recommended actions that general practitioners and practice nurses should consider, and these are shown in Table 15.1.

Table 15.1 Health risk assessment, prevention and health maintenance guidelines for patients aged 65 and over

Domains	Primary Prevention	Risk Assessment and Health Maintenance
Hypertension	Yearly screen	SBP ≥160 or DBP ≥100 – treat to achieve goal of BP ≤140/85 with thiazides first-line, aspirin if high cardiac risk *plus in all cases* diet, exercise, limit salt intake
Hyperlipidaemia	5-yearly screen / Coronary Risk Prediction chart	Total cholesterol ≥5.0 + high cardiac risk – if cholesterol still ≥5 after 3–6 months of lifestyle measures (diet, exercise, weight reduction, smoking cessation) – treat with statins
Diabetes mellitus	3-yearly screen with fasting blood glucose (FBG)	FBG ≥7.0mmol/l – treat with diet, glicazide is preferred sulphonylurea, multidisciplinary approach to promote compliance, modify individual treatment goals according to comorbidity
Colon cancer	Annual screening by FOBT	… but only if back-up with specialist investigations (e.g. colonoscopy) is available. High risk patients include those with previous polypectomy, ulcerative colitis, family history of bowel cancer
Prostate cancer	Screening in asymptomatic men not recommended	
Dental care	Recommend annual dental check	… to *all* patients
Eyesight testing	Recommend yearly eye test	… to *all* patients, specialist referral where undiagnosed problems identified
Hearing assessment	Annual whisper test	Auroscopy and audiometry referral to evaluate hearing loss
Exercise	Recommend regular exercise ± limits	Limits should not be age-dependent, encourage goal-setting based on prior activity level, physical functioning, patient motivation and preferences regarding exercise
Nutrition	Basic dietary advice	≥5 servings fruit and fibre daily, reduce saturated fats. Identify causes of malnutrition
Physical function	Periodic functional assessment for patients with co-morbidity	Multidisciplinary assessment for those needing help with one or more basic ADL
Pain	Routine enquiry each patient encounter	Thorough assessment to avoid both under-treatment, and over-treatment (e.g. with long-term NSAIDs)
Medication use	Monthly review for ≥3 medications	Prescribing appropriateness (both evidence-based prescribing e.g. bisphosphonates in fractured neck of femur, and inappropriate prescribing e.g. diuretics for dependent oedema), compliance aids
Injury prevention/falls	Annual falls risk assessment	Education re: falls and injury prevention, comprehensive assessment in fallers
Urinary incontinence	Routine enquiry	Assess for UTI, functional, drug-related UI – refer for diagnosis of overflow, stress, urge UI
Depression/dementia	Assess patients ≥75 years with symptoms using standardised instrument	Further evaluation for dementia and for depression according to patient history, informant history and assessment tool findings
Smoking	Cessation counselling for all smokers	Cognitive-behavioural approach ± nicotine replacement therapy
Alcohol use	Routine in-depth enquiry	Safe limit may be as little as 1 drink/day (less on neurotropic drugs)

S/DBP = systolic/diastolic blood pressure | LTC = long-term care | FOBT = faecal occult blood test | ADL = activities of daily living | UTI = urinary tract infection | UI = urinary incontinence

Hypertension

Hypertension, including isolated systolic hypertension (= ≥160/90 mm Hg), is found in more than half of all people aged over 60. Absolute benefit from treatment of diastolic hypertension and isolated systolic hypertension is greater in older people than younger age groups, particularly with respect to cardiovascular complications (including heart failure), and vascular dementia (**A**). Antihypertensive treatment is beneficial until at least age 80 (**A**), and regular screening of blood pressure should continue until this age. Once treatment is started, it should be continued after the age of 80.[3]

There is evidence, however, that current guidelines are not being implemented and the detection and management of hypertension remains suboptimal (**B**). As a rule of thumb, a minimum annual check is appropriate for older individuals with no history of hypertension and a quarterly check for those controlled on medication. For those with poor control, measures to achieve control (including specialist referral where necessary) and more frequent monitoring are appropriate. While the evidence is less robust for those over 80, the weighting is in favour of achieving control where there is no contraindicating co-morbidity.

There is no evidence base in the current literature on which to recommend firm guidelines on screening for hypertension, or on treating newly diagnosed hypertension in patients aged over 80. Consensus opinion regarding this age group, however, is that treatment of hypertension (with the same optimum levels as younger patients) is appropriate in the context of hypertensive complications or target organ damage. Antihypertensive treatment (even of borderline systolic hypertension) should also be considered in hypertensive patients over the age of 80, who are without complications and who are generally fit with reasonable life expectancy (**D**). Low-dose thiazides (e.g. bendrofluazide 2.5 mg) are the accepted first-line treatment for elderly people, and are well-tolerated (**A**). Beta-blockers are less effective than thiazides as first-line treatment, and meta-analysis suggests that they decrease stroke but no other cardiovascular events in this age group (**A**). Long-acting dihydropyridine calcium antagonists (e.g. amlodipine 5 mg) are suitable alternatives for elderly patients when thiazides are ineffective, contraindicated, or not tolerated (**A**). While ACE inhibitors may be useful in treating hypertension co-existing with heart failure or left ventricular dysfunction, they should be used with great caution in older hypertensives who have peripheral vascular disease (because of the association with renovascular disease), or established renal impairment. Angiotensin 2 receptor blockers may have a better tolerability profile.

Hyperlipidaemia

All older adults should have their total cholesterol levels tested every five years, in combination with an assessment for other cardiovascular risk factors. In addition to primary prevention, lowering cholesterol also delays progression of atherosclerotic cardiovascular disease (secondary prevention). In view of lack of evidence for individuals with hyperlipidaemia ages 75 years and above, current consensus agreement is that existing statin treatment should be continued in these patients, and de novo treatment should be considered on an individual patient basis (**D**). Non-pharmacological measures should, however, be appropriately applied in all older patients.[4]

Diabetes mellitus

The estimated prevalence of unrecognised diabetes in older people (5%), and the frequently asymptomatic or non-specific clinical presentation in this population provides the basis for consensus guidelines recommending screening every three years.[5]

Consensus opinion recommends screening for diabetes using a fasting blood glucose (FBG) test every three years in those over 45 years of age (**D**). Annual screening is recommended in older patients with first-degree family history, obesity, low HDL (= ≤0.9 mmol/L), high fasting triglycerides (= ≤2.8 mmol/L), or coronary heart disease (**D**). In treating diabetes, the same glucose targets (both FBG and HbA1c) apply to healthy older people as to younger people in order to lower the risk of complications (**A**). In elderly patients with co-morbidities, however, the goal of treatment should be to avoid symptoms of hyperglycaemia, and prevent hypoglycaemia (**D**). A multidisciplinary team approach to diabetes management, emphasising patient education by nurses and dieticians has been shown to improve blood glucose control in older patients (**B**).

Colon cancer

Neither colonoscopy nor testing for stool occult blood is yet part of routine screening in the United Kingdom, although there are strong pressures to move in the direction of routine occult blood testing.[6] Although many British gerontologists and gastroenterologists support the view that yearly faecal occult blood testing (FOBT) would be beneficial, neither this nor the necessary follow-up investigation is routinely available within the UK health care system. When individuals at low risk of bowel cancer request screening, they should be informed about the limitations and possible risks of the tests. Occult blood testing should only be offered when there are agreed protocols between primary and secondary care that are backed by the necessary resources for further investigation of individuals with a positive test. Mass screening for normal-risk individuals should await the results of ongoing trials, particularly the NHS pilot study of occult blood testing and the MRC/NHS trials of flexible sigmoidoscopy. Patients are encouraged to discuss the possible benefits of FOBT with their doctor on the basis of information that early detection of colon cancer increases the likelihood of cure.[7]

The United States Prevention Task Force recommendations are that all people over 50 should be screened annually with FOBT (**B**). For every ten people who test positive for faecal occult blood, one will be found to have cancer; three, an adenoma > 1 cm; one, a small adenoma; and five will have a negative examination. Three randomised trials have shown that screening by FOBT every two years has the potential to reduce mortality by up to 20% in patients between 50 and 80 years of age. Although 74% of bowel cancers found in patients testing positive on FOBT are distally located and therefore reachable by sigmoidoscopy, a distal lesion is associated with a greater than 10% chance of having another significant lesion proximally. Total colonoscopy is therefore regarded as the investigation of choice in patients with positive FOBT (**B**). There is insufficient evidence to determine whether the combination of FOBT and sigmoidoscopy produces greater benefits than either test alone.[8]

Prostate cancer

Early detection of prostate cancer by means of the prostate specific antigen (PSA) test is an area of active debate, but is not presently an agreed evidence-based screening strategy. High quality data are not as yet available as to whether early detection is beneficial in preventing mortality or symptomatic morbidity, or harmful in prompting unnecessarily aggressive treatment or over-diagnosis.[9] A cut-off value of 4.0 ng/ml has a sensitivity of 46% in identifying cancer in younger men (mean age 63 years)[10] and a specificity of only 54% in older men with benign prostatic hypertrophy.[11] A PSA level above 10.0 ng/ml increases the probability of prostate cancer to over 50%.[9] Primary screening in asymptomatic men over 75 years is generally not recommended, but consideration should be given to undertaking this test in older men presenting with symptoms, or with an abnormal prostate on digital rectal examination.

Dental care

Dental problems are a source of morbidity and suboptimal nutrition in late life. Numerous studies have demonstrated that many older adults have problems chewing, pain, difficulties in eating, and problems in social relationships because of oral disorders.[12] Periodontal diseases and recurrent caries are the predominant causes of tooth loss in older people; both problems are preventable. Oral mucosal lesions of all types are increasingly prevalent with age, affecting up to 30% of the elderly population. Individuals at greater risk of poor oral health are diabetics, smokers, and people taking medications with the side effect of reducing salivary flow (e.g. antidepressants, antihypertensives, diuretics). NHS dentistry is increasingly hard to locate and it is recognised that there are financial disincentives. Less than half of the community population in the UK are regular dental attenders, with non-attendance being associated with older age, fewer self-reported number of teeth possessed, edentulous status, and low income and other socio-demographic factors.[13] Every effort should be made to encourage each older patient to undergo an annual dental check.[14]

Eyesight

There is no evidence-based indication for routine ocular examination by physicians in all older people. Evidence for effectiveness of visual screening in older people who do not report visual impairment is lacking, but a small beneficial effect cannot be excluded.[15] There is evidence that visual impairment is prevalent in older people who fall.[16] Every effort should be made to encourage each older patient to undergo a yearly (or at least two-yearly) eye test, including a check on intraocular pressures. Conditions such as diabetes and regular steroid intake increase the importance of regular eye tests and should therefore also trigger examination.

Hearing

The commonest cause of hearing impairment in later life is presbyacusis (sensorineural high tone deafness). Hearing impairments are reported by 23% of people aged 65–74, 33% between age 75–84, and 48% by those aged 85 and over. Many older people are also not aware of having hearing loss. Although many older people with hearing loss may not report this symptom to their GP, screening for deafness in primary care (by whisper and vibrating fork tests) is suboptimal even within structured preventive health programmes.[17] Only 8% of hearing impaired people over 65 use a hearing aid, and 20% of users over 85 report impaired hearing despite adequate amplification. Hearing loss in later life can compromise ability to perform instrumental activities of daily living (e.g. shopping, using telephone, driving), and may lead to social withdrawal and depression.[18] There is some evidence to suggest that improvement of hearing may contribute to improvement in cognition in older people with cognitive impairment.[19] Referral for audiological assessment with pure-tone threshold audiometry is appropriate if hearing loss is having an impact on communication, socialisation, function, mood, or quality of life. Patients should be discouraged from spending large amounts of money on commercial hearing aids until they have had a formal assessment by an audiologist.

Exercise

Physical exercise in older people is beneficial both for primary and secondary prevention of cardiovascular morbidity and mortality, and on an individual basis as part of multifactorial measures for falls prevention in those indivi-dualy identified as at risk (see p. *301*). Where there are no contraindications, aerobic exercise should be promoted to enhance cardiopulmonary fitness (**A**) and general stamina, while resistance training should be advised to improve balance and muscular strength (**A**). Regular exercise programmes for older people can particularly benefit pain and disability related to knee osteoarthritis (**B**), weight loss in obese individuals (**A**), and control of hyperlipidaemia (**A**) and hypertension (**A**). Patients who are physically inactive receive written advice on exercise, but should also be advised to discuss this with their GP, particularly if they intend to make a significant increase in physical activity. Patients undertaking a new exercise programme should be advised to seek medical advice if they have new or worsening exercise-related symptoms such as breathlessness or joint pains.[20]

Nutrition

Poor nutrition in older people may result in obesity, or in protein-calorie malnutrition (commonly multifactorial in aetiology). Overall, people aged 65 and over living in the community in the UK meet dietary recommendations for total fat, vitamin and mineral intake, but not for saturated fat or fibre.[21] A healthy diet, as measured by an indicator based on WHO recommendations, has been associated with a reduction of 13% after 20 years in all-cause mortality for Western European men aged 50–70.[22] Dietary intervention has been shown to be effective in management of hyperlipidemia, hypertension, and cardiac disease (**A**). There is evidence, however, that while primary care practitioners recognise the value of dietary counselling in older people, multiple barriers to implementation exist, including lack of time, patient non-compliance, inadequate teaching materials, and lack of specialised knowledge.[23] Acute illness, especially when resulting in hospitalisation, accelerates nitrogen wasting and protein malnutrition in older people. Other modifiable causes of protein-calorie malnutrition in the elderly are depression, medications, congestive heart failure, malabsorption syndromes, chronic stool impaction, and social factors (immobility or isolation resulting in limited access to food, poverty).

Physical function and independence

Early multidisciplinary intervention in managing functional impairment in older people improves both functional and psychosocial outcomes (**B**). Recent work has focused on prevention by assessing early predictors of physical disability with ageing (so-called preclinical mobility disability).[24] Comprehensive multidisciplinary geriatric assessment (medical, nursing, physiotherapy, occupational therapy) (CGA) is indicated for patients newly reporting significant functional problems such as needing help with more than one basic activity of daily living.

A Canadian community-based study of screening for multidimensional functional capacity in patients aged 65 years and over, followed by appropriate referrals (e.g. to physiotherapy) showed an improvement in daily activities, mental health scores, and social functions in people aged over 75 years who were living alone or lonely. The intervention was less effective in improving total functional capacity of individuals without these sociodemographic factors.[25] A prospective study of women aged 70–80 without mobility problems showed that their self-report of how they carried out tasks was a strong predictor of future mobility limitations.

Pain

Chronic pain is a major problem among older people living in the community, reported by 46.5% of the primary care population, and is associated with a high level of primary care physician visits. Back pain and arthritis account for one third of all complaints.[26] Chronic pain in older people may lead to a downward spiral of depression, social isolation, sleep disturbance, and reduced mobility. Failure to evaluate pain in this age group is a critical factor leading to under treatment. Conversely, suboptimal assessment may also lead to inappropriate prescribing of analgesic medications such as non-steroidal anti-inflammatory drugs (NSAIDs) and opiates. Despite this high prevalence, people aged 65 and over have been systematically excluded from clinical trials of pain treatment, so current guidelines for the older population are largely based on consensus opinion. Use of the patient-administered pain assessment instruments in primary care patients has been shown to lead to greater patient satisfaction with physician–patient communication regarding pain complaints, regardless of the specific nature or cause of their pain.[27]

Routine inquiry about pain should be part of every new health care professional encounter with older patients. Any pain complaint that has an impact on physical or psychosocial function needs to be addressed as a significant problem, often involving early use of pharmacological treatment. Pain in older people should invariably trigger a careful diagnostic search, including a careful history, physical examination and any indicated investigations (e.g. for osteoporosis). Its control is most effective when the underlying cause of pain can be identified and treated and its consequences addressed through a careful multidisciplinary assessment. Where the cause remains in doubt, appropriate specialist referral should occur.

Simple patient self-assessment pain scales should be used to quantify pain (e.g. verbal or visual analogue scale: 'On a scale of zero to ten, with zero being no pain at all, and ten being pain as bad as you could possibly imagine, how much pain are you having now?') (**D**). Regular review of patients taking analgesic medications more than three times a week is recommended (**D**). Paracetamol (up to 1000 mg four times a day) is the drug of choice for most older people with mild-to-moderate pain, especially when the cause is identified as being osteoarthritic (**A**) or musculoskeletal (**D**).

Use of NSAIDs in older people should be limited to treating active inflammatory conditions or bone pain where there are no contraindications (renal impairment (**A**), upper gastrointestinal disease (**A**), congestive heart failure), and where alternative analgesic drug strategies (e.g. low-dose steroids or opiates) have failed (**D**). In older people, NSAIDs should only be used for short periods of time. Improved gastrointestinal tolerance with selective inhibitors of cyclo-oxygenase 2 inhibitors is unproven in older people, so a cautious approach to their use similar to NSAIDs, is recommended in this population. Constipation is a major problem for older people on any type of opiate analgesia (**C**), and a bowel programme should be started early on in a treatment course.

Injury prevention and falls

One-third of people over the age of 65 fall each year. Falls are the major cause of accidental death, particularly in this age group. Of these falls, 5–10% result in a fracture and 2.2% of injurious falls are fatal. Those not causing fractures are still associated with substantial morbidity and have considerable psychological consequences. Falls in older people are often a signal of underlying health-related problems or risk factors and are commonly due to a combination of these with environmental hazards.[28] Early and systematic assessment of risk with appropriate intervention can reduce the incidence of falls (**A**). Assessment of older people for multiple falls risk factors followed-up with appropriate intervention has been clearly shown to reduce the subsequent incidence of falling in robust randomised controlled clinical trials[29–30] (**A**). Using a postal questionnaire screen with follow-up assessment of those identified as at high risk resulted in a 30–40% reduction. Opportunistic specialist assessment of those presenting in accident and emergency within two weeks of a fall resulted in a 60–70% reduction in the number of falls in the subsequent year within the intervention group compared with controls.[31] Falls prevention is a major element of the current NHS National Framework for the Care of Older People and of a NICE clinical guideline. Most districts are developing specialist falls and syncope assessment clinics for referral as well as primary care guidelines.

Urinary incontinence

The prevalence of urinary incontinence increases with age affecting up to 44% of people aged 75 years and over living in the community.[32] Primary care physicians tend to have a low awareness of incontinence in older people. Overall the assessment and management of continence problems in older people continues to be inadequate in the majority of sufferers.

The high prevalence of urinary incontinence in older people is due largely to age-related changes (such as decreased bladder capacity, increased disinhibited bladder contractions, detrusor instability, increased nocturnal sodium and fluid excretion, decreased urethral resistance in post-menopausal women, increased urethral resistance in men with prostatic enlargement, and weakness of the pelvic floor in women) combined with predisposing factors such as co-morbidity, medications, and immobility.[33]

Assessment should aim to identify the type of incontinence – functional, drug-related, stress, urge or overflow, and to apply appropriate treatment plans. Such assessment commonly requires specialised techniques. Specialist assessment of older people with continence problems in the NHS is widely available but variably provided by departments of medicine for older people, urogynaecology, gynaecology or urology. GPs will need to ascertain the best line of referral in their locality.

Depression and dementia

The use by non-medical staff of a brief screening instrument – the Mini-Mental State Examination (MMSE) – to detect cognitive impairment among older people in primary care was described in 1170 patients aged 75 years and over in a UK primary care practice. The prevalence of cognitive impairment (score below 25 on the MMSE) was 12.8%. Six percent of patients scored below 19, yet less than one-third of this group had a diagnosis of dementia in their medical records. There was no association between low MMSE scores and gender or social class, but a relationship was observed with age – the proportion with dementia rose from 2.5% in those aged 75–9 years to 29.0% among those aged 90 years and over.[34] Similar prevalence of cognitive impairment was observed in a larger US survey of screening primary care patients aged over 60 years.[35] Moderate to severe impairment was associated with increased use of health services and increased mortality. However, there is insufficient evidence to support population screening for dementia in older populations.[36]

Despite positive attitudes about their skills for detecting and treating depression in the elderly, only one quarter of primary care physicians routinely used a screening tool in practice in a US study.[37] A UK survey of screening for depression in patients aged 75 and over found that 22% had some evidence of depression previously undiagnosed by the primary care physician.[38] There is insufficient evidence to support population screening for depression in later life.[39]

Smoking

Up to 30% of people over 65 years of age are current smokers. Respiratory problems, primarily due to smoking, are the second commonest cause of disability in old age. Smoking cessation strategies in young elderly have been shown to be efficacious and cost-effective in terms of cost per life year gained,[40] yet recent studies have shown that doctors are less likely to give advice on smoking cessation to older patients as compared with younger ones. As for younger people, the most important predictor of successful smoking cessation (i.e. for at least one year) in older individuals is motivation.[41] Counselling programmes can achieve a cessation rate of 15% in well-motivated older people, increasing to 20% when combined with nicotine replacement therapy (**A**). Concomitant exercise programmes have also been shown enhance the impact of cognitive-behavioural programmes on long-term smoking cessation in women (**A**). Where data is available, the benefits of smoking cessation appear to be comparable in young and in old. The beneficial impact of cessation on accelerated decline of lung function with smoking has been demonstrated up to the age of 80, especially in women. The decline in risk of myocardial infarction after stopping smoking (to virtually pre-smoking levels after 2–3 years) is also unaffected by ageing.

Data from the US suggests that older smokers are more likely to reject evidence that smoking is bad for the health, but whether these attitudes are prevalent in older smokers in Western Europe is unclear.

Alcohol use

The scale of alcohol problems amongst older people is widely underestimated. The continuation of a steady level of drinking may become problematic with ageing because of age-related changes in physiology and pharmacodynamics that increase sensitivity to the deleterious effects of alcohol. Between 5% and 12% of men and 1–2% of women in their 60s are problem drinkers. The rates are substantially higher among hospital outpatients and people attending clinics.[42] A study of 1070 older men and women selected from general practice lists showed that nearly one-fifth of both sexes who were regular drinkers exceeded the recommended limits.

Both the quantity of alcohol drunk and the frequency of drinking by elderly men – and so the frequency of problems related to alcohol – are higher than those in elderly women. On average older people drink less than younger people, but ageing does not always modify drinking behaviour, and excessive alcohol use may simply be carried into old age. The trend for older people to reduce alcohol consumption seems to be less noticeable in women.[43]

Older people may be less tolerant of the adverse effects of alcohol. The mechanisms are not clear, but may include an increase in distribution volume (due to an increase in the ratio of body fat to water), a reduction in hepatic first-pass metabolism and/or an increase in CNS sensitivity to alcohol. The current US National Institute on Alcohol Abuse and Alcoholism recommendations for safe limits of alcohol consumption have been adjusted downwards for people over 65 to no more than one drink a day, because of their particular vulnerability to its toxic effects.

Conclusion

The evidence base for health maintenance in later life is evolving slowly, and our proposals are in part based on consensus guidelines, some of which originate in a medical culture that is more defensive than that of British primary care. We do not claim that our suggestions are based on a systematic review of the evidence, but rather on a more pragmatic evaluation that favours a 'best buy' approach to clinical interventions. We do argue that the 17 domains described here allow general practitioners to recommend a systematic health promotion programme to their older patients, to organise their own approach to case finding, and to structure thinking about managing multiple pathologies and co-morbidities.

The available evidence in the domains we have reviewed does not support population screening, especially amongst asymptomatic individuals, but enhancement of clinical skills coupled to case finding appears a rational approach to timely identification of tractable problems. The second necessary component to comprehensive care for older people is systematic case management, in which practice nurses may play the central role, but this is beyond the scope of this chapter. The actions that we have suggested in Table 15.1 can be the basis for practice-based protocols, and as quality standards for auditing care. We hope that this chapter will help general practitioners with an interest in health care for older people to approach complex clinical scenarios with confidence.

References

1. Stuck A E, Elkuch P, Dapp U, Anders J, Iliffe S, Swift C. for the Pro-Age pilot study group. Feasibility and yield of a self-administered questionnaire for health risk appraisal in older people in three European countries. *Age & Ageing* 2002; **31**: 463–7

2. Eccles M, Freemantle N, Mason J and the North of England Aspirin Guidelines development group. North of England Evidence Based Guideline development group project: guidelines on the use of aspirin as secondary prophylaxis for vascular disease in primary care. *BMJ* 1998; **316**: 1303–9

3. Guidelines for Management of Hypertension: Report of the Third Working Party of the British Hypertension Society, 1999. *J Human Hypertension* 1999; **13**: 569–92. See: www.hyp.ac.uk/bhs (accessed 20/09/2004)

4. Scottish Intercollegiate Guidelines Network (SIGN) Lipids and the primary prevention of coronary heart disease 1999. See: www.show.scot.nhs.uk/sign/guidelines (accessed 20/09/2004)

5. Clinical practice guidelines for the management of diabetes in Canada. *Canadian Med Assoc J* 1998; **159 (8S)**: S1–28

6. Atkin W. Implementing screening for colorectal cancer. *BMJ* 1999; **319**: 1212–13

7. Rhodes J M. Colorectal cancer screening in the UK: Joint Position Statement by the British Society of Gastroenterology, Royal College of Physicians, and the Association of Coloproctology of Great Britain and Ireland. *Gut* 2000; **46**: 746–8

8. Colon cancer screening (USPSTF Recommendation). *J Am Geriatr Soc* 2000; **48 (3)**: 333–5

9. Barry M J. Prostate-specific-antigen testing for early diagnosis of prostate cancer. *N Engl J Med* 2001; **344 (18)**: 1373–7

10. Gann P H, Hennekens C H, Stampfer M J. A prospective evaluation of plasma prostate-specific antigen for detection of prostatic cancer. *JAMA* 1995; **273**: 289–94

11. Sershon P D, Barry M J, Oesterling J E. Serum prostate-specific antigen discriminates weakly between men with benign prostatic hyperplasia and patients with organ-confined prostatic cancer. *Eur Urol* 1994; **25**: 281–7

12. Locker D, *et al.* Self-perceived oral health status, psychological well-being, and life satisfaction in an older adult population. *J Dent Res* 2000; **79 (4)**: 970–5

13. McGrath C, *et al.* Factors influencing older people's self reported use of dental services in the UK. *Gerodontology* 1999; **16 (2)**: 97–102

14. Mandel I D. Preventive dental services for the elderly. *Dental Clin N America* 1989; **33**: 81–90

15. Smeeth L, Iliffe S. Effectiveness of screening older people for impaired vision in community setting: systematic review of evidence from randomised controlled trials *BMJ* 1998; **316**: 660–3

16. Reidy A, *et al.* Prevalence of serious eye disease and visual impairment in a north London population: population based, cross sectional study. *BMJ* 1998; **316**: 1643–6

17. Freedman A, *et al.* Preventive care for the elderly. Do family physicians comply with recommendations of the Canadian Task Force on Preventive Health Care? *Can Fam Physician* 2000; **46**: 350–7

18. Bess F H, *et al.* Hearing impairment as a determinant of function in the elderly. *J Am Geriatr Soc* 1989; **37**: 123

19. Gennis V, *et al.* Hearing and cognition in the elderly: new findings and a review of the literature. *Arch Intern Med* 1991; **151**: 2259–64

20. Christmas C, Andersen R A. Exercise and older patients: Guidelines for the Clinician. *J Am Geriatr Soc* 2000; **48**: 318–24

21. National Diet and Nutrition Survey of people aged 65 and over. Department of Health Food Safety Information Bulletin 1998; **103 (Dec)**

22. Huijbregts P, *et al.* Dietary pattern and 20 year mortality in elderly men in Finland, Italy, and the Netherlands: longitudinal cohort study. *BMJ* 1997; **315**: 13–17

23. Hushner R F. Barriers to providing nutrition counselling by physicians: a survey of primary care practitioners. *Prev Med* 1995; 24(6): 546–52

24. Freid L A, *et al.* Preclinical mobility disability predicts incident mobility disability in older women. *J Gerontology* 2000; **55A (1)**: M43–52

25. Hay W I, *et al.* Prospective care of elderly patients in family practice. Is screening effective? *Can Fam Physician* 1998; **44**: 2677–87

26. Elliot A M, *et al.* The epidemiology of chronic pain in the community. *Lancet* 1999; **354**: 1248–52

27. Radecki S E, *et al.* Randomised clinical trial of diagnostic intsrument for pain complaints. *Fam Med* 1999; **31**: 713–21

28. Tinetti M E, Speechley M, Ginter S F. Risk factors for falls among elderly people living in the community. *N Engl J Med* 1988; **319**: 1701–7

29. Tinetti M E, Baker D I, McAvay G, *et al.* A multifactorial intervention to reduce the risk of falling among elderly people living in the community. *N Engl J Med* 1994; **331**: 821–7

30. Campbell J A. Randomised controlled trial of a general practice programme of home based exercise to prevent falls in elderly women. *BMJ* 1997; **315**: 1065–9

31. Close J, Ellis M, Hooper R, Glucksman E, Jackson S, Swift C. Prevention of Falls in the Elderly Trial (PROFET). A Randomised Controlled Trial. *Lancet* 1999; **353**: 93–7

32. Prosser, *et al.* Case-finding incontinence in the over-75's. *Br J Gen Pract* 1997; **47**: 498–500

33. Ouslander J G, Johnson T M. Incontinence. Ch 126 pp1595–614. In: *Principles of Geriatric Medicine and Gerontology*: Hazzard W, *et al.* 4th edition. New York: McGraw-Hill, 1999

34. Iliffe S, *et al.* Screening for cognitive impairment in the elderly using the Mini-Mental State Examination. *Br J Gen Pract* 1990; **40**: 277–9

35. Callahan C M, *et al.* Documentation and evaluation of cognitive impairment in elderly primary care patients. *Ann Intern Med* 1995; **122**: 422–9

36. Iliffe S, Manthorpe J. Dementia in older people in the community: the challenge for primary care development. *Reviews in Clinical Gerontology* 2002; **12**: 243–52

37. Banazak D A. Late-life depression in primary care. How well are we doing? *J Gen Intern Med* 1996; **11**: 163–7

38. Iliffe S, *et al.* Assessment of elderly people in general practice. 1. Social circumstances and mental state. *Br J Gen Pract* 1991; **41 (342)**: 9–12

39. Iliffe S, Manthorpe J. Depression, anxiety & psychosis in older people: more challenges for primary care. *Reviews in Clinical Gerontology* 2002; **12**: 327–41

40. Vetter N J, Ford D. Smoking prevention among elderly people aged 60 and over: a randomised controlled trial. *Age & Ageing* 1990; **19**: 164–8

41. Connoly J M. Smoking cessation in old age: closing the stable door? *Age & Ageing* 2000; **29**: 193–5

42. Dunne F J. Misuse of alcohol or drugs by elderly people. *BMJ* 1994; **308**: 608–9

43. Dufour M C, Archer L, Gordis E. Alcohol and the elderly. *Clin Geriatr Med* 1992; **8**: 127–41

CHAPTER 16

Cancer

David Weller

RECENT ADVANCES ▼

- DoH guidelines on cancer referral have been an important step towards helping GPs identify patterns of presentation that require prompt attention, although early diagnosis remains a considerable challenge.

- Interest is growing in diagnostic algorithms that allow clinicians to estimate how much symptom patterns predict cancer, and should help to refine cancer referral guidance.

- Screening for colorectal cancer is to be introduced from 2006, and GPs will have important roles in information provision and co-ordination.

- Management of demand for prostate-specific antigen (PSA) testing is an emerging issue for general practice, and there is an increasing emphasis on developing improved strategies for providing informed consent.

- Liquid-based cytology for cervical screening will grow in usage over the next several years, which has the potential to considerably benefit patients.

► KEY MESSAGES

- Although the role of GPs in cancer detection and management has not been strongly emphasised in the past, this is changing and the concept of 'primary care oncology' is gaining recognition.

- GPs are involved in all stages of the cancer patient's journey, and have an important role in providing comprehensive and continuing care.

- There are substantially increased consultation rates in primary care in patients with a diagnosis of cancer; psychosocial problems figure prominently in these consultations.

- New screening programmes, such as faecal occult blood test (FOBT) screening, will have important implications for general practice – particularly in terms of workload, capacity, and information needs of patients.

- Many emerging technologies, such as genetic testing and oral chemotherapy treatments, will further underline the role of primary care.

Introduction

Cancer is responsible for one-quarter of all deaths in England and Wales, and incidence of new cases of cancer increased by 12% in males and 28% in females between 1960 and 1997.[1] Significant delays between the onset of symptoms and diagnosis can be associated with worse survival rates.[2] Survival rates in the UK for some cancers are lower than in other countries in Europe, reflecting more advanced disease at the time of diagnosis or treatment.[3-4]

This chapter examines the role of GPs in the early detection, screening and management of cancer. The importance of this role is widely acknowledged.[5] NHS Cancer Plans recognise that primary care has an important role in all stages of the patient's journey, and recommend increased roles in leading cancer services.[6-7]

Most patients with cancer present, with symptoms, in primary care.[8] All GPs are aware that diagnosing cancer early is difficult, particularly when symptoms are non-specific and poorly predictive.[9-10] Our challenge in general practice is to respond to these symptoms appropriately, make judgements about the likelihood of cancer or other serious illness, and make referrals selectively – otherwise there is the risk of swamping expensive and limited diagnostic services. Unfortunately, there is little supporting evidence to help practitioners in their diagnostic decisions, although recent efforts in developing referral guidelines and recommendations have helped. There is more evidence to support the role of primary care in cancer screening, with clearly identifiable roles in optimising and ensuring equitable uptake.[11]

The involvement of primary care continues through all stages of the 'cancer journey'. Increasingly, patients are making use of primary care services in the immediate post-diagnosis period.[12] This will increase as more oral therapies become available, and pressure on secondary care services continues to rise. Ideally, specialist and primary care services should be integrated, as this has significant benefits for patients, including less time spent travelling to and waiting in hospital.[13] Furthermore, rates of co-morbidity are high amongst cancer patients,[14] and many common illnesses managed in general practice, including vascular disease, asthma, chronic bronchitis, diabetes, and renal disease, are associated with high early mortality rates from cancer.[15]

Current priorities for cancer services include early detection, faster access to specialist treatment, improved support for patients living with cancer (including good communication and palliative care), and reducing inequalities. General practice has a critical role in all of these areas.

Referral guidance

The NHS Cancer Plan[6] recognised the need for improved guidance on referral of patients with suspected diagnoses of cancer, and the DoH produced referral guidelines outlining key symptoms and other patient-related factors that might prompt referral.[16] These guidelines aim to facilitate 'appropriate referral between primary and secondary care for patients whom a GP suspects may have cancer'. They are intended to help GPs to identify those patients who are most likely to have cancer and who therefore require urgent assessment in secondary care. The guidelines are presented in 12 tumour groups – for each tumour group the guidelines set 1) key points about the characteristics of patients with the relevant cancers, and 2) guidelines for urgent referral. The National Institute for Clinical Excellence (NICE) is in the process of updating this referral guidance.

Organisation of services

There has also been much activity to improve cancer services as part of the NHS Cancer Plan. For example, the Cancer Services Collaborative (CSC), part of the NHS Modernisation Agency is a national NHS programme designed to improve the way in which cancer services are provided. Its goal is to 'improve the experience and outcomes for patients with suspected or diagnosed cancer by optimising care delivery systems across the whole pathway of care'.[17] It offers practical approaches to delivering the improvement targets laid out in the Cancer Plan. Since April 2001 all 34 cancer networks in England have been taking part in the CSC programme. The programme encourages local clinical teams to look at their own services and supports them in making significant improvements by redesigning the way that care is delivered. The involvement of general practice and primary care teams in these efforts varies throughout the UK, but increasing engagement in these activities is an important priority.

Primary prevention

There is evidence that some lifestyle choices can increase the risk of cancer, and it is widely argued that GPs are well placed to encourage patients to modify their behaviour in order to minimise risk.[18] However, beyond smoking and alcohol, evidence suggests that GPs can bring about only modest lifestyle changes. Ideally, there should be a broader approach, which involves shifting the distribution of risk factors across a whole population in a favourable direction, combined with a further approach that targets individuals at increased risk due to genetic, environmental or other factors. Primary prevention features in the NHS Cancer Plan,[6] which tackles a number of key areas including smoking, diet and nutrition, obesity, physical activity, alcohol and exposure to sunlight. All of these are areas in which activities based in general practice could make a profound difference.

Smoking

Smoking causes about one in three cancer deaths in the UK. Furthermore, 90% of deaths from lung cancer among men and nearly 75% among women are estimated to have been caused by smoking.[19] Cancers of the mouth, oesophagus, bladder, kidney and pancreas are also strongly linked to smoking.[20] In addition to this, it is associated with many other conditions commonly seen in general practice, including heart disease, stroke, chronic obstructive lung disease, asthma and peripheral vascular disease. Smoking prevalence in the UK has fallen from 40% of adults aged 16 and over in 1978 to 27% in 2000,[21] although quit rates in middle-aged smokers are now only about 2% per year. There is evidence that GPs can reduce smoking rates by providing appropriate advice,[21] and PCTs are being actively encouraged to take the lead in commissioning and providing smoking cessation services. NICE has recommended the use of bupropion and nicotine replacement therapy for smokers who wish to quit, adding that these therapies should normally be prescribed as part of a commitment by smokers to stop smoking by a certain date and continue to remain smoke-free.[22]

Diet and nutrition

It has been estimated that around one third of cancers are related to diet.[23] Diet has a particularly close association with cancers of the colon, rectum, stomach, lung, and prostate. Improving diet is an important issue for general practice, not only to reduce the rates of cancer but other diet-related chronic conditions such as coronary heart disease, stroke, Type 2 diabetes and obesity. For GPs and their patients there are a number of sources of dietary recommendations to reduce the risk of cancer in the UK. The former Health Education Authority has produced a useful summary of evidence linking dietary factors and various cancers[24] (available at www.hda-online.org.uk). The report recommends:

- ▶ increasing the consumption of a wide variety of fruits and vegetables

- ▶ increasing intakes of dietary fibre from bread and other cereals (particularly wholegrain varieties), potatoes, fruit and vegetables

- ▶ maintaining a healthy body weight (within the BMI range 20–25) and avoiding an increase during adult life

- ▶ avoiding an increase in the average consumption of red and processed meat, current intakes of which are about 90 g / day

- ▶ avoiding the use of beta-carotene supplements to protect against cancer and being cautious in using high doses of purified supplements of other nutrients.

Increasing the population's average intake of fruit and vegetables to at least five portions a day is considered to be the second most important strategy in preventing cancers after reducing the rates of smoking[25] and primary care teams need to use whatever resources they have to help their patients bring about these dietary changes. In England, the DoH has funded 'Five-a-day' pilot sites across the country in the hope of promoting healthier diets and developing further community initiatives.

Physical activity

The importance of promoting physical activity is highlighted in The NHS Plan.[26] Evidence for a link between inactivity and a range of cancers has grown over several decades;[27] for example, regular physical activity is associated with a decreased risk of colon cancer (although there is no such association between physical activity and rectal cancer). Current evidence cannot draw conclusions regarding a relationship between physical activity and endometrial, ovarian or testicular cancers. Further, despite numerous studies, existing data are inconsistent regarding an association with breast or prostate cancers.

A recent systematic review concluded that there is evidence that interventions in primary care can increase physical activity in the short term.[28] Notably, brief interventions appear to be as likely to succeed as intensive interventions, although there is insufficient evidence to identify other attributes of successful interventions.

Alcohol

Alcohol is causally related to cancers of the oral cavity and pharynx, larynx, oesophagus and liver.[29-30] Hazardous alcohol consumption is thought to be a major cause in about 3% of all cancers in England.[31] GPs have the potential to reduce hazardous drinking in their patients, and numerous brief intervention strategies are available.[17] While brief advice can reduce excessive drinking, a recent systematic review suggests that routine screening in general practice does not seem to be an effective precursor to brief interventions targeting excessive alcohol use.[32]

Sun exposure

Both malignant melanoma and non-melanoma (basal cell carcinoma, squamous cell carcinoma and rarer cancers) are associated with sun exposure. There are approximately 6000 new cases of melanoma skin cancer diagnosed each year in the UK,[33] and well over 40,000 new cases of non-melanoma skin cancer each year.[34] The main risk factor for skin cancer is overexposure to sunlight in people with sensitive skin types (e.g. people with fair or freckled skin who burn easily and tan with difficulty)[35], and excessive sun exposure in childhood.[36]

Relatively small behavioural changes in the way people behave in the sun, can lead to a considerable decrease in personal risk. There is growing interest in promoting a greater role for primary prevention in general practice,[37] particularly targeting high-risk groups such as those with fair skin and red hair.

Breast cancer

Background

Breast cancer remains the most common cancer in women, although mortality rates in women under the age of 70 have fallen.[38-9] The reasons for this are not completely clear, but probably reflect the cumulative effects of a range of measures including better treatments, and more effective screening strategies.[39] A major pan-European study showed that survival rates in England and Scotland were lower than in other European countries in the 1980s;[40]

comparative data such as these have prompted many of the screening and treatment initiatives in breast cancer.

Early detection and screening
Screening for breast cancer began in the UK in 1988 and the prevalent screening round was completed in 1995. Currently, all women aged 50–64 are invited for mammograms every three years; the age range is to be expanded to women aged 70 by 2004.[6] There has been recent debate in the literature about the effectiveness of breast screening following the publication of a systematic review from the Nordic Cochrane Centre;[41] in response, evidence based on long-term follow-up of screening participants has been presented to support the case for mammography.[42] Such debates highlight the importance of the role of GPs in providing guidance to support informed decision making. There is limited evidence of benefit for routine breast self-examination or clinical examination,[43] although there is general acceptance of a policy of promoting 'breast awareness', and reporting suspicious symptoms early.

Management and follow-up
GPs are not generally involved in the primary treatment of breast cancer, which usually involves surgery, either breast conservation (wide local excision) or mastectomy. This is usually followed by adjuvant treatment such as radiotherapy, chemotherapy or hormone therapy or a combination of these. Adjuvant treatment choice depends on age, risk of relapse, potential benefits, oestrogen receptor status and acceptability to the patient. Tamoxifen is the most commonly used form of hormonal treatment. Metastatic breast cancer can affect many parts of the body, especially bones, lungs, soft tissue and liver. It causes a range of symptoms, particularly pain and fatigue. GPs are, however, involved in post-treatment management, and it is known that consultation rates increase following a diagnosis of breast cancer.[12] Although long-term follow-up is not routinely recommended, previous studies have demonstrated that GPs can provide follow-up with equal effectiveness to secondary care.[44]

Since 1999, the Cancer Services Collaborative has been developing practical ways of changing services to improve the experience and outcomes of care for people with breast cancer[45] and it is important for primary care teams to engage in these multidisciplinary management approaches.

Guidance
NICE is producing guidance on all aspects of breast cancer detection and treatment, building on the widely-used 'Improving Outcomes' breast guidance, which was published by the DoH in 1996 and has been very influential in

shaping service delivery.[46] Key recommendations in the draft NICE guidance include:

Multidisciplinary team working

▶ All patients with breast cancer should be managed by multidisciplinary teams and all multidisciplinary teams should be actively involved in network-wide audit of processes and outcomes.

▶ Multidisciplinary teams should consider how they might improve the effectiveness of the way they work. Some units should consider working together to increase the number of patients managed by the team.

Minimising delay

▶ No patient should have to wait more than four weeks for any form of treatment or supportive intervention.

Follow-up

▶ The primary aims of clinical follow-up should be to identify and treat local recurrence and adverse effects of therapy, not to detect metastatic disease in asymptomatic women. Long-term routine hospital-based follow-up should cease, except in the context of clinical trials.

The breast cancer component of the DoH Referral guidelines[16] is summarised below; the majority of patients present with lumps in the breast or axilla, which can be detected by clinical examination – overall, about 10% of lumps assessed in breast clinics are found to be malignant.

Urgent referral (within two weeks)

▶ Patients aged 30 or over (the precise age criterion to be agreed by each network) with a discrete lump in the breast.

▶ Patients with breast signs or symptoms which are highly suggestive of cancer. These include:
  ▷ ulceration
  ▷ skin nodule
  ▷ skin distortion
  ▷ nipple eczema
  ▷ recent nipple retraction or distortion (< 3 months)
  ▷ unilateral nipple discharge which stains clothes.

Conditions that require referral, not necessarily urgent

- ▶ Breast lumps in the following patients, or of the following types:
  - ▷ discrete lump in a younger woman (age < 30 years)
  - ▷ asymmetrical nodularity that persists at review after menstruation
  - ▷ abscess
  - ▷ persistently refilling or recurrent cyst
  - ▷ intractable pain which does not respond to simple measures such as wearing a well-fitting bra and using over-the-counter analgesics such as paracetamol.

Women with a family history of breast cancer

The level of risk for most women who have relatives with breast cancer will be only slightly higher than for others in the same age group; such women should normally be reassured and managed by primary care teams. An information pack to facilitate risk assessment in primary care is available from Cancer Research UK.[47] This pack includes suggested referral guidelines, a management guide and information booklets for patients.

At present, genetic testing is restricted to high-risk families after assessment by the regional clinical genetics service, but NICE is currently producing a guideline on the care of women at risk of familial breast cancer in primary, secondary and tertiary care.

Colorectal cancer

Background

GPs have important roles in early detection and screening for colorectal cancer, as well as follow-up post treatment. Colorectal (large bowel) cancer is the second most common cancer after lung cancer, both in terms of both incidence and mortality, in England and Wales.[48] Although prostate cancer is more common in men and breast cancer more common in women, colorectal cancer affects both sexes. Each year, over 30,000 new cases of colorectal cancer are diagnosed, and colorectal cancer is registered as the underlying cause of death in about half this number.[49] The incidence of colorectal cancer is gradually increasing. One reason for this is the ageing of the population: as with most forms of cancer, the probability of developing colorectal cancer rises sharply with age.

Early detection and screening

There is current widespread interest in strategies to improve recognition of potential symptoms of colorectal cancer in primary care and in the community. There is considerable evidence in the research literature of delays, often lasting a year or more, between the onset of symptoms of colorectal cancer and diagnosis and treatment.[50-1] This arises through a combination of patient-related factors and delays in both primary and secondary care. Some GP and hospital delay is due to inadequate investigation of symptoms, misdiagnosis, and false negative results of diagnostic tests.

A national survey of NHS patients carried out in 1999–2000 (just before the publication of two-week referral guidelines for colorectal cancer) found that 34% of patients with colorectal cancer had had an appointment with a hospital doctor within two weeks of visiting their GP with symptoms.[52] However, a substantial proportion, 37%, had to wait over three months for their first hospital appointment – 13% waited seven or more months.

The most common presenting symptoms and signs of cancer or large polyps are rectal bleeding, persisting change in bowel habit, and anaemia; more advanced tumours are likely to cause weight loss, nausea and anorexia, and abdominal pain. These symptoms are common in the general population, and GPs face considerable challenges in discriminating between those symptoms that carry increased risk of cancer and those that do not. In some patients symptoms do not become apparent until the cancer is far advanced. There is considerable interest in developing systems of improved discrimination of symptoms in primary care,[53] possibly through the use of patient-completed questionnaires about symptoms, which could be used to derive estimates of predictivity. The feasibility of such approaches is still not known.

By comparison, evidence supporting screening for bowel cancer is convincing. Trials have demonstrated about 17% reductions in groups that are offered screening using the FOBT.[54] A UK pilot of screening using the FOBT has just been completed; it demonstrated that screening is feasible in the general population, and can achieve uptake and detection rates that are similar to those observed in randomised studies.[55] There is also growing interest in the use of flexible sigmoidoscopy – particularly as this is a screening modality which could be delivered in primary care. A randomised study of flexible sigmoidoscopy screening will report in the near future.[56] Health ministers in both England and Scotland have committed to a national programme of screening for colorectal cancer, and this will have important implications for workload and capacity in primary care. At present there is considerable activity in increasing capacity for colonoscopy, pathology and other services associated with the provision of colorectal cancer screening.

Management and follow-up

Surgery to remove the primary tumour is the principal first-line treatment for approximately 80% of patients, after which about 40% will remain disease-free in the long term. In 20–30% of cases, the disease is too far advanced at initial presentation for any attempt at curative intervention; many of these patients die within a few months.

Results from meta-analyses show that follow-up can increase the probability of long-term survival after surgery; more intensive follow-up appears to be associated with significant improvements in five-year survival rates, although there are methodological concerns about these analyses.[57] A randomised controlled trial (the 'FACS' trial)[58] is on-going, and will assess the cost-effectiveness of intensive versus no scheduled follow-up in patients who have undergone resection for colorectal cancer with curative intent.

Guidance

Existing DoH guidance[59] has been updated by NICE.[60] Identification and management of high-risk groups is a particularly important issue for GPs; for high-risk groups it is recommended that cancer networks should develop guidelines on the nature and frequency of surveillance (based on the British Society of Gastroenterology (BSG) and the Association of Coloproctology), which can be found on the BSG website (www.bsg.org.uk). Several disease groups are associated with increased risk, of which the largest are patients who have had colorectal cancer, those found to have multiple or large (> 1 cm) adenomatous polyps, and patients with longstanding colitis. Regular colonoscopy is recommended for people in all these groups, but the frequency with which this should be carried out depends on the particular condition. People with two first degree relatives with colorectal cancer, or one first degree relative whose colorectal cancer is diagnosed before the age of 45, have a lifetime risk of death from colorectal cancer of 1 in 6 or 1 in 10 respectively. The BSG/ACPGBI guidelines suggest that people who meet these criteria should be referred for colonoscopy at 35–40 years of age, or as soon thereafter as the risk is recognised.

DoH referral guidance for urgent referral[16] indicates that the following symptom and sign combinations when occurring for the first time should be used to identify patients for urgent referral:

All Ages

- ▶ rectal bleeding WITH a change in bowel habit to looser stools and/or increased frequency of defecation persistent for six weeks

- ▶ a definite palpable right-sided abdominal mass

▶ a definite palpable rectal (not pelvic) mass

▶ rectal bleeding WITH a change in bowel habit to looser stools and/or increased frequency of defecation persistent for six weeks.

Over 60 years

▶ rectal bleeding persistently WITHOUT anal symptoms

▶ change of bowel habit to looser stools and/or increased frequency of defecation, WITHOUT rectal bleeding and persistent for six weeks.

Any age

▶ iron deficiency anaemia WITHOUT an obvious cause (Hb < 11 g/dl in men or < 10 g/dl in postmenopausal women).

Prostate cancer

Background

Cancer of the prostate is a leading cause of male cancer-related mortality in Western countries such as the UK and Australia, and its incidence is rising in the UK and internationally.[61-2] Prostate cancer is particularly common among elderly men, and death from prostate cancer is relatively uncommon under the age of 65.[47] Autopsy studies demonstrate that the majority of men over 80 years old have areas of malignant tissue in their prostate glands; most die *with* it, not *of* it.[63]

Early detection and screening

Lower urinary tract symptoms (such as frequency, hesitation, poor stream) are suggestive of obstructive disease of the prostate or bladder neck, and are common in general practice. Digital rectal examination (DRE) remains a useful examination; if the prostate feels normal, the option of PSA testing may be discussed with patients, but this should be in the context of providing informed consent about the limitations in accuracy of the test. Prostate cancer may produce no symptoms until it has reached an advanced stage, but early cancer can be detected by DRE. In older men, these symptoms are often caused by benign prostatic hyperplasia, with which cancer may co-exist.

PSA testing in asymptomatic men offers the prospect of early detection and treatment of the disease, but has not been shown conclusively to lead to observable improvements in mortality from prostate cancer.[64-5] Trials are currently underway in North America and Europe to examine this question,[66] but results will not be available for some years. Testing of asymptomatic men for prostate cancer is not widespread in the UK,[67] although recent NHS guidance promotes a policy of 'informed consent' in response to requests for PSA tests, replacing an active policy of discouragement;[68] this may lead to increased awareness and activity.[69] Recent analyses of trends suggest increasing rates of PSA testing in England,[69] and it is likely that demand for PSA testing will rise in the UK over the next few years, following trends in the US and Australia. Recent evidence suggests that PSA testing rates can be reduced by educational strategies targeting GPs.[70]

Management and follow-up

There is no consensus on the optimum form of management for patients with localised prostate cancer. Although observational studies suggest that radical treatment can improve long-term survival rates in particular patient groups, this evidence is by its nature subject to bias. In addition, the uncertain benefits of radical interventions must be balanced against the risk of lasting adverse effects. Research – both randomised controlled trials and audit of outcomes outside the context of clinical trials – is essential to clarify the role of each form of treatment and should be supported.

Large-scale prospective randomised trials are essential to resolve uncertainty about the relative effectiveness of different forms of treatment. A new trial, ProtecT, has been established by the Health Technology Assessment programme to compare outcomes in men with screen-detected prostate cancer treated with radiotherapy, radical prostatectomy or active monitoring.[71] In the meantime, GPs need to be aware that evidence for the various treatment options for localised cancer is still limited, and as more cancers are detected through PSA testing this is likely to become an issue of growing importance.

Guidance

An important recent initiative is the NHS Prostate Cancer Programme and a Prostate Cancer Risk Management Programme, which places an emphasis on information provision in response to requests for PSA testing.[70] This should include clear information about the test and the uncertainty surrounding the balance of benefits and risks of screening for prostate cancer.

Symptoms featuring in DoH guidelines for urgent referral[16] (within two weeks)
for urological cancers, including prostate cancer, are:

► macroscopic haematuria in adults

► microscopic haematuria in adults over 50 years

► swellings in the body of the testis

► palpable renal masses

► solid renal masses found on imaging elevated age-specific PSA in men
with a ten-year life expectancy, a high PSA (> 20 ng / ml) in men with a
clinically malignant prostate or bone pain.

Lung cancer

Background

With 33,390 deaths due to lung cancer in the UK in 2001, mortality rates are
higher than colorectal, breast and prostate cancers combined.[33] Lung cancer
accounts for 15% of new cases of invasive cancer (38,880 new cases in 1998).
These rates compare unfavourably with international figures, as does five-year
survival.[40] Despite projected decreases in the number of cases, lung cancer
will continue to be a major health issue in the UK for the next two decades.
Any attempt to comprehensively tackle this disease must address three critical
areas: health promotion, timely diagnosis of disease, and best practice in the
management of patients. The relative paucity of research into lung cancer was
highlighted in a recent strategic analysis of UK cancer research.[72]

Although the total number of people diagnosed with lung cancer is falling,
the rate of decrease is very small and is among men only.[53] Furthermore, numbers
continue to rise in women, with increased tobacco consumption particularly
among teenage girls.

Early detection and screening

In common with many other cancers, it is often difficult to distinguish
between those respiratory symptoms that carry increased risk of lung cancer
and those that do not. Many lung cancer patients in the UK are not diagnosed
early enough and/or are not referred to a specialist team and thus do not
receive treatment adequate treatment. Although lung cancer is the most common malignancy that GPs will encounter, lung cancer develops in a group
of patients with common respiratory symptoms, the majority of whom will

not have cancer.[73] Delays have been identified at two stages in the diagnostic process: delay in presentation by the patient to the GP, and delay in first investigation by the GP for chest X-ray or referral to secondary care.[74-80] The DoH Referral Guidelines for Suspected Cancer[16] note the paucity of evidence in this area.

There are few studies into the role of primary care in early lung cancer diagnosis. Several features worthy of systematic evaluation in symptom assessment have been noted.[77-9] These include the use of 'dynamic evidence' in primary care: i.e. the onset of new symptoms, the persistence of a symptom, or changes in the characteristic of a problem, change in patient behaviour, or the presence of 'symptom clusters'.

Difficulties in early diagnosis and the poor survival associated with lung cancer have helped maintain interest in screening for lung cancer. Low-dose spiral computed tomography (CT) of the chest is being evaluated in several centres around the world,[80] but results won't be available for some years.

Management and follow-up

Evidence suggests that the standards of management for lung cancer vary widely across the UK.[81] It is possible that more patients may benefit from surgery and existing guidelines in this area call for improved accuracy of the selection process of lung cancer patients suitable for surgery.[82]

Guidance

The National Collaborating Centre for Acute Care is developing a clinical guideline on lung cancer for use in the NHS in England and Wales (commissioned by NICE). The guideline will provide recommendations for good practice that are based on the best available evidence of clinical and cost effectiveness.

Skin cancer

Skin cancer is the most common type of cancer, accounting for half of all new cancers in Western populations. It occurs more often in people with light coloured skin who have had a high exposure to sunlight. The two most frequent types of skin cancer are basal cell carcinomas and squamous cell carcinoma. The third most frequent skin cancer is melanoma, although there are other, less common cancers starting in the skin including merkel cell tumours, cutaneous lymphomas, and sarcomas. Skin cancer is increasingly prevalent in the UK population[83-4] and this presents significant diagnostic challenges to GPs. Early diagnosis is associated with good prognosis.[85–90] Screening for melanoma by GPs appears to have low specificity, which would lead to high rates of excision of benign lesions.[87] International studies have shown that for every melanoma that is excised, between approximately ten and 30 benign lesions are removed,[88–93] hence the need for improved diagnostic techniques. There is growing interest in using techniques such as photography to assist in diagnosis.[90]

The Scottish Intercollegiate Guidelines Network (SIGN) has produced a clinical guideline for cutaneous melanoma.[91] This includes extensive reviews of evidence for diagnostic and screening strategies (highlighting the limitations in current evidence), and for long-term follow-up (emphasising that specific frequency and duration of follow-up should be determined from the timing and rate of recurrence of the individual patient's melanoma).

NICE has commissioned the National Collaborating Centre for Cancer to develop service guidance on skin tumours for use in the NHS in England and Wales. The guidance will address key areas of clinical management, including:

- diagnostic services (excluding referral guidelines) including the roles of:
  - ▷ GPs and other members of the primary care team
  - ▷ telemedicine
  - ▷ dermatologists
  - ▷ pathologists
  - ▷ radiologists

- treatment services, to include treatment in the following settings:
  - ▷ primary care – surgery, cryotherapy
  - ▷ dermatology centres – surgery, Mohs surgery, cryotherapy, photodynamic therapy, topical chemotherapy and immunotherapy
  - ▷ plastic surgery units
  - ▷ cancer centres – radiotherapy, chemotherapy and immunotherapy
  - ▷ other specialised units such as maxillofacial surgery and ENT

- follow-up

- supportive care of patients with disfigurement.

Cervical cancer

Although rare in the population, primary care invests very considerable resource and time in screening for cervical cancer. It has been estimated that the cervical screening programme has been responsible for averting an estimated 800 deaths annually in women under 55 years in England and Wales.[92] There is widespread recognition that screening also leads to harmful effects,[93] and the need for fully-informed choice is emphasised in national guidance.[94-9]

Because of the resources involved and the potential to do harm, quality assurance for cervical screening is critical. With this in mind, there has been an initiative to modernise the NHS Cervical Screening Programme. A key component of this process has been the examination of newer, potentially more accurate, technologies, of which the most promising appears to be liquid-based cytology (LBC). NICE has appraised LBC and recommends that LBC techniques be introduced across the NHS Cervical Screening Programme. It is expected that it will take up to five years to complete roll-out of LBC across the programme in England. Important issues will include frequency of cervical screening, workforce and skill mix development and pathology modernisation. It is hoped that through the implementation of LBC around 300,000 women a year will not have to have a repeat test due to inadequate samples, with all the associated anxiety and inconvenience.

Familial and genetic aspects of cancer

Increasingly, GPs have taken on a central role in identifying individuals at high risk of cancer. Using genetic tests within high-risk families and/or screening entire populations are vital to the possibility of preventing cancer. Genetic risk factor prediction could potentially lead to individually-tailored prevention programmes, as well as the more generic use of anti-cancer vaccines and drugs.[96] Advances in genetics may eventually profoundly affect assessment of disease risk, diagnosis and management. Eventually, genetic risk assessment may be integrated into primary care to assist in the early detection of common familial cancers such as breast and bowel cancer.[97]

Evidence suggests that GPs lack confidence in risk assessment based on genetics and family history, and that more adequate guidance and education is required.[98] Computerised decision support may be able to assist primary care in these areas by simplifying pedigree drawing and implementing management guidelines,[99-104] although such systems are still not in widespread use in the UK.

Palliative care

While GPs and primary care teams have traditionally had extensive involvement in the care of patients dying from cancer, there is considerable interest in improving and better co-ordinating primary care-based palliative care in the UK. Most people with an advanced, progressive incurable disease wish to spend their final days in their own home, although this need is often not met.[101-7] The demand on palliative care resources will increase markedly in the next two decades. Furthermore, the ageing population and changes in work patterns of general practice will lead to significant challenges in providing high quality palliative care.[104] While a range of experiences are reported, in general patients appreciate the care received from their GP, particularly when he or she takes time to explain what is happening and makes extra efforts in symptom control.[105-11]

Initiatives such as the Macmillan GP Facilitator Programme in Palliative Care have had a substantial impact on provision of palliative care services in the UK and have also influenced GPs' knowledge, attitudes and confidence in symptom control. Improving communication between primary and specialist palliative care is an integral component of high quality programmes.

It is widely advocated that palliative care should be an integral part of the GP's role and palliative care teaching and training should be available for GP registrars during vocational training.[108] Supportive and palliative care guidance is currently being developed by NICE. General principles that emerge:

- ▶ palliative care should be an integral part of patient management

- ▶ specialist palliative care teams should be available to arrange the provision both of relief from symptoms and social and psychological support for patients and their carers when these needs cannot be met by primary care teams

- ▶ patients with advanced cancer may require care from specialist cancer treatment teams, specialist palliative care teams and primary care teams

- ▶ palliative care teams should work closely with primary care teams and hospital services; rapid and effective communication and information-sharing between teams is essential

- ▶ primary care teams should assess patients' needs regularly and accurately, to ensure that patients who require specialist palliative care or interventions are referred quickly and appropriately.

The Gold Standards Framework,[109] developed by Dr Keri Thomas, helps primary health care teams in England, Scotland and Northern Ireland to deal with issues such as communication breakdowns, symptom management, out-of-hours care, and how best to support patients and carers. The framework includes tools to enable primary care teams to:

- ▶ work as a team and ensure continuity of care

- ▶ plan in advance for developments in a patient's illness

- ▶ provide patients with the best symptom control

- ▶ give support to patients and carers.

Psychosocial support

Cancer has profound effects on the lives of patients and their families. There are high rates of psychological morbidity amongst cancer patients and this is mainly dealt with in primary care. Social support and psychotherapeutic or psycho–educational interventions can improve patients' quality of life. The diagnosis of cancer leads to a significant emotional burden, which current health services often fail to address. There is a paucity of behavioural and social science research to underpin approaches to more effective, behaviourally-focused preventative strategies for cancer, and improved psychosocial support for cancer patients. Patients whose needs are not met typically show higher psychological and symptomatic distress. Furthermore, this extends well beyond the patient; issues of cancer survivorship have equal salience for carers and family members. Family carers frequently lack support, are given to feelings of isolation, and experience considerable anxiety.

There is a growing recognition that primary care has a vital role to play in the provision of psychosocial care to patients with cancer.[110] In the future, strategies for psychosocial support for cancer patients will need to take into account the ageing population of cancer patients, and the growing perception that cancer is a chronic illness. It is likely there will be a much greater need for better psychosocial care, particularly with the breakdown of community and family structures, and the growing number of people living alone. There will be a growing emphasis on quality of life (and death), with demands for greater choice in when and how to die.

Future focus

By 2020 it is predicted that one in two people will be affected by cancer in the UK; trends suggest that more people are going to be diagnosed with cancer in the UK in the future, but that they are going to live longer with the disease.[111] As a result, they are more likely to experience multiple, chronic health conditions.

There are predictions that technological advances, such as gene therapies, will eventually lead to the development of tailored treatments that target particular gene mutations within an individual's tumour.[113] While such developments are some way off, they will have a profound effect on the way in which GPs diagnose cancer, and their role in its management.

In the future, our patients will have even greater access to health information. The internet will vastly increase opportunities for both patients and health professionals to access health information.[113] As a result, patients will be better equipped to take responsibility for their own health and to have more say in their choice of treatment.[114] However, patients are also likely to want help in finding high-quality information and primary care will play a crucial role in providing such support. Remote diagnostic and monitoring technology (e.g. heart monitors, electronic stethoscopes and blood-testing devices) will also become more widely available.

This chapter has provided a brief overview of current issues and evidence in important areas of cancer prevention, diagnosis and management by GPs. In many ways, it is difficult to predict how future technologies and health care trends will impact on these activities. What seems inevitable, though, is that the role of the GP and the primary care team will continue to expand, at all stages of the patient's journey.

References

1. Swerdlow A, Silva I dos S, Doll R. *Cancer Incidence and Mortality in England and Wales. Trends and Risk Factors.* Oxford: Oxford University Press, 2001

2. Richards M A, Westcombe A M, Love S B, Littlejohns P, Ramirez A J. Influence of delay on survival in patients with breast cancer: a systematic review. *Lancet* 1999; **353**: 1119–26

3. Gatta G, Capocaccia R, Sant M, Bell C M, Coebergh J W, *et al.* Understanding variations in survival for colorectal cancer in Europe: a EUROCARE high resolution study. *Gut* 2000; **47 (4)**: 533–8

4. Sant M, Capocaccia R, Coleman MP, Berrino F, Gatta G, *et al.* Cancer survival increases in Europe, but international differences remain wide. *Eur J Cancer* 2001; **37 (13)**: 1659–67

5. Campbell NC, MacLeod U, Weller D. Primary care oncology: essential if high quality cancer care is to be achieved for all. *Fam Pract* 2002; **19**: 577–8

6. Department of Health. *The NHS Cancer Plan.* London: HMSO, 2000

7. Scottish Executive Health Department. *Cancer in Scotland: Action for Change.* Edinburgh: Scottish Executive, 2001

8. Ferguson R J, Gregor A, Dodds, Kerr G. Management of lung cancer in south east Scotland. *Thorax* 1996; **51**: 569–74

9. Jones R, Rubin G, Hungin P. Is the two week rule for cancer referrals working. *BMJ* 2001; **322**: 1555–6

10. Summerton N. Cancer recognition and primary care. *Br J Gen Pract* 2002; **52**: 5–6

11. Hermens R P, Hak E, Hulscher M E, Braspenning J C C, Grol R. Adherence to guidelines on cervical screening in general practice: programme elements of successful implementation. *Br J Gen Pract* 2001; **51**: 897–903

12. Macleod U, Ross S, Twelves C, George W D, Gillis C, Watt G C M. Primary and secondary care management of women with early breast cancer from affluent and deprived areas: retrospective review of hospital and general practice records. *BMJ* 2000; **320**: 1442–5

13. Campbell N C, Ritchie L D, Cassidy J, Little J. Systematic review of cancer treatment programmes in remote and rural areas. *Br J Cancer* 1999; **80**: 1275–80

14. Ogle K S, Swanson G M, Woods N, Azzouz F. Cancer and comorbidity: redefining chronic diseases. *Cancer* 2000; **88**: 653–63

15. Yancik R, Wesley M N, Ries L A, Havlik R J, Edwards B K, Yates J W. Effects of age and comorbidity in postmenopausal breast cancer patients aged 55 years and older. *JAMA* 2001; **285**: 885–92

16. Department of Health. Referral Guidelines for Suspected Cancer. London: HMSO, 2000 Available on www.dh.gov.uk/assetRoot/04/01/44/21/04014421.pdf (accessed 20/09/2004)

17. NHS Modernisation Agency. Cancer Services Collaborative. www.modern.nhs.uk/scripts/default.asp?site_id=26&id=5620

18. Ashenden R, Silagy C, Weller D. A systematic review of the effectiveness of promoting lifestyle change in general practice. *Fam Pract* 1997; **14 (2)**: 160–76

19. Callum, C. *The UK smoking epidemic: deaths in 1995.* London: Health Education Authority, 1998

20. US Department of Health and Human Services. *Women and smoking: a report of the Surgeon General.* US Department of Health and Human Services, Centers for Disease Control and Prevention, National Centers for Chronic Disease Prevention and Health Promotion, Office on Smoking and Health. Rockville, MD: CDC, 2001 www.cdc.gov/tobacco/sgr_forwomen.htm

21. Office for National Statistics. *Living in Britain – results from the 2000/01 General Household Survey.* London: HMSO, 2001

22. National Institute for Clinical Excellence. *Technology Appraisal Guidance No. 39. Nicotine replacement therapy (NRT) and bupropion for smoking cessation.* London: NICE, 2002

23. Doll, R, Peto, R. The causes of cancer: quantitative estimates of avoidable risks of cancer in the United States today. *J Natl Cancer Inst* 1981; **66**: 1191–308

24. Health Education Authority. Nutritional aspects of the development of cancer: nutrition briefing paper. London: Health Education Authority, 1999

25. Day, N. Cancer mortality target. Paper prepared for the Department of Health. Unpublished, 2000

26. Department of Health. *The NHS Plan. A plan for investment, a plan for reform*. London: HMSO, 2000

27. Thune, I. and Furberg, A. S. Physical activity and cancer risk: dose-response and cancer, all sites and sitespecific. *Med Sci Sports Exerc* 2001; **33(S6)**: S530–50

28. Smith B J, Merom D, Harris P, Bauman A E. Do physical activity interventions to promote physical activity work? A systematic review of the literature. Melbourne: National Institute of Clinical Studies, 2003.
Available at: www.cpah.unsw.edu.au/NICS.pdf (accessed 20/09/2004)

29. Royal College of Physicians. Alcohol – can the NHS afford it? A report of a working party of the Royal College of Physicians. London: RCP, 2001

30. Seitz, HK Homann, N. Alcohol – can the NHS afford it? A report of a working party of the Royal College of Physicians. London, 2001

31. Department of Health. The NHS Cancer Plan. London: HMSO, 2000

32. Beich A, Thorsen T, Rollnick S. Screening in brief intervention trials targeting excessive drinkers in general practice: systematic review and meta-analysis. *BMJ* 2003; **327**: 536–42

33. Office for National Statistics. Office for National Statistics, Mortality Statistics: Cause. England and Wales 1999; General Register Office for Scotland, Annual Report 1999; General Register Office for Northern Ireland, Annual Report 1999. London: HMSO, 2000

34. Cancer Research Campaign. www.cancerresearchuk.org (accessed 20/09/2004)

35. English D, Armstrong B, Kricker A, *et al*. Sunlight and cancer. *Cancer causes control* 1997; **8**: 271–83

36. Urist M, Miller D, and Maddox W. Malignant melanoma. In: Murphy G, Lawrence W, Lenhard R (eds). *Clinical Oncology*. Washington, D.C.: American Cancer Society, 1995

37. Jackson A, Wilkinson C, Pill R. Moles and melanomas – who's at risk, who knows, and who cares? A strategy to inform those at high risk. *Br J Gen Pract* 1999; **49**: 199–203

38. Purushotham AD, Pain SJ, Miles D, *et al*. Variations in treatment and survival in breast cancer. *Lancet* Oncol 2001; **2**: 719–25

39. Peto R, Boreham J, Clarke M, Davies C, Beral V. UK and USA breast cancer deaths down 25% in year 2000 at ages 20–69 years. *Lancet* 2000; **355**: 1822

40. Berrino F, *et al*. *Survival of Cancer Patients in Europe: The EUROCARE-2 Study*. IARC Scientific Publications No 151. Lyon, 1999

41. Gotzsche P C, Olsen O. Is screening for breast cancer with mammography justifiable? *Lancet* 2000; **355**: 129–34

42. Tabar L, Dean P B. Mammography and breast cancer: the new era. *Int J Gynaecol Obstet* 2003; **82**: 319–26

43. Kosters J P, Gotzsche P C. Regular self-examination or clinical examination for early detection of breast cancer. Cochrane Database Syst Rev 2003; CD003373

44. Grunfeld E, Mant D, Yudkin P, *et al.* Vessey M. Routine follow up of breast cancer in primary care: randomised trial. *BMJ* 1996; **313**: 665–9

45. Cancer Services Collaborative. Breast Cancer Service Improvement Guide. London: NHS Modernisation Agency, 2001

46. Cancer Guidance Sub-Group of the Clinical Outcomes Group. *Improving Outcomes in Breast Cancer: Guidance for Purchasers: the Manual.* Leeds: NHS Executive, 1996

47. CRC Primary Care Education Research Group. *Familial breast and ovarian cancer: an information pack for primary care.* Available on request from CRC Primary Care Education Research Group, University of Oxford; tel: 01865 226788, fax: 01865 226784

48. Quinn M, Babb P, Brock A, Kirby L, Jones J. *Cancer trends in England and Wales, 1950–1999.* London: HMSO, 2001

49. Source: data on ONS website (www.statistics.gov.uk)

50. Cockburn J, Paul C, Tzelepis F, *et al.* Delay in seeking advice for symptoms that potentially indicate bowel cancer. *Am J Health Behav.* 2003; **27**: 401–7

51. Robertson R, Campbell N C, Smith S, *et al.* Factors influencing time from presentation to treatment of colorectal and breast cancer in urban and rural areas. *Br J Cancer* 2004; **90**: 1479–85

52. Airey C, Becher H, Erens B, Fuller E. *National Surveys of NHS Patients – Cancer: National Overview 1999/2000.* London: HMSO, 2002

53. Selvachandran S N, Hodder R J, Ballal M S, *et al.* Prediction of colorectal cancer by a patient consultation questionnaire and scoring system: a prospective study. *Lancet* 2002; **360**: 278–83

54. Towler B, Irwig L, Glasziou P, Kewenter J, Weller D, Silagy C. A systematic review of the effects of screening for colorectal cancer using the faecal occult blood test, Hemoccult. *BMJ* 1998; **317**: 559–65

55. Weller D, Alexander F, Orbell S, *et al.* Evaluation of the UK Colorectal Cancer Screening Pilot. A report for the UK Department of Health. London: Department of Health, June 2003. See: www.cancerscreening.nhs.uk/colorectal/finalreport.pdf (accessed 20/09/2004)

56. Atkin W S, Edwards R, Wardle J, *et al.* Design of a multicentre randomised trial to evaluate flexible sigmoidoscopy in colorectal cancer screening. *J Med Screen* 2001; **8 (3)**: 137–44

57. Renehan A G, Egger M, Saunders M P, O'Dwyer S T. Impact on survival of intensive follow up after curative resection for colorectal cancer: systematic review and meta-analysis of randomised trials. *BMJ* 2002; **324**: 813

58. National Cancer Research Network Trials Portfolio. www.ncrn.org.uk/portfolio/data.asp?ID=762 (accessed 20/09/2004)

59. Department of Health, Clinical Outcomes Group, Cancer Guidance Sub-group. Guidance on commissioning cancer services: improving outcomes in colorectal cancer, the research evidence. London: HMSO, 1997 www.dh.gov.uk/assetRoot/04/01/13/60/04011360.pdf (accessed 20/09/2004)

60. National Institute for Clinical Excellence. Guidance on Cancer Services: Improving Outcomes in Colorectal Cancer. London: NICE, manual update, May 2004

61. Australian Institute of Health & Welfare & Australasian Association of Cancer Registries 2000. Cancer incidence in Australia 1997: Incidence and mortality data for 1997 and selected data for 1998 and 1999. AIHW cat. no. CAN 10. Canberra: AIHW (Cancer Series no. 15)

62. Majeed A, Babb P, Jones J, Quinn M. Trends in prostate cancer incidence, mortality and survival in England and Wales 1971–1998. *Br J Urol* 2000; **85**: 1058–62

63. Selley S, Donovan J, Faulkner A, *et al*. Diagnosis, management and screening of early localised prostate cancer. *Health Technol Assess* 1997; **1 (2)**: i 1–96

64. Chamberlain J, Melia J, Moss S, Brown J. Report prepared for the Health Technology Assessment panel of the NHS Executive on the diagnosis, management, treatment and costs of prostate cancer in England and Wales. *Br J Urol* 1997; **79 (S3)**: 1–32

65. Australian Health Technology Advisory Committee (AHTAC). *Prostate Cancer Screening.* Canberra: AGPS, 1996

66. International Prostate Screening Evaluation Group (IPSTEG). Rationale for randomised trials of prostate cancer screening. *Eur J Cancer* 1999; **3 S**: 262–71

67. Melia J, Moss S. Survey of the rate of PSA testing in general practice. *Br J Cancer* 2001; **85 (5)**: 656–7

68. NHS Executive. *The NHS Prostate Cancer Programme.* London: NHS Executive, 2000

69. Donovan J, Neal D, Hamdy F. Screening for prostate cancer in the UK. *BMJ* 2001; **323**: 763–4

70. Weller D, May F, Rowett D, Esterman A, Pinnock C, Nicholson S, Doust J and Silagy C. Promoting better use of the PSA test in general practice: randomized controlled trial of educational strategies based on outreach visits and mailout. *Family Practice* 2003; **20**: 655–61

71. National Cancer Research Network Trials Portfolio. www.ncrn.org.uk/portfolio/data.asp?ID=760 (accessed 20/09/2004)

72. National Cancer Research Institute. Strategic Analysis 2002. London: NCRI, 2002

73. Summerton N. *Diagnosing Cancer in Primary Care.* Oxford: Radcliffe Medical Press, 1999

74. Koyi H, Hillerdal G, Branden E. Patients' and doctors' delays in diagnosis of chest tumours. *Lung Cancer* 2002; **35**: 53–7

75. Krishnasamy M, Wilkie E. *Lung cancer: patients', families', and professionals' perceptions of health care needs. A national needs assessment study.* London: MacMillan Cancer Relief, 1997

76. Dische S, Gibson D, Parmar M, *et al*. Time course from first symptom to treatment in patients with non-small cell lung cancer referred for radiotherapy: a report by the CHART Steering Committee. *Thorax* 1996; **51**: 1262–5

77. Summerton N. Diagnosis and general practice. *Br J Gen Pract* 2000; **50**: 995–1000

78. Brashers V L, Haden K. Differential diagnosis of cough: focus on lung malignancy. *Lippincotts Prim Care Pract* 2000; **4**: 374–89

79. Love N. Emergent signs of cancer. Recognizing them early in the office or ER. *Postgrad Med* 1990; **88**: 125–32

80. Swensen S J, Jett J R, Hartman T E, *et al*. Lung cancer screening with CT: Mayo Clinic experience. *Radiology* 2003; **226 (3)**: 756–61

81. Royal College of Physicians of London (Peake M D, Thompson S, eds). *National audit of lung cancer in the UK 1999; cancer treatment policies and their effects on survival.* Key sites study No 2: Lung Cancer. Northern and Yorkshire Cancer Registry and Information Service (NYCRIS), 1999

82. British Thoracic Society and Society of Cardiothoracic Surgeons of Great Britain and Ireland Working Party. Guidelines on the selection of patients with lung cancer for surgery. *Thorax* 2001; **56**: 89–108

83. Lens M B, Dawes M. Global perspectives of contemporary epidemiological trends of cutaneous malignant melanoma. *Br J Dermatol* 2004; **150**: 179–85

84. Pearce M S, Parker L, Cotterill S J, *et al*. Skin cancer in children and young adults: 28 years' experience from the Northern Region Young Person's Malignant Disease Registry, UK. *Melanoma Res* 2003; **13**: 421–6

85. Breslow A. Thickness, cross-sectional areas and depth of invasion in the prognosis of cutaneous melanoma. *Ann Surg* 1970; **172**: 902–8

86. Shaw H M, Balch C M, Soong S J, Milton G W, McCarthy W H. Prognostic histopathological factors in malignant melanoma. *Pathology* 1985; **17**: 271–4

87. Burton R C, Howe C, Adamson L, Reid A L, Hersey P, Watson A, *et al*. General practitioner screening for melanoma: sensitivity, specificity, and effect of training. *J Med Screen* 1998; **5**: 156–61

88. Marks R, Jolley D, McCormack C, Dorevitch A P. Who removes pigmented skin lesions? *J Am Acad Dermatol* 1997; **36**: 721–6

89. DeCoste S D, Stern R S. Diagnosis and treatment of nevomelanocytic lesions of the skin. A community-based study. *Arch Dermatol* 1993; **129**: 57–62

90. English D, Burton R, del Mar C, *et al*. Evaluation of aid to diagnosis of pigmented skin lesions in general practice: controlled trial randomised by practice. *BMJ* 2003; **327**: 375

91. Scottish Intercollegiate Guidelines Network. Cutaneous Melanoma: A national clinical guideline. No. 72. Edinburgh: SIGN, 2003 www.sign.ac.uk

92. Sasieni P, Adams J. Effect of screening on cervical cancer mortality in England and Wales: analysis of trends with an age period cohort model. *BMJ* 1999; **318**: 1244–5

93. Raffle A E, Alden B, Quinn M, *et al*. Outcomes of screening to prevent cancer: analysis of cumulative incidence of cervical abnormality and modelling of cases and deaths prevented. *BMJ* 2003; **326**: 901

94. General Medical Council. *Seeking patients' consent: the ethical considerations*. London: GMC, 1998

95. UK National Screening Committee. Second report. London: Department of Health, 2000

96. Sikora K. The impact of future technology on cancer care. *Clin Med* 2002; **2**: 560–8

97. Kinmonth A L, Reinhard J, Bobrow M, Pauker M. The new genetics. Implications for clinical services in Britain and the United States. *BMJ* 1998; **316**: 767–70

98. Fry A, Campbell H, Gudmunsdottir H, *et al*. GPs' views on their role in cancer genetics services and current practice. *Fam Pract* 1999; **16**: 468–74

99. Gill M, Richards T. Meeting the challenge of genetic advance. *BMJ* 1998; **316**: 570

100. Kay C, ed. *Genetics in primary care A report from the North West England Faculty Genetics Group*. (Occasional paper 77). London: Royal College of General Practitioners, 1998

101. Tiernan E, O'Connor M, O'Siorain L, Kearney M. A prospective study of preferred versus actual place of death among patients referred to a palliative care home-care service. *Ir Med J* 2002; **95**: 232–5

102. Hinton J. Can home care maintain an acceptable quality of life for patients with terminal cancer and their relatives? *Palliat Med* 1994; **8**: 183–196

103. Bruera E, Russell N, Sweeney C, *et al.* Place of death and its predictors for local patients registered at a comprehensive cancer center. *J Clin Oncol* 2002; **20**: 2127–33

104. Yuen K J, Behrndt M M, Jacklyn C, Mitchell G K. Palliative care at home: general practitioners working with palliative care teams. *MJA* 2003; **179 (6S)**: S 38–40

105. Lecouturier J, Jacoby A, Bradshaw C, *et al.* Lay carer's satisfaction with community palliative care: results of a postal survey. *Palliat Med* 1999; **13**: 275–83

106. Hanratty B. Palliative care provided by GPs: the carer's viewpoint. *Br J Gen Pract* 2000; **50**: 653–4

107. Grande G E, Todd C J, Barclay S I. Support needs in the last year of life: patient and carer dilemmas. *Palliat Med* 1997; **11**: 202–08

108. Lloyd-Williams M, Carter Y H. General practice vocational training in the UK: what teaching is given in palliative care? *Palliat Med* 2003 Oct; **17(7)**: 616–20

109. Macmillan Cancer Relief. Gold Standards Framework. Contact: gsf@macmillan.org.uk Tel: 020 7840 4673.

110. Campbell N C, MacLeod U, Weller D. Primary care oncology: essential if high quality cancer care is to be achieved for all. *Fam Pract* 2002; **19**: 577–8

111. The Nuffield Trust, the RIBA Future Studies Group, Medical Architecture Research Unit (SBU). *2020 Vision: Our future healthcare environments.* Norwich: HMSO, 2003

112. Breast Cancer Care. Breast cancer in the UK: what's the prognosis? London: Breast Cancer Care, 2003

113. Wanless D. *Securing our future health: Taking a long-term view.* London: HMSO, 2002

114. Robert G. Science and Technology: Trends and issues forward to 2015: Implications for healthcare. In: Dargie C (editor). *Policy futures for UK Health.* London: The Nuffield Trust, 1999

CHAPTER 17

Palliative Care

Christina Faull, Alex Nicholson

▶ **KEY MESSAGES**

- The application of the principles and knowledge base of palliative care to new clinical scenarios.

- Quality and inequalities.

- Success relies on a partnership between primary and secondary care.

RECENT ADVANCES ▼

- NICE guidance on supportive and palliative care.

- Understanding issues related to dying at home and services to address these such as Hospice at Home.

- Frameworks for quality assurance: Gold Standards Framework and Liverpool Care of the Dying Pathway.

- Drug options in pain and other symptom management.

- Guidance on the place of complementary therapies.

Introduction

The majority of care received by patients during the last year of life is delivered by GPs and community teams. A systematic review of GP involvement in this care, which included analysis of the nature, perceptions of and training for that care reported that:[1]

▶ GPs value this work and it is appreciated by patients

▶ the bereaved in some studies feel that community palliative care is delivered less well than in other settings

▶ some GPs are unhappy with their competence in this field.

▶ with specialist support, GPs demonstrably provide sound, effective care

▶ the confidence of GPs and their understanding of the potential of team members increases through working with specialist teams.

This chapter provides GPs with some new information but also presents concepts and areas of debate that challenge both personal and team practice, leading to a heightened quality of palliative care delivered by primary teams in conjunction with specialist services.

Tackling inequalities and improving access

Recent advances

- A focus on people with non-malignant illness through National Service Frameworks.
- Service developments in working with people from minority ethnic communities.
- Development of assessment tools and professional networking for people with learning disabilities.
- Enhancement of choice in manner and place of death and care after death.

This key theme within the NHS has very specific challenges for the delivery of palliative care. There are defined groups of patients who have poor outcomes, who under utilise specialist palliative care services, who have insufficient access to services and for whom service models should develop to meet their needs in an appropriate way.

Patients with non-malignant illness

Studies discussed in more detail on *p. 338* indicate that these patients are considerably disadvantaged compared to those with cancer. Initiatives that are enabling this to be tackled include:

▶ National Service frameworks: those for heart disease[2] and older people[3] include sections on palliative care provision

▶ New Opportunities Fund health grants programme

▶ disease-specific charities such as the British Heart Foundation.

The National Council for Hospices and Specialist Palliative Care Services has begun to focus the national debate and help specialist services to consider how to develop new models of service, quality assurance, commissioning and fundraising.[4–5] As yet there is little literature on the implementation of these strategies.

Ethnic diversity

Whilst there are greater similarities than differences between white and, for example, South Asian patients living and dealing with cancer[6] we know that it is more difficult for people from ethnically diverse communities to access or obtain information, support and services that will meet their needs. Issues of communication, cultural diversity, appropriateness of information, discrimination, organisational and staff attitudes, are all contributing factors across the spectrum of health and illness contexts[7–8] and it seems that having cancer is no exception to this experience.[6,9–12] For example, services such as counselling and psychological interventions in appropriate languages may not be available.[6] There may be difficulties in accessing self help and support groups, Asian or African-Caribbean wig types or prostheses and holistic pain control.[13] Compounding this disadvantage and poor quality of life is that people from diverse ethnic communities are more likely to be poor and have financial and housing difficulties.[6] In addition, evidence, although limited by inadequacy of ethnicity monitoring, suggests people with cancer from diverse ethnic communities have poorer survival rates than others.[14]

Given the above, it is unsurprising that people with cancer who are from ethnically diverse communities consistently wish for:[15]

▶ more information about cancer, cancer treatments and cancer care services

▶ improved open communication and awareness about their condition

▶ reduced feelings of stigma, isolation and fear

▶ greater control and choice in their care

▶ more effective care.

Innovations in practice around the UK to address these needs and inequalities have largely been – at least initially – funded by the New Opportunities Fund and Cancer Research UK (Box 17.1).

Box 17.1 **Examples of initiatives to tackle disadvantage related to ethnicity**

- Community advocacy in Birmingham.

- South Asian palliative care awareness project in the West Midlands.

- Development of training for primary care health professionals to respond effectively to cancer and ethnic diversity, University of Nottingham.

Learning disabilities

An NHS Beacon service in Northumberland and a recent conference in Scotland[16] are both initiatives that have addressed the palliative care needs of people with learning disabilities. Particular challenges in practice are those who do not use verbal communication and those with challenging behaviour. A tool to aid non-verbal assessment of pain has been developed[17] and there is a national network aiming to reduce practitioner isolation, and to enhance practice.

Natural death

The Natural Death Centre (www.naturaldeath.org.uk) aims to support those dying at home and their carers and to help people to pre-plan for dying and after death and arrange inexpensive, Do-It-Yourself and environmentally-friendly funerals. There are over 120 woodland burial sites around the UK.[18] It has a more general aim of helping to improve the quality of dying.

Service developments to enable the dying to be at home

Recent advances

- NICE guidance on supportive and palliative care.[19]

- Understanding issues related to dying at home and services to address these such as Hospice at Home.

- Frameworks for quality assurance: Gold Standards Framework[20] and Liverpool Care of the Dying Pathway.[21]

The biggest changes in the focus and organisation of palliative care have stemmed from the National Cancer Plan 2000.[22] Formalised Networks provide support to the commissioning process, and drive and co-ordinate improvement in service quality.

High quality care at home for people with advanced disease is a key focus of the Plan and of the NICE guidance on supportive and palliative care (Box 17.2).[19]

Box 17.2 **Some recommendations of the NICE guidance for supportive and palliative care 2004**[19]

Mechanisms need to be implemented within each locality to ensure medical and nursing services are available on a 24-hour, seven-days–a-week basis for patients with advanced cancer, and that equipment can be provided without delay. Those providing generalist medical and nursing services should have access to specialist advice at all times.

Primary care teams should institute mechanisms to ensure that the needs of patients with advanced cancer are identified and their needs assessed, and that this is communicated within the team and with other professionals as appropriate. *The Gold Standards Framework* provides one mechanism for achieving this.

In all locations, the particular needs of patients who are dying from cancer should be identified and addressed. The *Liverpool Care Pathway for the Dying Patient* provides one mechanism for achieving this.

Dying at home

In the UK about 24% of deaths occur at home – the preferred place of death for the majority of the population. Surveys of patients with terminal illness generally concur but also indicate that people may change their minds depending on the reality of the situation for them and their carers. Dying can, despite great symptom management and lots of support, turn out to be much more difficult than people anticipate. Our understanding of this time and its struggles for patients and carers is becoming more sophisticated.

The palliative care provided for patients with cancer or cardiopulmonary disease was studied recently in two cancer accredited practices in Leicestershire, one urban, the other rural.[23] Roughly 1:5 people died at home, 1:2 people in hospital and 15% of cancer patients died in the hospice. In this retrospective study 41% of relatives indicated that the patients had expressed a preference in where they wanted to die, 95% indicating home. Although less than half of those that expressed a preference were able to achieve this, 77% of carers felt that, on balance, the place that the patient had died had been the best place for them to die, irrespective of whether it was their preferred place of death or not.

Other significant factors in this 'home is best' debate are:

▶ although many people may have clear views about their choice of place they may be unwilling to believe that they are dying here and now

▶ the views of many patients cannot be established.[24]

However, even allowing for a change of heart and the difficulties of accurate prognostication there is a big gap between what patients seem to want and what is achieved. Key factors enabling home care include:[25]

► adequate nursing care

► night-sitting service

► good symptom control

► confident committed GPs

► access to specialist palliative care

► effective co-ordination of care

► financial support

► education.

Recent advances show ways to improve these.

The Gold Standards Framework

Thomas[26] has developed seven standards (Box 17.3) to help general practices improve their delivery of palliative care. Clear benefits have been demonstrated: more patients dying in the place of their choice, fewer crises, better communication and co-working, increased staff morale.[20] Communication with, and the quality of, out-of-hours primary care services is of critical importance in achieving the goals of care. The Cancer Services Collaborative is enabling the implementation of this framework within all cancer networks (www.modern.nhs.uk/cancer).

Box 17.3 **The seven 'C's: Gold standards for palliative care in primary care**

Communication: practice register; regular team meetings for information sharing, planning and reflection/audit; patient information; patient-held records.

Co-ordination: nominated co-ordinator maintains register, organises meetings, audit, education symptom sheets and other resources.

Control of symptoms: holistic, patient-centred assessment and management.

Continuity out-of-hours: effective transfer of information to and from out-of-hours services. Access to drugs and equipment assured.

Continued learning: audit/reflection/critical incident analysis. Use of PLT.

Carer support: practical, financial, emotional and bereavement support.

Care in the dying phase: protocol-driven care addressing physical, emotional, spiritual needs. Care needs around and after death acted upon.

Care of people in their last days

The care of people who are dying often requires a change of gear to provide high quality care and raises particular challenges and responsibilities.[27-8] The *Liverpool Care Pathway for the Dying Patient* (LCP) is a systematic approach to defining and monitoring the needs of patients together with guidance for interventions that are commonly required.[21,29] Review of its implementation has assisted development of standards for symptom management: one study demonstrated that 80% of patients had either complete symptom control or only one episode of loss of control.[30]

Initiation of the LCP for a patient requires joint medical and nursing agreement that the patient's condition has progressed to the dying (terminal) phase. Meeting at least two of four criteria indicates that death is likely within 48 hours (range of zero to five days):[31]

▶ bedbound

▶ semiconscious

▶ only able to take sips of fluid

▶ no longer able to take tablets.

The LCP prompts decision making:

▶ discontinuation of inappropriate medication, interventions and investigations

▶ conversion of essential symptom control medication to drugs administrable via subcutaneous route at correct doses

▶ anticipatory prescribing of medication for breakthrough pain, nausea and vomiting, agitation and retained respiratory secretions.

The pathway also focuses on carers' needs: communication about the changes that are occurring; and discussion around place of care for the final phase of life. A multi-professional record is used; the combined approach to monitoring and measurement of outcome facilitates the audit of care quality and identification of areas where improvement in treatment, co-ordination and communication may be needed. Use of the LCP has been implemented in Wales. Analysis of the first 500 patients across all care settings identified inadequate symptom control in half of the patients.[32]

Hospice at Home

Hospice at Home services are developing nationwide but vary in composition, availability and referral criteria. Research into their benefits has had severe methodological impediments and there is no absolute clarity as to whether they do increase the home death rate or improve patient experience.[33-4] On balance it seems that they can do both these things.

Advances in pharmacotherapy

Recent advances
• Successful symptom control relies on a partnership between primary and secondary care including shared knowledge of the drugs available.
• Oxycodone, buprenorphine and fentanyl – three opioids, seven formulations, each with potential in pain management.
• COX-2 inhibitors – the new NSAIDs – increasing experience indicates they must be prescribed with care.
• Gabapentin – licensed for neuropathic pain.
• Levomepromazine – antiemetic at low dose orally and parenterally.
• Bisphosphonates – expanding remit in bony metastatic disease.

These recent advances are summarised in Table 17.1

Use of drugs beyond licence

Management of complex and refractory symptoms may involve use of a drug for a purpose or by a route for which a licence has not been granted. Licensed drugs can be used legally in such situations ('off label'). The Association for Palliative Medicine and the Pain Society published a joint position statement in 2002 to clarify the associated clinical and legal implications.[52]

Non-malignant illness and end-stage organ failure

Undoubtedly palliative care is needed by patients with a spectrum of terminal diseases. High-quality care for patients with motor neurone disease and AIDS is well established.[53-4] For some other diagnoses, both experience and an evidence base are accumulating. This section discusses the most recent developments. In the ageing Western population the burden of both coronary heart disease (CHD) and chronic obstructive pulmonary disease (COPD) will continue to rise but that of cancer is expected to plateau.[55] Recent studies have exposed the degree of unmet need in these patients with advanced-stage disease:[23,56]

► compared with cancer patients, they have a larger burden of symptoms that are longer lasting and less likely to be resolved

► they seldom receive a holistic approach to their care

► they access less support from primary care and other services

► the illness has a high psychological impact

► the illness has a much greater social impact than cancer

► they may not access sources of financial support such as attendance allowance.

Compared with cancer patients they are:

► less likely to be aware of prognosis

► less likely to be knowledgeable about disease progression and its management

► less likely to have discussed end of life issues with doctors.

The additional challenges of providing high quality palliative care for patients with CHD and COPD are that many patients:

► have multiple organ problems due to common aetiologies of smoking and diabetes

► are on multiple drugs

► run a course of illness characterised by acute, life-threatening episodes that are not predictably terminal.

In these and other non-malignant illnesses an amalgam of preventive, active and palliative care is the norm. For some there is also the consideration of transplantation, which may challenge the palliative care focus for a dying patient.[57]

Table 17.1 **An overview of recent advances in drug treatment of pain and other symptoms in palliative care**

(Further guidance: Palliative care formulary)[35]

Drug	Where does it fit in?	Useful features	Dosing issues				Other points
Oxycodone Strong semi-synthetic opioid analgesic SR; IR; O; SC;	Moderate/severe cancer pain. Step 3 of WHO analgesic ladder Possible additional effect in neuropathic pain[36] Useful in patients who cannot tolerate morphine	Normal release formulation may be given 6-hourly[37] Similar efficacy to morphine Less itching,[38] nausea,[38] hallucination[37] Parenteral preparation now available	oxycodone oral : morphine oral = 1 : 2 oxycodone oral : oxycodone sc = 2:1 oxycodone oral: diamorphine sc = 2:1 oxycodone sc: diamorphine sc = 1:1				Consider dose reduction in severe hepatic or renal impairment Parenteral formulation is compatible in syringe drivers with hyoscine (butyl and hydrobromide), midazolam, metoclopramide, haloperidol, or levomepromazine[39]
Buprenorphine Opioid analgesic SL·TD	Moderate/severe cancer pain Severe non-malignant pain Steps 2–3 of WHO ladder	Transdermal and sublingual formulations available – role in patients with head and neck tumours, dysphagia, risk of aspiration Safe in renal impairment	Dose equivalences[40]				Extensive first pass metabolism therefore oral administration inappropriate Transdermal formulation not appropriate for management of severe unstable pain (takes 60hrs to achieve steady state plasma levels) Possible ceiling dose
			Transdermal buprenorphine	35 μg/hr	52.5 μg/hr	70 μg/hr	
			Oral morphine (per 24hrs)	30–60 mg	90 mg	120 mg	
			Transdermal fentanyl		25 μg/hr	25 μg/hr	
			Treating breakthrough pain[41]				
			Patch strength	35 μg/h	52.5 μg/h	70 μg/h	
			SL dose (4-hourly)	200 μg	200–400 μg	400 μg	
Oral transmucosal fentanyl citrate Strong semi-synthetic opioid analgesic SL	For episodic pain in patients whose background pain is well controlled	Lozenge consists of drug matrix mounted on a 'stick' Rapid onset (5–10 mins) short duration (2hrs) analgesic effect. Half bio-available dose directly absorbed via buccal mucosa Inactive metabolites safe in renal failure	Six lozenge strengths – 200, 400, 600, 800, 1200, 1600 (μg) Individualised dose titration (start low) – effective dose is **not** related to dose of regular opioid[42] Patient compliance maximises efficacy; patient must actively suck lozenge for 15 minutes whilst matrix dissolves Some work using sublingual fentanyl citrate injection: well tolerated, safe and effective[43]				Dose titration may tax patient's confidence Dry mouth will reduce efficacy and tolerability. Oral ulcers occasionally occur Studies show 69–75% patients achieve satisfactory analgesia[42,44]

Key: **SR** = sustained release | **IR** = immediate release | **SL** = sublingual | **TD** = transdermal | **O** = oral | **SC** = subcutaneous | **IV** = intravenous.

Drug	Where does it fit in?	Useful features	Dosing issues	Other points
COX-2 inhibitors COX-2 selective: celecoxib COX-2 specific: rofecoxib* O	Analgesic; potential opioid sparing role used at any step of WHO ladder NSAID uses in palliative care: bone, soft tissue and neuropathic pain, bladder spasm, sweating, biliary and ureteric colic	Trials against other NSAIDs or placebo in OA/RA patients suggest reduced (not absent) GI toxicity[45] No platelet effect (useful if ulcerating tumour at risk of bleeding, or thrombocytopenia) Rofecoxib (and probably celecoxib) do not cause bronchospasm	See BNF for dose guidance Extra notes on gastric toxicity: Most palliative care patients have enhanced risk of GI events;[35] corticosteroids (10x), anticoagulation (13x); age and co-morbidities (aspirin use) (3–13x) Addition of PPI to any NSAID prescription is recommended[46]	Theoretical increased risk of thromboembolic events May affect renal function as other NSAIDs therefore caution advised in patients with renal disease[47]
Gabapentin[48] O	Anticonvulsant licensed for neuropathic pain Adjuvant for use at any step of WHO ladder	No significant drug interactions Tolerable side-effect profile (commonest: drowsiness, dizziness, ataxia, fatigue)	Different titration schedules are described. Frequent and regular clinical review is essential Rapid (robust, inpatients): 300 mg OD, BD, TDS, 400 mg QDS on consecutive days Slow (elderly, frail, outpatients): 100mg OD to TDS week 1, 300mg TDS wk 2, 600mg TDS wk 3 Maximum licensed dose 1800 mg/day – higher doses may be needed	Absorption reduced by Al/Mg antacids (give 2 hrs apart) Reduce dose in renal failure Evidence drawn from studies in diabetic neuropathy and post-herpetic neuralgia
Levomepromazine[49] Phenothiazine Formerly called methotrimeprazine O; SC;	Potent broad spectrum antiemetic Antipsychotic providing effective relief of agitation (including terminal restlessness)	Long half-life and duration of action allows once daily dosing Antiemetic at low dose with few sedative and hypotensive side effects Parenteral tolerated sc Compatible with diamorphine in syringe driver	Antiemetic doses are LOW: Oral: 6.25–25 mg nocte (6.25 = quartered tablet) 5–25 mg/24hrs via syringe driver or as single sc bolus Doses higher than 12.5mg have dose-related sedative effect (which may be desirable) Terminal agitation: 25–200mg/24hrs titrated against response	New low dose oral formulation (6mg tablet) currently on trial to obtain licence. Available on named patient basis (Link pharmaceuticals)
Bisphosphonates[50-1] O; IV	Bone metastases (breast, lung, prostate, myeloma, renal): Significant reduction in hypercalcaemia and pathological fracture; prolonged time to radiotherapy. May delay development of bone mets	Parenteral forms are more potent and effective than oral, and better tolerated. Newer drugs permit rapid administration In trials, follow up of at least 6 months was needed to demonstrate significant morbidity reductions	Disodium pamidronate 60–120 mg ivi or zoledronic acid 4mg ivi are typical doses given monthly. Monitoring for recurrent hypercalcaemia ensures timely re-treatment (effect may be less than 1 month). Anecdotal reports of hypocalcaemia associated with treatment for bone mets; guidance on management and monitoring is awaited	Intravenous drugs are more expensive but may be more cost effective; economic appraisal needed Caution in renal impairment Brief 'flu'-like syndrome may follow IV treatment

Key: **SR** = sustained release | **IR** = immediate release | **SL** = sublingual | **TD** = transdermal | **O** = oral | **SC** = subcutaneous | **IV** = intravenous.

* Note: **Withdrawn, September 2004**

Respiratory failure

In the UK, 32,000 people die of COPD annually and it is increasingly recognised that they have significant problems in addition to their breathlessness (Box 17.4). In addition, 7750 people have cystic fibrosis.

Box 17.4 **The symptom burden in patients with advanced COPD**

Breathlessness	Fear	Sleep difficulties	Thirst	Social isolation
Cough	Anxiety	Fatigue	Anorexia	
Pain	Depression	Reduced exercise tolerance	Constipation	

A study comparing the experience of lung cancer and COPD[56] patients showed that there was little numerical difference in the symptom burden between the two. Pain may be worse in cancer patients but perhaps better managed. For patients with COPD:

▶ breathlessness is worse

▶ standard of daily life is worse with hugely diminished social, emotional and physical function

▶ 90% suffered clinically relevant anxiety or depression compared with 52% of patients with lung cancer.

Pulmonary rehabilitation

This describes a multidisciplinary programme of exercise, education, physiotherapy and psychotherapy that focuses on factors that reduce quality of life and potentially heighten the sense of dyspnoea (anxiety, depression, sense of loss and low self-esteem). In patients fit enough to get to hospital, evidence suggests that symptoms, performance, exercise endurance and quality of life improve although survival, lung function and arterial blood gases do not. Patients often need permission and encouragement to exercise. By experiencing dyspnoea in a controlled environment it becomes less anxiety provoking and disabling. Patients get fitter and have more confidence. However, those with more profoundly reduced function appear not to benefit.[58-9] There is similar evidence from a more relaxation-orientated approach for patients with cancer-related dyspnoea.[60] This may be of more relevance to patients with very severe COPD.

Additional points to consider:

▶ Low-flow oxygen > 15 hours per day improves survival but the jury is out on quality of life for patients with severe hypoxia.

▶ Assisted ventilation such as NIPPV may be useful and used in a few patients but is more effective and more commonly used in the UK in patients with motor neurone disease.[61]

Cystic fibrosis (CF)

Like AIDS there are some very distinct features about patients dying from CF. They are young; hope for a cure one day or at least a transplant; have multiple prior experiences with illness and death of friends, which may be primary factors in shaping views, concerns and choices about end of life care; have close bonds with fellow patients and with clinical teams. In addition families live with the illness and its practical demands for a long time. There is an enormous gap in time and emotion when a child with CF dies.[58]

Heart failure

The incidence and prevalence of heart failure is increasing as the population ages and more people survive an acute myocardial infarction.[62] Stage IV failure imparts a 40% risk of dying within one year and an 80% risk of dying within two years. The Framingham study found that 30–40% of patients have a sudden death and 60–70% have a gradual deterioration in cardiac function[63] although more recent treatments may have altered this picture. A study in primary care in London in patients with a new diagnosis of heart failure found that 25% died within three months and nearly half within 18 months.[64] Patients with heart failure constitute about 5% of medical admissions and an audit of 139 of such patients in Birmingham found that 42% died in hospital during that admission. Features indicating poor prognosis are: clinical stage IV; low left ventricular ejection fraction; high plasma noradrenaline and natriuretic factor concentrations; age; cachexia; other organ impairment (renal, liver, respiratory).

Two large studies (one retrospective, one prospective) have examined symptom burden utilising carers' perceptions.[24,65] In the UK, McCarthy found a broad range of symptoms that were distressing, poorly controlled and lasted greater than six months: breathlessness, pain, nausea, constipation and low mood. Pain and low mood were about 10% less common in the last year of life than in cancer patients but much more likely to last over six months. Open communication with health professionals about dying was rare[66] and quality of life for those with advanced heart failure was worse than for those with lung cancer. In the US, Lynn identified that patients suffered severe symptoms in the last three days of life (breathlessness and pain). In this hospital-based study there was also conflict between the level of clinical intervention, the clinical outcomes, patients' quality of life and in some cases patients' wishes for treatment approach.[24]

The National Service Framework for heart disease chapter 6 (heart failure) indicates (Box 17.5):[2]

Box 17.5 **The National Service Framework for heart disease**[2]

Primary care teams, PCTs and hospitals should work together to agree and put in place models of care so that they use a systematic approach to:
• identify people at high risk of heart failure (e.g. people who have had a heart attack)
• assess and investigate people with suspected heart failure
• provide and document the delivery of appropriate advice and treatment (including palliative care)
• offer regular review to people with established heart failure.

Heart failure specialist nurses were shown to help prevent hospital readmission, first in the USA[67] and then the UK.[68] Work in Australia has shown they also reduce costs.[69] Their development, as part of the multidisciplinary team and heart failure network, has been supported in the UK by the British Heart Foundation and the New Opportunities Fund. A key opportunity for the future is their integration with specialist palliative care services.

Creutzfeldt-Jakob disease (CJD)

Creutzfeldt-Jakob disease (CJD) is a prion disease causing progressive physical and cognitive deterioration, leading to death. Variant CJD (vCJD), which emerged in the 1990s, is related to bovine spongiform encephalopathy and predominantly affects young people. At mid-October 2003, 137 people had died from vCJD in the UK contributing, since 1998, about a quarter of the monthly deaths from CJD. Their disease presentation is different from other forms of CJD; patients typically present with psychiatric features, with or without sensory disturbance. Prognosis for sporadic CJD is a few months but longer (6–36 months) for vCJD. Useful overviews of issues in caring for patients with CJD are given by Weller[70] and de Vries.[71] The CJD education website is also valuable: www.cjd.ed.ac.uk.[72] Key issues in the care of patients are outlined in Box 17.6

Box 17.6 **Key issues in the care of patients with CJD**

- place of care
- carer support: stigma, psychiatric diagnosis
- psychiatric symptoms: depression, anxiety, delusions, hallucinations, personality change
- Movement disorders: myoclonus and other
- pain difficult to assess
- speech loss
- swallowing loss
- pyrexia
- mouth care: difficult because of myoclonic jerking
- cause of death usually respiratory infection
- post mortem not obligatory: no restrictions in burial or cremation

Place of care presents a problem because of the relatively long prognosis, complexity of problems – including psychiatric disturbances – and the young age of patients. Primary care teams, hospices, hospitals, psychiatric wards and nursing homes may all feel ill-equipped to provide the care needed. Non-pharmacological means are best used to manage behaviour and movement disorders (minimal stimulation, touch and noise) but if this proves difficult consider:

► risperidone or olanzapine (less likely to cause Parkinsonian side-effects) for hallucinations and delusions

► benzodiazepines for anxiety and insomnia

► clonazepam, sodium valproate or piracetam for myoclonus

► tetrabenazine, haloperidol or other antipsychotics for chorea

► baclofen for spasticity or dystonia.

Pain may be difficult to assess because of loss of speech and because patients may adopt postures that appear painful or to indicate pain and may cry out as part of the disease process. Dysaesthesia and allodynia may be features: gabapentin, sodium valproate and carbamazepine are therapeutic options.

The loss of swallowing requires assessment and discussion about interventions such as subcutaneous fluids and nasogastric or percutaneous endoscopic gastrostomy (PEG) feeding.

Complementary therapies for patients with advanced cancer

Recent advances

- Significant numbers of patients access complementary therapies.

- Despite the absence of a substantial scientifically-controlled evidence base to inform commissioners[73] service provision must answer the demands of clinical governance.

- Research is very challenging;[74] nevertheless the best available guidance has recently been published.[75]

Therapies supported by published work and considerations for safe, appropriate referral, are summarised (Table 17.2).

Complementary therapies aim to relieve symptoms and enhance quality of life, with no claim to cure disease or prolong life expectancy. They may be offered alongside oncological and palliative medicine interventions. Surveys suggest 30% of patients access complementary therapies provided by two-thirds of hospices and hospitals.[19]

A House of Lords report has reviewed available medical and scientific opinion on complementary methods and identified a need for '*a critical mass of scientifically controlled evidence to support the claims of benefit*'.[73] The Research Council for Complementary Medicine is undertaking a systematic review of the evidence.

Service provision

The NICE guidance on Supportive and Palliative Care[19] recommends that partnerships of commissioners, NHS and voluntary providers, and user groups collaborate to establish ways of meeting patients' needs for complementary therapies. Practical guidance on issues such as accreditation, clinical supervision, indemnity, appraisal and review is provided by the new National Guidelines.[75]

Regulation and accreditation

Registration issues for most complementary therapies are overseen by two umbrella bodies:

Council for Complementary and Alternative Medicine (acupuncture, homeopathy) • 63 Jeddo Road, London W12 6HQ

British Complementary Medicine Association (reflexology, aromatherapy, hypnotherapy) • 249 Fosse Road South, Leicester LE3 1AE

Table 17.2 Recent advances in complementary therapy use for palliative care

Therapy	Role	Cautions	Regulation & accreditation
Acupuncture	Nausea, vomiting, pain Respiratory symptoms (COPD and cancer) Xerostomia Hot flushes	Knowledge of sites to avoid Contraindications: clotting disorders, immunocompromise, risk of bacter-aemia (valvular heart disease/valve replacement)	British Medical Acupuncture Society (BMAS) www.medical-acupuncture.org.uk British Acupuncture Council (BAcC) www.acupuncture.org.uk Acupuncture Association of Chartered Physiotherapists www.aacp.uk.com Acupuncture Regulatory Working Group working towards recommendations for statutory regulation in England
Aromatherapy	Reduce anxiety, tension, pain, depression Improve concentration, mood, self-perception, thoughts of future	Knowledge of essential oil safety (opinions vary widely, evidence lacking) Risk of local skin sensitivity especially if recent (<6 weeks) radiotherapy	Aromatherapy Organisations Council. www.aromatherapy-uk.org Aromatherapy Regulatory Working Group has published national occupational standards
Healing and energy therapies (including Reiki)	Pain, tension, stress and anxiety Promote sleep and relaxation Chemo and radiotherapy side effects	Danger of misunderstanding of notion of 'healing' with emotional and psycho-logical consequences Fully-informed consent is crucial	Confederation of Healing Organisations represents several groups Working groups (the UK Reiki Foundation, UK Healers) each working towards National Occupational Standards
Homeopathy	Skin effects of radiotherapy after surgery in breast cancer Chemotherapy induced stomatitis Fatigue Hot flushes	Published cautions relate to indirect risks (i.e. practitioners' competence)	Faculty of Homeopathy (www.trusthomeopathy.org) for medical practitioners (registration with GMC) Others trained and governed by Society of Homeopaths www.homeopathy-soh.org Council of Organisations Registering Homeopaths has published national occupational standards
Hypnotherapy	Emotional well-being Adjunct to psychotherapy Chemotherapy side effects Coping with scanning and radiotherapy	Indirect risks (inexpert practitioner) Vulnerable clients (severe emotional or psychiatric problems)	Health care professionals trained by British Society of Medical & Dental Hypnosis or British Society of Experimental & Clinical Hypnosis Registration with GMC or Nursing & Midwifery Council. Psychotherapists trained by the United Kingdom Council for Psychotherapists. Universities and others provide training; no standardised curriculum. National occupational standards published
Massage	Anxiety, pain, nausea Relaxation Adjustment to mastectomy	Tumour sites, ascitic abdomen, bone metastases Thrombocytopoenia Venous thrombosis Lymphoedema (unless trained therapist) Skin areas subject to recent radiotherapy (within 6 weeks)	The British Massage Therapy Council (umbrella organisation) Working group is General Council for Massage Therapy – draft national occupational standards out to consultation
Reflexology	Anxiety, pain, nausea Relaxation Improved 'quality of life'	Thrombocytopoenia Venous thrombosis Lymphoedema Peripheral neuropathy	Several organisations. Largest: Association of Reflexologists & International Federation of Reflexologists. Reflexology Forum (10 member organisations) published national standards

Conclusion

Two significant themes that inspire modern palliative care are exemplified within this chapter:

▶ application of the principles of patient-centred, holistic, detailed and individualised care to new clinical scenarios

▶ modification of existing therapies to meet the needs of complex symptom control.

These themes embrace two challenges:

▶ the provision of relevant, accessible education for all clinicians who need to apply these principles to their field of expertise

▶ the routine adoption of rigorous systems of critical appraisal into the practice of palliative care so that use and recommendation of novel interventions may be founded upon the most secure evidence base that is practicably possible.

References

1. Mitchell G K. How well do general practitioners deliver palliative care? A systematic review. *Palliat Med* 2002; **16**: 457–64

2. Department of Health. *National Service Framework for Coronary Heart Disease*. London: Department of Health, 2000. www.dh.gov.uk/assetRoot/04/04/90/70/04049070.pdf (accessed 20/09/2004)

3. Department of Health. National Service Framework for Older People. London: Department of Health, 2001. www.dh.gov.uk/assetRoot/04/07/12/83/04071283.pdf (accessed 20/09/2004)

4. Tebbit P. *Palliative Care for Adults with Non-malignant Diseases: Developing a National Policy.* London: National Council for Hospices and Specialist Palliative Care Services, 2003

5. Addington-Hall J. *Reaching Out: Specialist Palliative Care for Adults with Non-Malignant Diseases*. Occasional Paper 14. London: National Council for Hospices and Specialist Palliative Care Services, 1998

6. Chattoo S, Ahmad W, Haworth M, Lennard R. *South Asian and White Patients with Advanced Cancer: Patients' and Families' Experiences of the Illness and Perceived Needs for Care. Final Report to Cancer Research UK*. Leeds: Centre for Research in Primary Care, University of Leeds, January 2002

7. Smaje C. *Health race and ethnicity: making sense of the evidence*. London: King's Fund, 1995

8. Atkinson M, Clark M, Clay D, *et al. Systematic review of ethnicity and health service access for London*. Centre for Health Service Studies, University of Warwick, 2001

9. Hill D, Penso D. *Opening doors: Improving access to hospice and specialist palliative care services by members of the black and ethnic minority communities.* London: The National Council for Hospice and Specialist Palliative Care Services, 1995

10. Firth S. *Wider Horizons: Care of the Dying in a Multicultural Society.* London: The National Council for Hospice and Specialist Palliative Care Services, 2001

11. Karim K, Bailey M, Tunna K H. Non-white ethnicity and the provision of specialist palliative care services: factors affecting doctors' referral patterns. *Palliat Med* 2000; **14**: 471–8

12. Gunarantum Y. Ethnicity and palliative care. In: Culley L and Dyson S (eds). *Ethnicity and Nursing Practice.* Basingstoke: Palgrave, 2001

13. Faull C. Cancer and palliative care In: Kai J (ed). *Ethnicity, Health and Primary Care.* Oxford: Oxford University Press, 2003

14. Selby P. Cancer clinical outcomes for minority ethnic groups. *British Journal of Cancer* 1996; 74: (suppl. XXIX) S54–S60

15. Johnson M R D, Bains J, Chauan J, *et al. Improving palliative care for minority ethnic communities in Birmingham.* A report for the Birmingham Specialist and Community NHS Trust and Macmillan Trust, 2001

16. Common Knowledge. *Palliative care and people with learning disabilities.* Edinburgh: SHS Trust, 2003. www.ckglasgow.org.uk (accessed 20/09/2004)

17. Regnard C, Matthews D, Gibson L, & Clarke C. Difficulties in identifying distress and its causes in people with severe communication problems. *Int J Pall Nurs* 2003; **9**: 173–6

18. Weinrich S. Do-it-yourself funerals and The Natural Death Centre. *Eur J Palliat Care* 2001; **8**: 70–2

19. National Institute for Clinical Excellence. *Guidance on Cancer Services: Improving Supportive and Palliative Care for Adults with Cancer.* London: NICE, 2004

20. Thomas, K. The Gold Standards Framework in community palliative care. *Eur J Palliat Care* 2003; **10**: 3, 113–15

21. Ellershaw J, Foster A, Murphy D, *et al.* Developing an integrated care pathway for the dying patient. *Eur J Palliat Care* 1997; **4**: 203–7

22. Department of Health. *The NHS Cancer Plan: a plan for investment, a plan for reform.* London: Department of Health, 2000

23. Exley C, Field D, McKinley R K, Stokes T. *An evaluation of primary care based palliative care for cancer and non-malignant disease in two cancer accredited primary care practices in Leicestershire.* University of Leicester, Department of Epidemiology and Public Health, 2003

24. Hofmann J C, Wenger N S, Davis R B, *et al.* Patient preferences for communication with physicians about end-of-life decisions: SUPPORT Investigators: Study to Understand Prognoses and Preference for Outcomes and Risks of Treatment. *Ann Intern Med* 1997; **127**: 1–12

24. Lynn J, Teno J M, Philips R S, *et al.* Perceptions by family members of the dying experience of older and seriously ill patients: SUPPORT Investigators. *Ann Intern Med* 1997; **126**: 97–106

25. Thorpe G. Enabling more people to die at home. *BMJ* 1993; **307**: 915–8

26. Thomas K. *Caring for the Dying at Home: companions on a journey.* Oxford: Radcliffe Medical, 2003

27. Faull C and Nyatanga B. Terminal care and dying In: Faull C, Carter Y, Daniels L W. *Handbook of Palliative Care*. (2nd ed.) Oxford: Blackwell Publishing, 2004 (In press)

28. Clinical Guidelines Working Party. *Changing Gear: Guidelines for Managing the Last Days of Life*. London: National Council for Hospice and Specialist Palliative Care Services, 1997

29. Ellershaw J, Wilkinson S. *Care of the Dying: A pathway to excellence*. Oxford: Oxford University Press, 2003

30. Ellershaw J, Smith C, Overill S, *et al*. Care of the dying: setting standards for symptom control in the last 48 hours of life. *J Pain Symptom Manage* 2001; **21**: 12–17

31. Ellershaw J, Sutcliffe J M, Saunders C M. Dehydration and the dying patient. *J Pain Symptom Manage* 1995; **10**: 192–7

32. Fowell A, Finlay I, Johnstone R, Minto L. An integrated care pathway for the last two days of life: Wales-wide benchmarking in palliative care. *Palliat Nurs* 2002; **8**: 566–73

33. Grande G E, Todd C J, Barclay S I G, Farquhar M C. Does hospital at home for palliative care facilitate death at home? Randomised controlled trial. *BMJ* 1999; **319**: 1472–5

34. Grady A, Travers E. Hospice at Home 2: evaluating a crisis intervention service. *Int J Palliat Nurs* 2003; **9**: 326–35

35. Twycross R, Wilcock A, Charlesworth S, Dickman A. *Palliative care formulary*. (2nd ed.) Oxford: Radcliffe Medical, 2002

36. Shah S, Hardy J. Oxycodone: a review of the literature. *Eur J Palliat Care* 2001; **8**: 93–6

37. Mucci-LoRusso P, Berman B S, Silberstein P T, *et al*. Controlled-release oxycodone compared with controlled-release morphine in the treatment of cancer pain: a randomised, double-blind, parallel-group study. *Eur J Pain* 1998; **2**: 239–249.

38. Heiskanen T, Kalso E. Controlled-release oxycodone and morphine in cancer related pain. *Pain* 1997; **73**: 37–45

39. S P C oxycodone. Napp laboratories, 2003

40. S P C buprenorphine transdermal patch (Transtec). Napp laboratories, 2002

41. Twycross R. *Course handbook. Advanced course in pain and symptom management*. Oxford: Sobell Study Centre, 2003

42. Portenoy R K, Payne R, Coluzzi P, Raschko J W, *et al*. Oral transmucosal fentanyl citrate (OTFC) for the treatment of breakthrough pain in cancer patients: a controlled dose titration study. *Pain* 1999; **79**: 303–12

43. Zeppetella G. Sublingual fentanyl citrate for cancer-related breakthrough pain: a pilot study. *Palliat Med* 2001; **15**: 323–28

44. Coluzzi P H, Schwartzberg L, Conroy J D, Charapata S, *et al*. Breakthrough cancer pain: a randomised trial comparing oral transmucosal fentanyl citrate and morphine sulphate immediate release. *Pain* 2001; **91**: 123–30

45. National Institute for Clinical Excellence. *Guidance on the use of cyclo-oxygenase (COX-2) selective inhibitors, celecoxib, rofecoxib, meloxicam and etodolac for osteoarthritis and rheumatoid arthritis*. Technology appraisal. No. 27. London: NICE, 2001

46. Rostom A, Wells G, Tugwell P, Welch V, *et al*. *Prevention of NSAID-induced gastroduodenal ulcers (Cochrane review)*. Oxford: The Cochrane Library, Issue 4. Update Software, 2000

47. Brune K. COX-2 inhibitors and the kidney: a word of caution. *Pain Clin Updates* 2003; **11**: Number 4

48. Rocafort J, Viguria J. Gabapentin as an analgesic. *Eur J Palliat Care* 2001; **8**: 54–6

49. Skinner J, Skinner A. Levomepromazine for nausea and vomiting in advanced cancer. *Hosp Med* 1999; **60**: 568–70

50. Ross J R, Saunders Y, Edmonds P M, Patel S, *et al*. Systematic review of role of bisphosphonates on skeletal morbidity in metastatic cancer. *BMJ* 2003; **327**: 469–72

51. Neville-Webbe H L, Coleman R E. The use of zoledronic acid in the management of metastatic bone disease and hypercalcaemia. *Palliat Med* 2003; **17**: 539–53

52. Bennett M, Simpson K. The use of drugs beyond licence in palliative care and pain management. *Palliat Med* 2002; **16**: 367–68

53. Jones G, Faull C and Carter Y. Palliative Care for People with Acquired Immune Deficiency Syndrome. In: Faull C, Carter Y, Woof R (eds). *Handbook of Palliative Care*. Oxford: Blackwell Science, 1998

54. Hicks F. Motor Neurone Disease. In: Faull C, Carter Y, Woof R (eds). *Handbook of Palliative Care*. Oxford: Blackwell Science, 1998

55. Murray C J, Lopez A D. Global mortality, disability and the contribution of risk factors: global burden of disease study. *Lancet* 1997; **349**: 1436–42

56. Gore J M, Brophy C J, Greenstone M A. How well do we care for patients with end stage chronic obstructive pulmonary disease (COPD)? A comparison of palliative care and quality of life in COPD and lung cancer. *Thorax* 2000; **55**: 1000–6

57. Lowton K. Can we provide effective palliative care for adults with cystic fibrosis? *Eur J Pall Care* 2002; **9**: 142–4

58. Lacasse Y, Wong E, Guyatt G H, King D, Cook D J, Goldstein R S. Meta-analysis of respiratory rehabilitation in chronic obstructive pulmonary disease. *Lancet* 1996; **348**: 1115–9

59. Skillbeck J, Mott L, Page H. Palliative care in chronic obstructive pulmonary disease: a needs assessment. *Palliat Med* 1998; **12**: 245–54

60. Bredin M, Corner J, Krishnasamy M, Plant H, Bailey C, A'Hern R. Multicentre randomised controlled trial of nursing intervention for breathlessness in patients with lung cancer. *BMJ* 1999; **318**: 901–4

61. Wijkstra P J, Avendano M A, Goldstein R S. Inpatient chronic assisted ventilatory care: a 15-year experience. *Chest* 2003; **124**: 850–6

62. Davis R C, Hobbs F D R, Lip G Y H. ABC of Heart Failure: History and epidemiology. *BMJ* 2000; **320**: 39–42

63. Ho K K, Pinsky J L, Kannel W B Levy D. The epidemiology of heart failure: The Framingham study. *J Am Coll Cardiol* 1993; **22**: 6a–13a

64. Cowie M R, Wood D A, Coats A J S. Survival of patients with new diagnosis of heart failure: a population based study. *Heart* 2000; **83**: 505–10

65. McCarthy M, Lay M, Addington-Hall J. Dying from heart disease. *J R Coll Physicians Lond* 1996; **30**: 325–8

66. McCarthy M, Addington-Hall J M, Lay M. Communication and choice in dying from heart disease. *J R Soc Med* 1997; **90**: 128–31

67. Rich M W, Beckham V, Wittenberg C, Leven C L, Freedland KE, Carney R M. A multidisciplinary intervention to prevent the readmission of elderly patients with congestive heart failure. *N Engl J Med* 1995; **333**: 1213–14

68. Blue L, Lang E, McMurray J J V, *et al*. Randomised controlled trial of specialist nurse intervention in heart failure. *BMJ* 2001; **323**: 715–18

69. Stewart S, Blue L, Walker A, Morrison C, McMurray J J. An economic analysis of specialist heart failure nurse management in the UK; can we afford not to implement it? *Eur Heart J* 2002; **231**: 369–78

70. Weller B, Knight R, Will R. An overview of the care issues for Creutzfeldt-Jakob disease. *Eur J Pall Care* 2003; **10**: 5–8.

71. De Vries K. Nursing patients with variant Creutzfeldt-Jakob disease. *Eur J Pall Care* 2003; **10**: 9–12

72. Douglas M J, Campbell H, Will R G. *Patients with new variant Creutzfeldt-Jakob disease and their families: care and information needs*. Edinburgh: The National Creutzfeldt-Jakob Disease Surveillance Unit, 1999 www.cjd.ed.ac.uk (accessed 20/09/2004)

73. House of Lords Select Committee on Science and Technology. *Complementary and Alternative Medicine: HL Paper 123*. London: HMSO, 2000

74. Mason S, Tovey P, Long A F. Evaluating complementary medicine: methodological challenges of randomised controlled trials. *BMJ* 2002; **325**: 832–4

75. *National Guidelines for the Use of Complementary Therapies in Supportive and Palliative Care.* London: Foundation for Integrated Health and National Council for Hospice and Specialist Palliative Care Services, 2003

CHAPTER 18

Nursing

Rosemary Cook

▶ KEY MESSAGES
- Primary care nursing, and nursing in general, has developed in response to three influences: professional, policy and pragmatic.

- The degree of congruence between these influences in recent years means that nursing has moved well beyond traditional professional boundaries, and has led to nurses developing discrete new roles, to the expansion of both vertical and horizontal skill mix in nursing/multi-disciplinary teams, and to changes in the traditional division of tasks such as referral and admission of patients.

- Primary care organisations, at practice or primary care trust (PCT) level, can exploit these new developments to get the best from their workforce by focusing on the key issues of recruitment, capacity development and funding.

- The challenges for the future of primary care are likely to include staffing patient care pathways that cross primary and secondary care boundaries, rather than staffing specific sites; and maintaining safe patient services while exploiting the possibilities of a more diverse workforce that includes growing numbers of workers who are not professionally regulated.

Introduction

This chapter looks at the causes and effects of the significant changes to nursing practice in primary care that have taken place in recent years. These include changes to the ways that nurses are employed, the development of skill mix and team working, and the widening range of tasks and skills undertaken by nurses. It also considers the potential future contribution of nursing to the delivery of health services, and some of the key issues that deserve debate.

The stimuli for change

Most change in the nursing profession comes about as a result of three principal influencing factors:

- ▶ Professional – the collective result of internal debate in the profession, the policies and campaigns of professional organisations, individual ambition, and regulatory decisions

- ▶ Policy – the influence of government decisions on the structure, funding, management and workforce of the health services, and related issues such as drugs policy and public health measures, as well as policies relating directly to nursing, midwifery and health visiting as professions

- ▶ Pragmatic – ad hoc local changes to roles and ways of working that come about in response to a changing external environment.

All the significant developments in primary care nursing over the last decade or so have resulted from one or a combination of these factors. For example, policy-driven changes to the services provided by general practitioners (GPs), following changes to their national contract, the advent of National Service Frameworks defining care for specific conditions, and the shift of care for many conditions from secondary to primary care, have led to more nurses being employed in primary care and taking on a wider range of skills to provide a new range of services – a pragmatic response. Similarly, demographic and sociological factors, such as increasing local populations in many areas, rising expectations of convenient and flexible service provision, and growing demand for appointments for preventive and follow-up care in the community, have led to the establishment of new kinds of services, and the need for some to be led by nurses rather than GPs.

The development of the nurse telephone helpline NHS Direct from 1998, the opening of nurse-led NHS walk-in centres in 1999 and the bringing together of general practices and community trusts in PCTs, completed in April 2002 – all policy developments – widened the options for employment for nurses in primary care, and enabled some to combine clinical and corporate roles, thus fulfilling professional ambitions to diversify roles, develop autonomy and increase nurses' contribution to the leadership of NHS organisations.

The degree of congruence between professional, policy and pragmatic influences has been key to the extent of change that has taken place over the last 15–20 years. In that time, primary care nursing has been transformed from the traditional treatment room nurse working for a GP in the surgery, plus patch-based district nurses and health visitors visiting patients at home, to a much wider range of models characterised by:

▶ skill-mixed teams that include support workers, as well as qualified nurses ranging from newly registered to nurse consultants

▶ a spectrum of care provided by nurses that covers public health, health promotion and disease prevention, as well as highly specialised investigative and therapeutic interventions previously undertaken in hospital settings by doctors

▶ more autonomous practice that includes geographically separate, nurse-led centres and services, as well as nurse-run clinics, drop-in sessions and direct access appointments

▶ more flexible employment that allows the combination of clinical and other responsibilities – such as teaching or corporate governance roles – and rotational posts between different employment settings.

Professional-policy alignment

If professional development had not been largely aligned with the direction of policy, it is doubtful if such radical change could have taken place. One key example of the cumulative power of such alignment is the development of nurse prescribing, championed by the Royal College of Nursing (RCN) in a sustained campaign of support and encouragement designed to speed up and extend incrementally-developing government policy. Another example is the promotion of non-medical roles in public health work, set out in the Standing Nursing and Midwifery Advisory Committee report *Making it Happen* (Department of Health)[1] and supported by the Community Practitioners' and Health Visitors' Association (CPHVA) over many years. These roles are now a mainstream reality, with the appointment of health visitor-qualified public health specialists or nurse consultants in public health in some PCTs.

On a broader scale, the publication of a document called *The Scope of Professional Practice* by the nursing regulatory body, then the United Kingdom Central Council for Nursing, Midwifery and Health Visiting (now Nursing and Midwifery Council) in 1992 (UKCC),[2] freed nurses from the need to obtain individual certificates of competence for every additional skill they acquired following registration. This professionally-led change enabled nurses and their employers to respond more readily to the developing roles and additional skills that characterised the direction of government nursing policy from the late 1990s, including nurse-led services and Personal Medical Services pilots, nurse prescribing and nurse consultants. It also provided a supportive regulatory framework for the pragmatic development of 'extended' nursing roles that had been taking place in primary care since the 1980s, with the employment of nurse practitioners working alongside general practitioners, in particular to deal with minor illness.

Given the dividend to be gained from harmony between the direction of government policy and of professional developments, it is worth examining in more detail those government policies relating specifically to the nursing profession, and how the profession has responded to them.

Policies on nursing

A closer look at nursing policy

The most comprehensive recent statement of policy was the government's strategy for nursing, midwifery and health visiting, *Making a Difference* (Department of Health)[3], launched by the Prime Minister in 1999. It set out plans to strengthen nurse education, for example by providing longer clinical placements, and to introduce the nurse consultant as the top clinical grade for nurses. These developments, and changes to professional regulation, leadership programmes and quality of care initiatives for nurses, were intended to support a further set of developments, described collectively as 'working in new ways'.

These included public health roles for health visitors and school nurses, roles for nurses in fast access services such as NHS Direct and NHS walk-in centres, and in Personal Medical Services (PMS) pilots, nurses' contribution to the governance arrangement of (then) Primary Care Groups and Primary Care Trusts, and the expansion nationally of district nurse and health visitor prescribing. The strategy – which had been preceded by a national consultation exercise – received a lot of attention in the nursing press, and appeared to be welcomed by the profession as providing a necessary blueprint for change and progression.

Further definition was given to the 'new' roles to be undertaken by nurses when The NHS Plan, launched in 2000 (Department of Health),[4] included the Chief Nursing Officer's 'Ten key roles for nurses' (see Box 18.1).

Box 18.1 **The Chief Nursing Officer's ten key roles for nurses (from The NHS Plan)**

To order diagnostic investigations such as pathology tests and x-rays
To make and receive referrals direct e.g. to a therapist or pain consultant
To admit and discharge patients for specified conditions and within agreed protocols
To manage patient caseloads e.g. for diabetes or rheumatology
To run clinics e.g. for ophthalmology or dermatology
To prescribe medicines and treatments
To carry out a wide range of resuscitation procedures including defibrillation
To perform minor surgery and outpatient procedures
To triage patients using the latest IT to the most appropriate healthcare professional
To take the lead in the way local health services are organised and the way that they are run

While The NHS Plan did not suggest that every nurse must undertake each role, there was a clear statement that,

'NHS employers will be required to empower appropriately qualified nurses, midwives and therapists to undertake a wider range of clinical tasks including the right to make and receive referrals, admit and discharge patients, order investigations and diagnostic tests, run clinics and prescribe drugs.' (para 9.5)

For nurses who had previously met resistance from managers or employers when they wanted to take on these roles, or who looked for professional 'permission' to extend their roles, this endorsement from the Department's Chief Nurse provided legitimacy for their arguments. Two subsequent reports illustrate the extent to which nurses are reported to have taken up these 'key roles' (DoH).[5-6]

The NHS Plan also focused on the need to speed up patients' access to care. In secondary care, this further encouraged growth of nurse triage and treatment roles in accident and emergency and minor injury units, to reduce waiting times for emergency treatment; and stimulated growth in the number of nurses with endoscopy, colposcopy and other diagnostic skills in outpatient clinics, in order to reduce waiting times for in-patient treatment. Outside of the hospital sector, NHS Direct and NHS walk-in centres mirrored provision that had already been developed in many general practices, where practice nurses or nurse practitioners provided direct access appointments for patients.

Liberating the Talents

In 2002, another DoH document, *Liberating the Talents*,[7] identified three core functions for nurses and health visitors in primary care, that defined their contribution to delivering The NHS Plan, regardless of who employed them or where they worked. These were:

- ▶ first contact/acute assessment, diagnosis, care treatment and referral

- ▶ continuing care, rehabilitation, chronic disease management and delivering National Service Frameworks

- ▶ public health/health protection and promotion programmes that improve health and reduce inequalities.

Liberating the Talents explicitly takes the approach that 'it is what gets done and the skills needed that matter not the title of the person delivering the service or who employs them'(p8). This is a very significant recognition that traditional titles such as 'health visitor' and 'practice nurse' are no longer sufficient to encompass the wide-ranging scope of nursing work in primary care, and the increasingly flexible way in which it is delivered. While this principle is generally acknowledged by the professions involved, there is some support for preserving the traditional titles, which are both valued by their holders and understood by the public.

Changes in nursing practice

The response to the alignment of these policy, professional and pragmatic stimuli for change has been a significant expansion in the boundaries of nursing practice that are particularly visible in primary care:

- ▶ some specific and significant roles have been developed that cross traditional professional boundaries, such as nurse prescribing, and the diagnosis and treatment of minor illness by nurses

- ▶ the skill mix of nursing teams has expanded both vertically (greater range from support worker to consultant) and horizontally (wider range of skills at each level)

- ▶ individual tasks that traditionally belonged to doctors – such as referral or admission of patients, or requests for investigations – are increasingly being undertaken by nurses.

Specific roles

Nurse prescribing

The development of nurse prescribing has been one of the most obvious examples of cross-boundary roles supporting changes to services. The first district nurse (DN) and health visitor (HV) prescribers began piloting non-medical prescribing in 1994, and the national roll-out of DN/HV prescribing was completed when around 23,000 were trained by 2001. Training to prescribe from the *Nurse Prescriber's Formulary for District Nurses and Health Visitors* is now integrated into the degree-level course for DN and HV qualifications, making primary care currently the only setting in which the nursing team routinely includes nurse prescribers. Evaluation of the original pilots showed that the move to nurse prescribing of dressings, appliances and some medicines did not increase prescribing costs, and appeared to be both safe and acceptable to patients (Luker *et al*).[8]

Since 2001, a longer and more comprehensive training programme for prescribing has been available to all first-level registered nurses and registered midwives, and a new *Nurse Prescriber's Extended Formulary* (NPEF) is available to these prescribers. The focus of 'extended formulary' prescribing is the treatment of minor illness, minor injury, health promotion and palliative care, and recent additions have expanded this further to include emergency treatment of conditions such as asthma and diabetes. Many of the early cohorts training as 'extended formulary' nurse prescribers were nurse practitioners in primary care, running open access minor illness clinics. Although more limited than some nurses would like, this formulary allowed them for the first time to sign their own prescriptions for many of the conditions that they had assessed and diagnosed. Evaluation of the extension to nurse prescribing is currently being undertaken by a team at the University of Southampton.

In 2003, 'supplementary prescribing' – that is, prescribing following diagnosis and in partnership with a doctor – was introduced for nurses and pharmacists. There is no 'limited list' formulary for supplementary prescribing, and the prescriber can prescribe any medicine (except, at the time of writing, controlled drugs and unlicensed medicines) that is included in the patient's clinical management plan, drawn up and agreed with the independent prescriber (the doctor). When supplementary prescribing is fully implemented, it will enable nurses who run chronic disease management clinics to take on the bulk of prescribing for patients with asthma, diabetes, heart disease and a wide range of longer-term conditions.

Skill mix

Traditionally, all health visitors were employed on the same grade, and each worked at the same level of competence. While there was some grade mix in the practice nursing team, this often reflected time served rather than different levels of skills. By contrast, district nursing teams have long included nurses without the district nursing qualification, who are employed on a lower grade to deliver care in accordance with care plans drawn up by a qualified district nurse team leader who is employed on a higher grade. This pattern – a mix of grades of staff within a team, reflecting clearly-identified competencies and/or qualifications – allows the development of far more diverse teams. So, in recent years it has become more common for health care assistants or support workers to be employed in providing clerical, administrative or basic clinical assistance to nursing teams (in both district and practice nursing), and for nursery nurses to join teams of health visitors. At the other end of the competency scale, some primary care teams have expanded to include nurse practitioners, nurse consultants and so-called Nurses with Special Interests,[9] who may work across more than one team to provide specialist input.

At the same time as increasing the 'vertical' spread of skill mix in the team, it has become commoner to increase the 'horizontal' spread, by including other professionals such as physiotherapists, community mental health nurses, or social workers in the core team. In addition, entirely new roles in primary care are being established that do not fit in to traditional definitions, or existing types of services. One example is the development of (Associate) mental health practitioners in a joint project by the University of Southampton and the West Hampshire NHS Trust (see Box 18.2).

Box 18.2 **The (Associate) Mental Health Practitioner**

'The (Associate) Mental Health Practitioner is an innovative new role, designed to complement and work alongside psychologists, nurses, social workers, occupational therapists and psychiatrists. As a trainee, you will be fully employed by the NHS whilst also working towards a Postgraduate Diploma in Mental Health Studies at the University of Southampton. You will spend one day a week studying at the University, one day a week on a 'community' placement and three days a week working in an adult mental health setting.

This innovative new project is designed to respond to … changes in health service delivery by preparing (A)MHP trainees to work across traditional professional and organisational boundaries, within mental health and social care in tomorrow's NHS.

The Postgraduate Diploma is a nationally recognised academic qualification. The professional recording/registration of a health care qualification is the responsibility of various professional regulatory bodies. There is ongoing consultation with these organisations and it is envisaged that, in time, the (A)MHP will become a nationally recognised health profession.'

Source: '(Associate) Mental Health Practitioner – A new way of working' published by the West Hampshire NHS Trust and the University of Southampton, February 2003

Some of the more innovative developments, involving new roles for nurses, therapists and pharmacists, are being led by the Changing Workforce Programme (CWP) of the Modernisation Agency, which has published a booklet on role redesign in primary care (Modernisation Agency).[10] The CWP helps the NHS and other health and social care organisations to test and implement new ways of working to improve patient services, tackle staff shortages and increase job satisfaction by:

▶ redesigning staff roles – either by combining tasks differently, expanding roles or moving tasks up or down a traditional uni-disciplinary ladder

▶ removing any obstacles to change to ensure new ways of working become embedded as a new way of life within the NHS.

Specific tasks

The increasing autonomy of nurses providing direct access services or appointments to patients has also helped to bring about changes to the 'ownership' of some tasks that, unlike, for example, prescribing, are not limited by law, but are reserved by custom, practice or local policy to particular groups. There are currently very different attitudes in different areas, and between different sites in the same area, to nurses undertaking tasks such as referring patients to secondary care, running clinics, requesting laboratory tests or radiological investigations, and admitting patients to hospital beds.

Where nurses have been enabled to undertake these tasks, it is usually the result of personal contact and negotiation with specific people in the Trust, hospital or laboratory service, rather than because of any agreed local policy. The persistence of such micro-control over these developments is surprising because there is a body of high-quality evidence to demonstrate the effectiveness of nurses in these roles. A systematic review[11] of 11 randomised controlled trials and 23 prospective observational studies, comparing nurse practitioners and doctors providing the first point of contact for patients with undifferentiated health problems in primary care, found that there were no differences in the health status of patients following consultation with each group, and that there were no differences in rates of prescriptions, referrals or return consultations.

Where we are now

All general practices are now part of local commissioning groups (PCTs in England) but retain the ability to employ their own staff, including nurses; community nurses formerly employed by community trusts are now generally employed by PCTs. At the level of deployment of nurses, and of clinical practice, however, there is now a wide spectrum of models of nursing in primary care.

In some places nursing provision has barely changed – there is limited team working between practice and other nurses, and traditional tasks are undertaken along traditional specialty lines. In others, some or all of the following developments have been incorporated into local primary care services:

- ▶ highly-qualified nurse practitioners or nurse consultants run their own clinics or services alongside GP services, in GMS or PMS practices

- ▶ nurses and pharmacists train as supplementary prescribers to prescribe from the full *British National Formulary*, and share the care of patients with longer-term conditions with GPs or hospital consultants

- ▶ practice-based teams include non-registered support workers who relieve nurses and others of administrative tasks, freeing up time for patient care

- ▶ there are full-time nurse directors on PCT boards and nurses and health visitors working in dedicated public health roles in PCTs

- ▶ NHS Direct nurses triage all out-of-hours calls to general practices in their area, and other nurses form the front-line staff in out-of-hours primary care centres and NHS walk-in centres

- ▶ rotational posts have been created that allow nurses to combine working in NHS Direct and general practice, or general practice and an NHS walk-in centre.

Exploiting the potential of nursing

Every practice or PCT locality has to choose the model of service provision that best meets the needs of its population, and the services it intends to provide (for example, under the new GMS contract – see Box 18.3).

Box 18.3 **Opportunities for change in nursing through the new GMS contract**

A much greater emphasis on a flexible team approach to meeting the needs of patients
More opportunities for nurses and others to take on new clinical roles
The chance to become equal members of the practice team holding the contract
Greater skill mix so that practitioners can be freed up to take on advanced and specialist roles
Closer cross-practice and PCT joint working
Opportunities for nurses and others to provide those services that local practices have opted out of providing.

Source: **'Liberating the talents – helping Primary Care Trusts and nurses to deliver The NHS Plan',
Department of Health 2002**

So it is inevitable that there will be variation in the way in which staff are deployed and services are delivered to local people. In order to exploit the potential of the whole workforce, there are some key practical issues for primary care planners at practice or PCT level.

1. Recruitment – attracting and keeping the right kind of staff, based on the services the organisation plans to provide.

2. Capacity development – developing staff skills to match the competencies required for the services, and preparing the next generation in anticipation of staff turnover.

3. Funding – exploiting central funding and flexible or shared posts to get the best value from investment in staff training.

Recruitment issues

▶ Identifying patient and service needs before deciding what roles need to be filled – for example, by using the Changing Workforce Programme's role redesign workshop, which tackles local services issues through role redesign.

▶ Ensuring that the right kind of workers are recruited, based on an analysis of the competencies required for the post. A support worker might be able to bring or develop a wide range of competencies that were once expected only of nurses, such as venepuncture or screening. A specialist nurse, or highly-skilled generalist nurse, might be a valuable investment if a service is to be nurse-led and free up GPs' time.

▶ Making posts attractive – the opportunity to develop professionally, work independently or rotate between bases or clinical posts can help attract and retain ambitious people.

Capacity development issues

▶ Matching the competencies required for the post with those offered by candidates – because staff without the requisite skills, or any plan to obtain them, will be anxious and unsettled and may find themselves professionally vulnerable; staff who are working below their skill level will be hard to retain.

▶ Ensuring that there is an appraisal and development planning system, and access to appropriate forms of skills training and education – these need not be formal academic courses, but 'transferability' is important to staff who will move on in future, and assessed and accredited skills are more valuable than those acquired informally 'in-house'.

▶ Succession planning – preparing for the inevitable turnover in skilled nursing staff by identifying other internal staff who can be developed in advance, using the skilled staff as mentors.

Funding issues

▶ Looking for opportunities to share posts between practices, across a locality or PCT-wide.

▶ Using the new 'Agenda for Change' (DoH)[12] pay system to ensure that increased skills are appropriately rewarded, and pay differentials between staff are justified.

▶ Identifying training and education for which central funding is available via Workforce Development Confederations (for example, currently there is central funding for nurses to train to prescribe.)

The wider issues

The changes described above, and the resulting changes to the employment and deployment of nursing and other staff in primary care, point to a number of bigger issues that deserve attention. These can be summarised in two key questions:

1. What is the future of primary care as an employer?

2. How far can skill mix be exploited without compromising the safety of patients or the quality of services?

The future of primary care as an employer?

The increasing focus on National Service Frameworks, and agreed local 'patient pathways' between primary and secondary care, setting out what should happen to a patient with a particular condition from first assessment, through in-patient treatment to recovery or stabilisation at home, diminishes the significance of the boundary between care that happens in a hospital, and that which happens outside. The development of nursing 'in-reach' services (primary care based nurses who visit patients in hospital) and 'out-reach' services (hospital-based nurses who visit patients at home) demonstrate early changes to the traditional employment separation between two sectors that match this trend.

An entire children's nursing service that is jointly managed by a PCT and a hospital trust is another example. It seems likely that such patient-focused, flexible posts and services will increase in future, allowing nurses (and other staff) to choose the specialty or patient group in which they want to develop their expertise, rather than choosing between acute and primary care as settings for their career. As a bonus, staff in these posts should have a better appreciation of the challenges of health care in each setting, and of the patient's experience of moving between home and hospital, that could help them to identify and address quality of care issues that are currently unrecognised.

Exploitation of skill mix without compromising patient safety and quality of services

The increase in the employment of support workers, and other practitioners in new or hybrid roles, brings more patients, more often, into direct contact with workers who are not governed by a professional regulatory body, or working to an agreed code of conduct. Increasingly, these contacts involve invasive and diagnostic procedures, the results of which determine the future course of treatment for the patient.

At the other end of the skill mix scale, nurses, therapists and others are undertaking tasks and exercising skills – such as assessment, diagnosis, referral and prescribing – that were formerly in the medical domain.

The key to maintaining patient safety under these circumstances lies in the transparency and quality of core elements of the role: of the competencies (knowledge as well as skills) that it is agreed are needed to perform the task; of the training and assessment that the practitioner has undergone to acquire these competencies; and of the lines of accountability and responsibility for the practitioner's actions on a day to day basis. For registered health care workers, the responsibility for these core elements lies with the professional regulatory body which sets and maintains the boundaries for entry into the profession and for the scope of professional practice. For non-registered workers, this responsibility lies directly with the employing organisation. For the protection of the patient, the worker and the employer (which has vicarious liability for the actions of its employees), it is essential that these core elements are explicitly agreed and understood, and that all skill mix developments are integrated into the clinical governance processes of the organisation.

Some groups of new practitioners will undoubtedly continue to seek the recognition and 'respectability' of registration with the Health Professions Council: at the time of writing, health care support workers are still awaiting the DoH's consultation on proposals that they should become registered workers. However, some workers in new roles believe that the lengthy and restrictive process of becoming a registered profession stifles the innovation, freedom and flexibility that they currently have to respond to service need. With the Agenda for Change pay system, and specifically its 'knowledge and skills framework', offering a single pay spine for most workers in the NHS that recognises and rewards additional skills, there may be less incentive than before to seek professional status.

Summary

The congruence between professional, policy and pragmatic influences on nursing in recent years has resulted in significant changes to nursing in primary care. Nurses are employed in an increasing variety of roles, including clinical, corporate and public health roles, and undertake a much wider range of responsibilities than previously. Research evidence suggests that these changes have been implemented without detriment to patients. It is increasingly difficult to consider nursing in isolation from the multi-disciplinary team of both registered and unregistered workers who contribute to the provision of care outside hospitals.

The focus on National Service Frameworks and patient pathways is also eroding the traditional division between primary care and acute care, and one challenge for the future is to reflect this in new ways of employing staff. The other major challenge is to exploit the flexibility of a more diverse workforce, including growing numbers of workers who are not members of regulated professions, while protecting patient safety and the quality of services. The principal mechanisms for this are competency-based role development, appropriate training and assessment, and clear lines of accountability and responsibility, overseen by the employer rather than a professional body, and using the national pay modernisation framework as a guide.

References

1. Department of Health. *Making it happen – public health – the contribution, role and development of nurses, midwives and health visitors. Report of the Standing Nursing and Midwifery Advisory Committee.* London: Department of Health, 1995

2. UKCC. *The scope of professional practice.* London: UKCC, 1992

3. Department of Health. *Making a difference – strengthening the nursing, midwifery and health visiting contribution to health and healthcare.* London: Department of Health, 1999

4. Department of Health. *The NHS Plan. A plan for investment, a plan for reform.* London: Department of Health, 2000

5. Department of Health. *Developing key roles for nurses and midwives – a guide for managers.* London: Department of Health, 2002

6. Department of Health. *Modern matrons in the NHS a progress report.* London: Department of Health, 2002

7. Department of Health. *Liberating the talents – helping primary care trusts and nurses to deliver the NHS Plan.* London: Department of Health, 2002

8. Luker K A, Hogg C, Austin L, Ferguson B, Smith K. Decision-making: the context of nurse prescribing. *J Adv Nur* 1998; 3: 657–65

9. Department of Health. *Practitioners with special interests in primary care: implementing a scheme for nurses with special interests in primary care – liberating the talents.* London: Department of Health, 2003

10. Modernisation Agency. Workforce matters – a good practice guide to role redesign in primary care. London: Modernisation Agency, 2002

11. Horrocks S, Anderson E, Salisbury C. Systematic review of whether nurse practitioners working in primary care can provide equivalent care to doctors. *BMJ* 2002; 324: 819–23

12. Department of Health. Agenda for Change associated three year pay deal. Leeds: Department of Health, 2003

Further reading

Humphris D, Masterson A (eds). *Developing new clinical roles – a guide for health professionals.* Edinburgh: Churchill Livingstone, 2000

Useful websites

Modernisation Agency Changing Workforce Programme • www.modern.nhs.uk/cwp

Department of Health website: for specific DH documents, search under 'Publications' • www.dh.gov.uk

Nursing and Midwifery Council • www.nmc-uk.org

Royal College of Nursing • www.rcn.org.uk

National Primary Care Development Programme • www.npdp.org

National Primary and Care Trust Development Programme • www.natpact.nhs.uk

Index